T0362452

# Environmental and Wilderness Medicine

*Editors*

CHEYENNE FALAT
STEPHANIE LAREAU

# EMERGENCY MEDICINE
# CLINICS OF NORTH AMERICA

www.emed.theclinics.com

*Consulting Editor*
AMAL MATTU

August 2024 • Volume 42 • Number 3

**ELSEVIER**

1600 John F. Kennedy Boulevard • Suite 1800 • Philadelphia, Pennsylvania, 19103-2899

http://www.theclinics.com

**EMERGENCY MEDICINE CLINICS OF NORTH AMERICA Volume 42, Number 3**
**August 2024 ISSN 0733-8627, ISBN-13: 978-0-443-12959-9**

Editor: Joanna Gascoine
Developmental Editor: Varun Gopal

© 2024 Elsevier Inc. All rights are reserved, including those for text and data mining, AI training, and similar technologies.

This periodical and the individual contributions contained in it are protected under copyright by Elsevier, and the following terms and conditions apply to their use:

**Photocopying**
Single photocopies of single articles may be made for personal use as allowed by national copyright laws. Permission of the Publisher and payment of a fee is required for all other photocopying, including multiple or systematic copying, copying for advertising or promotional purposes, resale, and all forms of document delivery. Special rates are available for educational institutions that wish to make photocopies for non-profit educational classroom use. For information on how to seek permission visit www.elsevier.com/permissions or call: (+44) 1865 843830 (UK)/(+1) 215 239 3804 (USA).

**Derivative Works**
Subscribers may reproduce tables of contents or prepare lists of articles including abstracts for internal circulation within their institutions. Permission of the Publisher is required for resale or distribution outside the institution. Permission of the Publisher is required for all other derivative works, including compilations and translations (please consult www.elsevier.com/permissions).

**Electronic Storage or Usage**
Permission of the Publisher is required to store or use electronically any material contained in this periodical, including any article or part of an article (please consult www.elsevier.com/permissions). Except as outlined above, no part of this publication may be reproduced, stored in a retrieval system or transmitted in any form or by any means, electronic, mechanical, photocopying, recording or otherwise, without prior written permission of the Publisher.

**Notice**
No responsibility is assumed by the Publisher for any injury and/or damage to persons or property as a matter of products liability, negligence or otherwise, or from any use or operation of any methods, products, instructions or ideas contained in the material herein. Because of rapid advances in the medical sciences, in particular, independent verification of diagnoses and drug dosages should be made.

Although all advertising material is expected to conform to ethical (medical) standards, inclusion in this publication does not constitute a guarantee or endorsement of the quality or value of such product or of the claims made of it by its manufacturer.

*Emergency Medicine Clinics of North America* (ISSN 0733-8627) is published quarterly by Elsevier Inc., 360 Park Avenue South, New York, NY, 10010-1710. Months of issue are February, May, August, and November. Business and Editorial Offices: 1600 John F. Kennedy Boulevard, Suite 1800, Philadelphia, PA 19103-2899. Customer Service Office: 6277 Sea Harbor Drive, Orlando, FL 32887-4800. Periodicals postage paid at New York, NY, and additional mailing offices. Subscription prices are $100.00 per year (US students), $388.00 per year (US individuals), $220.00 per year (international students), $505.00 per year (international individuals), $100.00 per year (Canadian students), $463.00 per year (Canadian individuals). For institutional access pricing please contact Customer Service via the contact information below. International air speed delivery is included in all *Clinics'* subscription prices. All prices are subject to change without notice. **POSTMASTER:** Send address changes to *Emergency Medicine Clinics of North America*, Elsevier Periodicals Customer Service, 11830 Westline Industrial Drive, St. Louis, MO 63146. Customer Service (orders, claims, online, change of address): Elsevier Periodicals **Customer Service, 11830 Westline Industrial Drive, St. Louis, MO 63146. Tel: 1-800-654-2452 (U.S. and Canada); 314-453-7041 (outside U.S. and Canada). Fax: 314-453-5170. E-mail: journalscustomerservice-usa@elsevier.com (for print support); journalsonlinesupport-usa@elsevier.com (for online support).**

*Reprints.* For copies of 100 or more of articles in this publication, please contact the Commercial Reprints Department, Elsevier Inc., 360 Park Avenue South, New York, NY 10010-1710. Tel.: 212-633-3874; Fax: 212-633-3820; E-mail: reprints@elsevier.com.

*Emergency Medicine Clinics of North America* is covered in *MEDLINE/PubMed (Index Medicus), Current Contents/Clinical Medicine, EMBASE/Excerpta Medica, BIOSIS, SciSearch, CINAHL, ISI/BIOMED,* and *Research Alert.*

# Contributors

## CONSULTING EDITOR

**AMAL MATTU, MD**
Professor and Vice Chair of Academic Affairs, Department of Emergency Medicine, University of Maryland School of Medicine, Baltimore, Maryland

## EDITORS

**CHEYENNE FALAT, MD**
Assistant Professor, Department of Emergency Medicine, University of Maryland School of Medicine, Baltimore, Maryland

**STEPHANIE LAREAU, MD, FAWM, FACEP**
Associate Professor, Department of Emergency Medicine, Virginia Tech Carilion School of Medicine, Roanoke, Virginia

## AUTHORS

**LAUREN ALTSCHUH, MD**
Emergency Medicine Physician, Department of Emergency Medicine, University of California San Diego, San Diego, California

**JONATHAN BAUMAN, MD**
Clinical Instructor, Department of Emergency Medicine, University of California San Francisco, Fresno, California

**MARK BINKLEY, MD**
Assistant Professor, Division of Undersea and Hyperbaric Medicine, Department of Emergency Medicine, University of Pennsylvania, Philadelphia, Pennsylvania

**JACE BRADSHAW, MD**
Resident, Department of Emergency Medicine, Johns Hopkins Medicine, The Johns Hopkins University School of Medicine, Department of Anesthesiology and Critical Care Medicine, Johns Hopkins Medicine, Baltimore, Maryland

**NATACHA G. CHOUGH, MD, MPH**
Board Certified in Emergency Medicine and Aerospace Medicine, Assistant Professor, Division of Aerospace Medicine, University of Texas Medical Branch (UTMB), Department of Global and Emerging Diseases, School of Public and Population Health, Galveston, Texas

**GEOFFREY COMP, DO, FACEP, FAWM**
Emergency Medicine Resident, Valleywise Health Medical Center (Phoenix); Assistant Professor, University of Arizona College of Medicine (Phoenix), Creighton University School of Medicine, Phoenix, Arizona

**CHRISTOPHER A. DAVIS, MD**
Assistant Professor of Emergency Medicine, Wake Forest University School of Medicine, Winston-Salem, North Carolina

**VERONICA DIEDRICH, DO**
Resident Physician, Department of Emergency Medicine, Kansas City, Missouri

**SOFIYA DIURBA, MD**
Emergency Medicine Resident, Department of Emergency Medicine, Atrium Health Carolinas Medical Center Main, Wake Forest University School of Medicine, Charlotte, North Carolina

**JENNIFER DOW, MD, MHA, FACEP, FAWM, DIMM**
Emergency Medicine Physician, Department of Emergency Medicine, National Park Service, Alaska Region, Alaska Regional Hospital, Anchorage, Alaska

**BRANDON ELDER, MD, FAAEM, FAWM**
Assistant Professor, Department of Emergency Medicine, Kansas City, Missouri

**CHEYENNE FALAT, MD**
Assistant Professor, Department of Emergency Medicine, University of Maryland School of Medicine, Baltimore, Maryland

**ANDREA FERRARI, MD**
Emergency Medicine Specialist, Valleywise Health Medical Center (Phoenix), Phoenix, Arizona

**ZACHARY GASKILL, DO**
Physician, Division of Undersea and Hyperbaric Medicine, Department of Emergency Medicine, University of Pennsylvania, Philadelphia, Pennsylvania

**JESSICA GEHNER, MD**
Wilderness Medicine Fellowship, Assistant Director, Department of Emergency Medicine, Virginia Tech Carilion School of Medicine, Roanoke, Virginia

**KYLE GLOSE, MD**
Resident Physician, Department of Emergency Medicine, University of Maryland Medical Center, Baltimore, Maryland

**MATT GOLUBJATNIKOV, MD**
Emergency Resident, St Joseph's Medical Center, Stockton, California

**GABRIELLE GOSTIGIAN, MD**
Emergency Medicine Physician, Department of Emergency Medicine, Atrium Health Carolinas Medical Center Main, Wake Forest University School of Medicine, Charlotte, North Carolina

**ERIC HAWKINS, MD, MPH, FAEMS, FAWM**
Clinical Associate Professor, Department of Emergency Medicine, Atrium Health Carolinas Medical Center Main, Wake Forest University School of Medicine, Charlotte, North Carolina

**SAMANTHA A. KING, MD**
Board Certified in Emergency Medicine, Aerospace Medicine Resident, University of Texas Medical Branch (UTMB), Division of Aerospace Medicine, Department of Global and Emerging Diseases, School of Public and Population Health, Galveston, Texas

**CRAIG J. KUTZ, MD, MPH, PhD**
Board Certified in Emergency Medicine and Undersea and Hyperbaric Medicine, Aerospace Medicine Resident, University of Texas Medical Branch (UTMB), Division of Aerospace Medicine, Department of Global and Emerging Diseases, School of Public and Population Health, Galveston, Texas

**DAVID LAMBERT, MD**
Chief, Division of Undersea and Hyperbaric Medicine, Department of Emergency Medicine, University of Pennsylvania, Philadelphia, Pennsylvania

**STEPHANIE LAREAU, MD, FAWM, FACEP**
Associate Professor, Department of Emergency Medicine, Virginia Tech Carilion School of Medicine, Roanoke, Virginia

**CHRISTOPHER LEMON, MD**
Assistant Professor, Department of Emergency Medicine, Johns Hopkins School of Medicine, The Johns Hopkins University School of Medicine, Baltimore, Maryland

**ANDREW PARK, DO**
Emergency Medicine Physician, Larner College of Medicine, University of Vermont, Burlington, Vermont

**NICHOLAS RIZER, MD**
Resident, Department of Emergency Medicine, Johns Hopkins Medicine, The Johns Hopkins University School of Medicine, Baltimore, Maryland

**SARAH SCHLEIN, MD**
Associate Professor, Larner College of Medicine, University of Vermont, Burlington, Vermont

**SAVANNAH SEIGNEUR, DO**
Emergency Medicine Resident, Valleywise Health Medical Center (Phoenix), Creighton University School of Medicine, Phoenix, Arizona

**SAMEER SETHI, MD**
Emergency Medicine Fellow, Larner College of Medicine, University of Vermont, Burlington, Vermont

**SUSANNE SPANO, MD**
Professor of Clinical Emergency Medicine, Department of Emergency Medicine, University of California San Francisco, Fresno, California

**MICHELLE STORKAN, MD**
Assistant Professor, Department of Emergency Medicine, University of California San Francisco, Fresno, California

**MICHAEL D. SULLIVAN, MD**
Resident Physician, Department of Emergency Medicine, University of Maryland Medical Center, Baltimore, Maryland

**DOUGLAS SWARD, MD**
Assistant Professor, Department of Emergency Medicine, University of Maryland School of Medicine, Baltimore, Maryland

**ANNE WALKER, MD, FAWM, DiMM**
Emergency Medicine Physician, Clinical Faculty, St Joseph's Medical Center, Stockton, California

**ELAINE YU, DO, MS**
Ultrasound Fellow, Department of Emergency Medicine, University of California
San Diego, San Diego, California

**KARA ZWEERINK, MD**
Resident Physician, Department of Emergency Medicine, Kansas City, Missouri

# Contents

There is a growing incidence of heat-related illnesses due to rising global temperatures. Heat-related illnesses range from mild to severe, with heat stroke being the most critical. The wet bulb global temperature index considers humidity and solar intensity; its use is recommended to estimate heat stress on an individual and mitigate risk. Efficient cooling methods, such as cold water immersion, are essential in severe cases. Prevention is through hydration, appropriate clothing, recognition of high risk medications, and awareness of environmental conditions. Recognizing heat-related illnesses early in the clinical course and implementing rapid cooling strategies reduces morbidity and mortality.

Although a rare diagnosis in the Emergency Department, hypothermia affects patients in all environments, from urban to mountainous settings. Classic signs of death cannot be interpreted in the hypothermic patient, thus resulting in the mantra, "No one is dead until they're warm and dead." This comprehensive review of environmental hypothermia covers the clinical significance and pathophysiology of hypothermia, pearls and pitfalls in the prehospital management of hypothermia (including temperature measurement techniques and advanced cardiac life support deviations), necessary Emergency Department diagnostics, available rewarming modalities including extracorporeal life support, and criteria for termination of resuscitation.

Cold injury has been documented for centuries and remains a concern for military personnel, winter recreationalists, and urban homeless populations. Treatment advances in the last decades have included thrombolytic and prostaglandin therapies however the mainstay remains early recognition and rapid rewarming. This chapter focuses on frostbite, with a brief overview of other cold related conditions.

> Endurance sports encompass a broad range of events from marathons and triathlons to ultramarathons, long-distance cycling, skiing, and swimming. As these events have experienced a surge in popularity, we have a greater need to understand the associated medical risks. This article reviews the history of endurance races, reviews the most critical and common causes of cardiovascular, heat, electrolyte, and musculoskeletal injuries/illnesses, and discusses considerations for medical directors/personnel associated with such events.

> This review highlights the causative organisms, clinical features, diagnosis, and treatment of the most common tick-borne illnesses in the United States, including Lyme disease, Rocky Mountain spotted fever, anaplasmosis, ehrlichiosis, tularemia, Powassan virus, and alpha-gal syndrome. Tick bite prevention strategies and some basic tick removal recommendations are also provided.

> Plant dermatitis is a common pathology that plagues those who work and recreate in the North American outdoors. The most common plant family to cause dermatitis is the Toxicodendron genus, which includes the plants known by the common names of poison ivy, poison oak, and poison sumac. While mortality is usually quite low for this pathology, the incidence and prevalence of the disease leads to substantial healthcare burden and financial implications across the population. The mainstays of treatment have focused on prevention, corticosteroids, and antihistamines.

> This text serves to familiarize readers with animal bites and attacks. Topics include appropriate management of animal bite wounds, postexposure prophylaxis for possible rabies exposures, and unique infectious diseases transmitted through animal vectors. Large mammal attacks are discussed, in addition to the management of smaller animal attacks and exposures.

> Envenomations are the 23rd most common reason for calls to US poison control centers, with over 35,000 incidents reported annually. Snake bites account for over 20% of those calls, while marine envenomations are likely underreported at 3% to 4%.[1] While these types of envenomations may not be encountered on a daily basis for many physicians, the different types of envenomations warrant unique management strategies based on the offending creature and symptom presentation. This text serves as a review

# EMERGENCY MEDICINE
# CLINICS OF NORTH AMERICA

---

## SERIES OF RELATED INTEREST

***Critical Care Clinics***
https://www.criticalcare.theclinics.com/
***Cardiology Clinics***
https://www.cardiology.theclinics.com/

---

**THE CLINICS ARE NOW AVAILABLE ONLINE!**
Access your subscription at:
**www.theclinics.com**

# Foreword

# Environmental and Wilderness Medicine

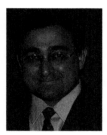

Amal Mattu, MD
*Consulting Editor*

"It's a dangerous world out there. And that's why we need emergency physicians." I recall these words from an emergency physician faculty member many years ago when I was a medical student, as he talked about why students should consider emergency medicine as a specialty. When pressed on what he meant by the statement, he responded that many other physicians are trained to deal with most maladies that afflict patients in the hospital—pneumonia, appendicitis, sepsis, myocardial infarctions, strokes, and so on—but there is only one type of physician to turn to when *the Earth itself* inflicts harm on patients. Heat-related illness, altitude illness, animal bites and envenomations, water or plant–induced illnesses, and so forth are conditions that generally only emergency physicians are trained to treat. "…That's why we need emergency physicians." Unfortunately, these environmental and wilderness–related ailments are often insufficiently taught in most residency curricula and continuing medical education (CME) conferences. Nevertheless, it is still the emergency physician we count on to care for these patients.

Fortunately, Drs Cheyenne Falat and Stephanie Lareau have stepped forward to advance our education in these fields. Both Drs Falat and Lareau have developed academic niches in environmental and wilderness medicine during their careers. They have taught numerous physicians personally and in CME conferences about the management of environmental and wilderness–related maladies. Now, they have assembled an outstanding group of additional experts in environmental and wilderness medicine, and together this group is bringing their expertise to us so that we *all* can gain increased knowledge in the proper care of these patients.

This group of editors and authors have provided cutting-edge discussions of heat and cold injuries, altitude illness, drowning and underwater accidents, plant and animal–related illnesses/injuries, and lightning strikes. An additional article is devoted

Emerg Med Clin N Am 42 (2024) xiii–xiv
https://doi.org/10.1016/j.emc.2024.04.001
0733-8627/24/© 2024 Elsevier Inc. All rights reserved.

to conditions associated with endurance sporting events, which is increasingly more common among fitness enthusiasts.

This issue of *Emergency Medicine Clinics of North America* is written not just for those with a passion for environmental and wilderness medicine; it is written for all of us in emergency medicine. Guest Editors Drs Cheyenne Falat and Stephanie Lareau deserve a great deal of credit for providing us with this valuable resource. Kudos to these editors and authors for putting together such a practical and informative issue, which reminds us once again why the House of Medicine needs emergency physicians.

Amal Mattu, MD
Department of Emergency Medicine
University of Maryland School of Medicine
Baltimore, MD, USA

*E-mail address:*
amattu@som.umaryland.edu

# Preface

# Entering the Extreme

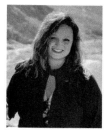 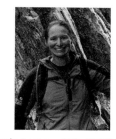

Cheyenne Falat, MD    Stephanie Lareau, MD, FAWM, FACEP
*Editors*

Emergency Medicine physicians around the world practice in a variety of settings—from academic tertiary care medicine to community and rural medicine. One thing that unites all Emergency Medicine physicians is that all care for patients who consistently try to push the limits of this world. In doing so, these patients are exposed to the extremes of temperature, altitude, terrain, physical activity, and flora and fauna, all in a changing climate. Some will even push past the limits of this world in their quest to explore outer space. The Emergency Medicine physician must be equipped with the knowledge to effectively care for all these patients.

Cheyenne Falat, MD
Department of Emergency Medicine
University of Maryland School of Medicine
110 South Paca Street
Sixth Floor, Suite 200
Baltimore, MD 21201, USA

Stephanie Lareau, MD, FAWM, FACEP
Department of Emergency Medicine
Virginia Tech Carilion School of Medicine
1 Riverside Circle
Roanoke, VA 24016-4962, USA

*E-mail addresses:*
cfalat@som.umaryland.edu (C. Falat)
salareau@carilionclinic.org (S. Lareau)

Emerg Med Clin N Am 42 (2024) xv
https://doi.org/10.1016/j.emc.2024.02.008
0733-8627/24/© 2024 Published by Elsevier Inc.

# Heat-Related Illnesses

Jonathan Bauman, MD, Susanne Spano, MD*,
Michelle Storkan, MD

## KEYWORDS

- Heat stroke • Heat exhaustion • Heat emergency • Environmental heat emergency

## KEY POINTS

- Heat-related illnesses are preventable through careful planning and risk mitigation, adequate hydration, and early recognition of developing symptoms.
- Rapid cooling is the most essential treatment for patients suffering from severe heat illness.
- Cold water immersion is the most effective way to rapidly cool a patient, though evaporation is likely more practical in the emergency department.
- Clear delineation between heat-related illnesses is less critical than recognition of the severity of the presentation, which will dictate treatment and care.
- Do not neglect to consider other possible causes of hyperthermia and altered mental status.

## INTRODUCTION

Heat-related illness has become an increasingly common global occurrence. The hottest average global temperatures have been during the last 7 years.[1] Extreme heat waves have become more frequent and intense.[2] As climate change causes global average temperatures to rise, the prevalence of such syndromes will only grow.[1] It is essential that clinicians are comfortable recognizing the symptoms, diagnosing them, and efficiently treating heat related illness.

Elevated ambient temperatures cause physiologic responses that can increase core body temperature and cause thermoregulatory disarray. This insult may be acute or insidious, and it can be life-threatening. The spectrum of heat-related illness includes heat exhaustion to heat stroke, with sequalae including organ failure and central nervous system dysfunction. There are specific definitions of heat-related illnesses, though the presentation is mainly based on a spectrum of symptoms, and reliance on strict definitions may not encompass the severity of the patient's presentation.

Four main mechanisms contribute to heat exchange: conduction, convection, evaporation, and radiation (**Table 1**). Conduction involves direct contact between

Department of Emergency Medicine, University of California San Francisco, 155 N. Fresno Street, Fresno, CA 93701, USA
* Corresponding author.
*E-mail addresses:* Susanne.Spano@ucsf.edu; sspano@gmail.com

Emerg Med Clin N Am 42 (2024) 485–492
https://doi.org/10.1016/j.emc.2024.02.010
0733-8627/24/© 2024 Elsevier Inc. All rights reserved.

emed.theclinics.com

| Table 1<br>Heat transfer mechanisms | | |
| --- | --- | --- |
| Mechanism | Definition | Example |
| Conduction | Direct contact between 2 surfaces | Laying on cold rock at night |
| Convection | *Moving* air or liquid | Wind chill factor |
| Radiation | Electromagnetic waves | Solar energy warming surfaces |
| Evaporation | Liquid to gas phase transition | Sweat evaporating from the skin |

surfaces, facilitating heat transfer. Heat transfer between a solid or liquid and a moving fluid or the air is called convection. Evaporation is the phase change of water from liquid to gas, decreasing the temperature of the surfaces on which this occurs. Heat transfer via electromagnetic waves is radiation; an example is the sun's warmth on exposed skin. When the body is warmer than the ambient surfaces, conduction and convection result in body heat loss. When the ambient surfaces are warmer than the body, these mechanisms result in net heat gain. Cold-water immersion, a treatment for extreme heat-related illness, employs conduction through the contact between cold water and the body. If the cold water is circulated, the addition of convection heat loss can significantly increase the effectiveness of rapid cooling.[3]

The hypothalamus is responsible for coordinating exogenous and endogenous signals to maintain thermoregulation. Humans maintain an average internal temperature of 37°C. The body generates heat independently through metabolism, though exogenous heat adds to the total heat burden. An increased metabolic rate is the most critical factor in the elevation of body temperature.[4] When an exogenous heat source or the body's excess metabolic heat raises the core temperature, the hypothalamus signals peripheral vasodilation, which can increase skin blood flow from approximately 250 mL/min to up to 6-8 L/min, allowing heat dissipation.[5] Peripheral vasodilation can result in decreased splanchnic and renal blood flow by 30%.[6] The average skin temperature is around 35°C, allowing a heat gradient to dissipate core body heat to the environment.[7] Sweat evaporation is the predominant cooling mechanism at high temperatures. Hypothalamic-signaled sweat production aids in evaporative cooling, relying on the convection of moving, cooler air to offload heat. When stagnant conditions exist, evaporative cooling is less effective. Sweat evaporation stops when humidity levels are greater than approximately 75%.

The heat index, which encompasses the relative humidity and temperature, is a commonly reported metric. However, a more physiologically sensitive measure is accomplished with the wet bulb global temperature (WBGT). The dry bulb temperature (DBT) is the ambient air temperature. Wet bulb temperature (WBT) is measured by covering a thermometer with a white cloth kept moist by wicking. Globe temperature (GT) measures the radiant heat from the sun and surrounding surfaces with a special thermometer. As a measure of the surrounding humidity, WBT has the largest impact on the WBGT index. The WBGT index takes into account the impact on the body's compensatory mechanisms and incorporates temperature, humidity, wind speed, sun angle, and cloud cover. The WBGT index is recommended to estimate heat stress on an individual and mitigate risk; the Occupational Safety and Health Administration, the US military, and professional athletics organizations endorse its use.

$$\text{WBGT index} = [\text{DBT} \times 0.1] + [\text{WB}T \times 0.7] + [\text{GT} \times 0.2]$$

The body can acclimatize to increased heat stress and elevated temperatures through 1 to 2 hours of heat-exposed daily exertion for 10 to 14 days.[4] Acclimatization results in an improved ability to dissipate heat. Mechanisms include a faster sweat response, increased volume of sweat, decreased sodium content of sweat to maintain intravascular volume, improved cutaneous blood flow, and reduced cardiovascular strain.[8] Physiologic heat acclimatization changes can persist for up to a month.

Hyperthermia, is an overarching term describing a rise in body temperature above the hypothalamic set point when heat-dissipating mechanisms are impaired (by clothing/insulation, drugs, and disease) or overwhelmed by external or internal factors such as environment and metabolism, respectively. Hyperthermia certainly exists in conjunction with many of the disease processes described below, though it can be solitary, transient, and ultimately benign.

## PRESENTATION

Heat stroke transpires when the internal core temperature rises above a certain threshold, (around 103°F to 104°F with other contributing external factors) and causes multiple systemic and cellular effects. These include a systemic inflammatory response similar to sepsis, causing increased mucosal permeability and allowing gut endotoxins into the systemic circulation, ultimately causing further tissue injury and impaired thermoregulation, worsening heat stroke, and hypotension.[4,5] Medications, chronic medical conditions, and the absence of heat acclimatization can negatively impact the body's ability to effectively respond to heat stress.

Exposure to elevated temperatures also increases exacerbations of chronic medical conditions including ischemic heart disease, stroke, asthma, chronic obstructive pulmonary disease (COPD), and kidney failure.[9] Hydration status is the most significant modifiable risk factor, especially during acute heat exposure or stress. Dehydration can cause electrolyte abnormalities, decrease the cardiac output via relatively reduced intravascular volume, decrease sweat rates, and increase core temperature.[10,11]

Heat stroke, the most severe heat-related illness, is a syndrome of symptoms occurring in individuals who exceed thermoregulatory boundaries, usually in conjunction with exposure to high ambient temperature.[9] The definition is a core body temperature greater than 40°C (104°F) with central nervous system involvement. Central nervous system involvement can include altered mental status, encephalopathy, seizures, or coma. There are 3 characteristic phases of heat stroke: (1) hyperthermic-neurologic acute phase, (2) hematologic-enzymatic phase with inflammation and coagulopathy, peaking at 24–48 hours, and (3) hepatorenal phase with organ failure, occurring at approximately 96 hours after onset.[12] Mortality due to heat stroke is high at about 10%, and increases to 33% when presenting with hypotension.[13,14]

There are 2 main types of heat stroke: exertional and classic. Exertional heat stroke usually affects healthy patients secondary to increased metabolic heat generation from physically demanding tasks. Physiologic malfunctions include the inability to dissipate excessive body heat, cellular and organ dysfunction, a systemic inflammatory response triggering, and ultimately, the core body temperature elevation.[9] Exertional heat stroke is often associated with elevated ambient heat exposure, though it can happen in its absence. Classic heat stroke, often seen within older patients with comorbidities, is instigated by exogenous factors and comes with a higher risk of mortality. These factors include certain medications, a lack of air conditioning, chronic diseases, decreased ability to sense or act regarding external temperatures, and dehydration.

Diagnosing this severe heat-related illness may be challenging due to the overlap between other pathologies causing altered mental status, such as sepsis with fever, drug-induced syndromes, or endocrine disorders. A comprehensive history is vital with an accurate core temperature (rectal is superior to oral, axillary, skin sensing, or tympanic membrane methods).[15] Indwelling temperature-sensing bladder and esophageal probes can also be used with no objective clinical difference in accuracy, though they are likely only useful in the hospital setting.[16] Recognize that the patient's core temperature may have decreased from the time of exposure.

Heat exhaustion, a moderate heat-related illness, encompasses fatigue, weakness, nausea, headache, or dizziness. Heat exhaustion almost uniformly occurs following recent exposure to high temperatures and stems from a combination of sodium depletion and dehydration.

Mild heat-related illness can be found in normothermic patients with exposures to elevated temperatures. These include heat syncope, heat edema, heat cramps, and heat rash. Heat syncope is a transient loss of consciousness with a rapid and spontaneous return to normal mentation. This diagnosis is highly dependent on the patient history, and other causes of syncope should be investigated if there is any doubt. Heat edema is a dependent extremity swelling secondary to interstitial fluid pooling due to increased peripheral vascular vasodilation from heat exposure. Heat cramps often occur in proximal large muscle groups (thighs, shoulder girdle) or abdominal wall muscles that spasm during or soon after activity in high-heat conditions. They are secondary to mild hyponatremia from excessive salt loss during perspiration. Heat rash, also known as lichen tropicus or miliaria rubra, usually manifests as small painless though often pruritic blister-like bumps after heat exposure. It occurs due to excessive sweating against blocked sweat glands, causing secondary inflammation, though it usually quickly resolves with cooling of the skin. There is an increased risk of secondary cellulitis involved, and appropriate treatment should be taken when signs of infection are present.

## RISK STRATIFICATION

Medication and drug use can significantly affect the risk of a patient developing a heat-related illness. These effects occur through 2 main mechanisms: compromised function of thermoregulatory centers and increased heat production from drug actions.[4] **Table 2** describes the mechanism by which many medications and drugs may alter the normal physiologic response to heat exposure.

| Table 2 Drug effects on heat transfer | |
|---|---|
| **Medication or Drug** | **Proposed Mechanism** |
| Alcohol | Decrease alertness as well as perception of heat, increased dehydration |
| Amphetamines | Increase metabolic heat production |
| Anticholinergics | Decrease sweat production |
| Antihistamines | Cause peripheral vasoconstriction |
| Antipsychotics | Interfere with hypothalamic thermoregulation |
| Benzodiazepines | Similar to alcohol, decreasing alertness and perception of heat |
| Beta blockers | Decreases heart rate and cardiac contractility |
| Calcium channel blockers | Decreases cardiac contractility and can effect vascular responses to heat |
| Cocaine | Increase metabolic heat production |
| Diuretics | Increase risk of dehydration and hypovolemia |
| Laxatives | Increase risk of dehydration and hypovolemia |
| Thyroid agonists: | Increase metabolic heat production |
| Tricyclic antidepressants: | Cause peripheral vasoconstriction |

Hydration status profoundly affects one's ability to tolerate heat. However, hyperhydration prior to strenuous activity or active body cooling before exercise has not been shown to mitigate heat stress or increase heat tolerance.[4]

Clothing can affect all 4 heat exchange methods. Insulated garments, constrictive base layers, or occluding sporting equipment compromise convection, radiation, conduction, or evaporation; the presence of these will increase the risk of heat illness. To mitigate this risk, close attention should be given to these factors when choosing uniforms, equipment, and clothing for potentially strenuous activities. An overweight body habitus, which insulates against heat loss, has also been associated with an increased risk of heat illness.

Utilizing the WBGT, knowledge of individual comorbidities, evaluating at-risk medications, and wisely choosing times of days or certain seasons for work or sports-related activities can significantly mitigate the incidence of heat-related illness.

## TREATMENT

Treatment for heat-related illness is similar in principle across the severity spectrum and is primarily based on clinical experience, observational studies, and consensus guidelines; evidence is limited. General recommendations are to remove the patient from heat and into a cool environment, expose them to allow increased convective and evaporative cooling, and implement cooling measures. The severity of the illness generally dictates the means and urgency of cooling.

Both exertional and classic heat stroke cause the same downstream effects, necessitating no difference in treatment. Rapid cooling should begin in the field with cold-water or ice-water immersion, as well as intravenous rehydration and evacuation or rapid transport to an emergency department for further treatment and eventual intensive-care unit (ICU) admission.[17] In the field, a natural body of water may be another safe and efficient option. Often, cooling should be initiated and planned for in the field prior to transportation to mitigate delays in decreasing core temperatures, as delays in cooling are associated with worse outcomes. However, immersion should always be conducted safely in the field, with a patient who is able to maintain their own airway and with supervising bystanders.

Heat stroke treatment necessitates an algorithmic approach, given the severity of the disease process, and should start with the management of the airway, breathing, and circulation (ABCs). Rapid cooling should be to a goal temperature of 38° to 39°C.[17] In a hyperthermic patient with signs of altered mental status and a history consistent with heat stroke, empiric cooling should be initiated regardless of a temperature reading below the classic diagnostic threshold of 40°C. Cooling in cold-water immersion or ice-water immersion is the preferred and fastest method. However, studies have not implicated inferiority between ice-water immersion and evaporative cooling.[4] If immersion is unavailable, large amounts of cold water are poured or sprayed on the patient with multiple fans to aid convection. Evaporation has been shown to achieve a cooling rate of approximately 0.10°C per minute.[9] Given the difficulty of immersing patients during hospital resuscitation and the widespread lack of this capability in most emergency rooms, evaporative cooling is likely most practical when initiating invasive testing or treatments such as IVs, cardiac monitoring, and central lines. However, there are multiple reports of improvised methods, such as the tarp-assisted cooling with oscillation (TACO) method and others with similar methodology in body bags that appear to be quite effecient.[18] The TACO method describes using a tarp with ice water and immersing the patient to mid chest for 10 to 15 minutes while using movements of the tarp to facilitate water oscillation, all of which can be accomplished with relative ease in most situations in the field.

Heat stroke patients often need fluid resuscitation, and when possible, cold fluids (4°C) should be used and can decrease the core temperature at a rate roughly double that of room temperature fluid. However, these should be combined with other active cooling methods, such as cold-water immersion or evaporative techniques, as this is an inadequate sole measure.[17] Additionally, given that some patients are euvolemic, the proposed fluid resuscitation should be careful at the risk of precipitating hypervolemia-related pathologies.

The 2019 Wilderness Medical Society practice guidelines on heat illness cite a small study that showed cold packs applied to the skin of the palms, soles, and cheeks to elicit twice the cooling rate of the traditional central vascular locations (axilla, groin, and neck).[4] If cold-water immersion and evaporative cooling techniques are not possible, and cold packs are the only option, they should be applied to the entire body and especially the areas whereby high-capacity subcutaneous arteriovenous anastomoses occur (palms, cheeks, soles of the feet). Ice packs were also found to be more effective than chemical cold packs and should be used whenever possible.[4] Antipyretics and other medications, such as dantrolene, are ineffective and may worsen coagulopathy and end-organ damage.[4]

Treating moderate heat illness, heat exhaustion, is similar to heat stroke. Remove the patient from hot environments, use various forms of cooling, and hydrate the patient. Heat illnesses exist on a spectrum; close monitoring of the patient's neurologic status is prudent to make sure the patient does not develop signs of heat stroke. Heat exhaustion patients can be safely discharged from the hospital if their symptoms improve after observation.[17]

Treatment with minor heat-related illness (heat syncope, heat edema, heat rash, and heat cramps) is essentially supportive, with removal from the heat source or environment, rehydration if necessary, and cooling techniques. Heat syncope requires investigation for other causes of syncope; it is a diagnosis of exclusion. Heat edema generally improves with elevating the affected limbs in a cooler environment. Diuretics are not indicated for heat edema. Heat rash is an inflammatory cutaneous disorder. Remove constrictive clothing, add evaporative cooling techniques, and evaluate for overlying infectious cellulitis. Antibacterial or topical corticosteroids may be helpful. Heat cramps usually improve with oral electrolytes and fluids, rest, and removal from the hyperthermic environment.

The best treatment for heat-related illness is prevention and risk reduction. Education, preparedness with a comprehensive cooling strategy, adequate hydration, and decreasing time outside when conditions are high risk for heat-related illness are necessary. Using the WBGT index as a guide can help estimate these conditions and implement guidelines for workers and athletes with predetermined plans for the above.

## SUMMARY

Interaction with high-temperature environments is becoming increasingly common. The incidence of heat-related illness and hyperthermia is expected to continue to rise in the era of global warming and climate change. Prevention and education are paramount to mitigate the risk of heat-related illness. Adequate hydration, avoiding high ambient temperatures, assessing one's risk with the WGBT, proper clothing, and recognition of unsafe features or signs of worsening heat illness can decrease morbidity and mortality. Recognition of heat-related illness is the first step in treatment. A thorough clinical history and examination are needed. In areas at high risk of heat stroke and heat-related illness, setting up specific protocols and equipment to allow rapid cooling for patients in the emergency setting is prudent. Primary care physicians can do much to warn and educate certain patients at risk of heat-related illness, such as those on certain medications or with specific medical pathologies.

## CLINICS CARE POINTS

- Exertional heat injury occurs in those partaking in exertional activities such as athletic events or physically demanding jobs and tends to affect younger, healthier individuals.
- Classic heat injury occurs in high ambient temperature environments and mainly affects both very young and very old individuals.
- Heat stroke is the most severe heat-related illness and is a medical emergency. It is defined as a core temperature greater than 40°C (104°F) with neurologic dysfunction, usually altered mental status.
- Other causes of elevated core temperature and altered mental status should be considered in patients with suspected heat stroke, such as infections, endocrine emergencies, toxicologic sources, neuroleptic malignant syndrome, malignant hyperthermia, and delirium tremens.
- The most important component of heat stroke treatment is rapid cooling, which can significantly decrease morbidity and mortality.
- Most minor heat illnesses can be treated by removing the patient from the hot environment with no specific treatment.
- Heat-related illness is preventable.
- Antipyretics or dantrolene play no role in the treatment of heat stroke.
- Patients with heat stroke require admission to the hospital, even if they seem to be improving.
- All heat-related illnesses other than heat stroke can be safely discharged from the hospital after symptoms improve after observation.

## DISCLOSURE

The authors have *no relevant financial or nonfinancial relationships* to disclose.

## REFERENCES

1. Romanello M, McGushin A, Di Napo- li C, et al. The 2021 report of the Lancet Countdown on health and climate change: code red for a healthy future. Lancet 2021;398:1619–62.
2. USGCRP (U.S. Global Change Research Program). In: Wuebbles DJ, Fahey DW, Hibbard KA, et al, editors. Climate science special report: Fourth National Climate Assessment, volume I. 2017. Available at: https://science2017.globalchange.gov. [Accessed 1 September 2023].
3. O'Connor JP. Simple and effective method to lower body core temperatures of hyperthermic patients. Am J Emerg Med 2017;35(6):881–4.
4. Lipman GS, Gaudio FG, Eifling KP, et al. Wilderness Medical Society Clinical Practice Guidelines for the Prevention and Treatment of Heat Illness: 2019 Update. Wilderness Environ Med 2019 Dec;30(4S):S33–46.
5. Leon LR, Helwig BG. Heat stroke: role of the systemic inflammatory response. J Appl Physiol (1985) 2010;109(6):1980–8.
6. Rowell LB. Cardiovascular aspects of human thermoregulation. Circ Res 1983; 52(4):367–79.

7. Atha WF. Heat-related illness. Emerg Med Clin North Am 2013;31(4):1097–108.
8. Périard JD, Racinais S, Sawka MN. Adaptations and mechanisms of human heat acclimation: Applications for competitive athletes and sports. Scand J Med Sci Sports 2015;25(1):S20–38.
9. Sorensen C, Hess J. Treatment and Prevention of Heat-Related Illness. N Engl J Med 2022;387(15):1404–13.
10. Sawka MN, Wenger CB. Physiological responses to acute exercise-heat stress. In: US Army Research Institute of Environmental Medicine. Defense Technical Information Center; 1988.
11. Sawka MN, Latzka WA, Matott RP, et al. Hydration effects on temperature regulation. Int J Sports Med 1998;19(2):S108–10.
12. Epstein Y, Yanovich R. Heatstroke. N Engl J Med 2019;380(25):2449–59.
13. Centers for Disease Control and Prevention (CDC). Heat-related illnesses and deaths-United States, 1994-1995. MMWR Morb Mortal Wkly Rep 1995;44(25): 465–8.
14. Austin MG, Berry JW. Observations on one hundred cases of heatstroke. J Am Med Assoc 1956;161(16):1525–9.
15. Smith JE. Cooling methods used in the treatment of exertional heat illness. Br J Sports Med 2005;39(8):503–7.
16. Bräuer A, Weyland W, Fritz U, et al. Determination of core body temperature. A comparison of esophageal, bladder, and rectal temperature during postoperative rewarming. Anaesthesist 1997;46(8):683–8.
17. Michelle S, Lori W. Heat-Related Emergencies. In: Mattu A, Swadron S, editors. CorePendium. Burbank, CA: CorePendium, LLC; 2021. Available at: https://www.emrap.org/corependium/chapter/recxgSvmWxwnxEZ8t/Heat-Related-Emergencies#h.dz5n6yrsefki. [Accessed 9 September 2023].
18. Luhring KE, Butts CL, Smith CR, et al. Cooling Effectiveness of a Modified Cold-Water Immersion Method After Exercise-Induced Hyperthermia. J Athl Train 2016; 51(11):946–51.

# Environmental Hypothermia

Cheyenne Falat, MD

## KEYWORDS

- Hypothermia • Rewarming • Osborn • Wave • HOPE • Score • ECLS • Avalanche

## KEY POINTS

- Classic signs of death, such as fixed and dilated pupils or muscle rigidity, cannot be interpreted in the profoundly hypothermic patient and are not contraindications to attempted resuscitation.
- Patients with severe hypothermia are at high risk of ventricular fibrillation and hypothermic cardiac arrest, but survival with full recovery is possible even in cases of prolonged downtimes.
- Perform only 1 to 3 defibrillation attempts (when indicated) until hypothermic patients have been rewarmed to 30°C. Do not administer vasoactive medications in patients with core temperatures below 30°C.
- Various rewarming modalities exist for hypothermic patients, but studies show improved survival when extracorporeal life support is used to rewarm patients in hypothermic cardiac arrest.
- Indications to terminate resuscitation in the hypothermic patient are an initial potassium level ≥12 mmol/L, injuries incompatible with life, or failure to achieve return of spontaneous circulation when rewarmed to 32 to 33°C.

## INTRODUCTION, MORTALITY, AND BACKGROUND

Accidental hypothermia is defined as an unintentional drop in core temperature below 35°C, whereas environmental hypothermia is a particular subset of accidental hypothermia attributed to environmental heat loss via convection, conduction, evaporation, and radiation.[1] Accidental hypothermia, environmental hypothermia, and hypothermia are used interchangeably during this review.

In the United States, there are 600 to 1500 annual deaths from hypothermia. Higher mortalities are seen in the western states with high elevations that experience considerable changes in nighttime temperatures (such as New Mexico), and in milder temperate climates that experience rapid temperature changes (such as North Carolina).[2,3]

Department of Emergency Medicine, University of Maryland School of Medicine, 110 South Paca Street, 6th Floor, Suite 200, Baltimore, MD 21201, USA
E-mail address: cfalat@som.umaryland.edu

Emerg Med Clin N Am 42 (2024) 493–511
https://doi.org/10.1016/j.emc.2024.02.011

emed.theclinics.com

0733-8627/24/© 2024 Elsevier Inc. All rights reserved.

Reported mortality among hypothermic patients ranges from 12% to 80%, with reported mortality for severe hypothermia ranging from 30% to 78%.[4,5] Trauma patients who develop hypothermia (<32°C) have a nearly 100% mortality.[2]

Appropriate recognition and resuscitation of hypothermic patients are important because hypothermic arrests can result in intact neurologic outcomes despite prolonged downtimes. At a core temperature of 20°C, cardiac arrest can be tolerated for up to 30 minutes without clinically significant neurologic deficits, largely because of a decrease in metabolic rate.[6] Generally, the duration of cardiac arrest after which full neurologic recovery is possible doubles for every 8°C decrease in core temperature.[7] The literature is full of almost unbelievable case reports with incredible stories of survival.

The lowest recorded temperature from which a patient with hypothermic cardiac arrest was successfully resuscitated is 13.7°C.[8] The patient made a full neurologic recovery.

The longest recorded successful combination of mechanical cardiopulmonary resuscitation (CPR) and extracorporeal life support (ECLS) is 8 hours and 42 minutes, after a suspected 28-minute low-/no-flow time.[9] The patient made a full neurologic recovery.

The highest reported serum potassium levels in hypothermic patients who were successfully rewarmed are 11.8 mmol/L in a child, 9.0 mmol/L in an adult, and 6.4 mmol/L in an avalanche patient.[10,11] The lowest recorded pH in a survived hypothermic cardiac arrest was 6.29.[12]

The highest number of simultaneous cases of hypothermic cardiac arrest took place at the Danish Præstø Fjord boating accident. All seven of the patients who received ECLS survived, only one of whom has persistent severe cognitive impairment.[13]

The longest avalanche burial duration leading to hypothermic cardiac arrest from which a patient survived was 7 hours.[14]

The longest period of submersion in icy water, of a hypothermic drowned cardiac arrest patient from which they were successfully resuscitated, was 83 minutes.[15,16] The child went on to make a full recovery.

## DEFINITIONS

Under normal physiologic conditions, humans maintain a core temperature of 37 ± 0.5°C.[17,18] Hypothermia is defined as a core temperature below 35°C. Hypothermia can be further stratified into mild hypothermia (core temperature 32–35°C), moderate hypothermia (core temperature 28–32°C), and severe hypothermia (core temperature <28°C).[19] Hypothermic cardiac arrests occur as a direct result of hypothermia, generally with a core temperature below 30°C.[20]

Primary accidental hypothermia is a decrease in core temperature (<35°C) that results from overwhelming environmental cold stress, such as in the stranded hiker.[2] Secondary accidental hypothermia is a decrease in core temperature (<35°C) occurring in patients with impaired heat production or thermoregulation who become hypothermic even in milder environmental cold stress.[2] Discussed further, this occurs with conditions such as older age, substance abuse, and neurologic impairment. Chronic hypothermia and induced hypothermia (such as with targeted temperature management) are not covered in this review.[21]

Human thermoregulation is a balance between heat production and heat loss. Heat loss occurs via 4 major mechanisms: conduction, convection, evaporation, and radiation.[17] Conduction is the direct transfer of heat between 2 touching objects. Convection is the transfer of heat from an object to a moving liquid or gas. A wet and windy environment will speed convective cooling.[18] Evaporation is heat loss owing to vaporization of water. Finally, radiation is heat loss via electromagnetic energy and accounts for 60% of total heat loss in humans under normal physiologic conditions.[22]

Exposure to cold increases activity at the peripheral cold receptors and triggers a hypothalamus-mediated direct reflex vasoconstriction.[20] Once colder blood reaches the temperature-sensing neurons in the hypothalamus, the hypothalamus also initiates various responses via the autonomic nervous system, the endocrine system, adaptive behavioral responses, extrapyramidal skeletal muscle stimulation, and shivering.[20] Notably, shivering can increase endogenous basal heat production up to 5 times the baseline rate.[18] However, exercise-induced thermogenesis produces the greatest heat gain, approximately 15 to 20 times the baseline metabolic rate.[18]

## RISK FACTORS

There are certain populations of patients that are at higher risk of developing accidental hypothermia. Primary hypothermia is oftentimes found in patients participating in recreational activities, such as climbing, hiking, skiing, snowboarding, or boating.[23] Secondary hypothermia is more complex and can be thought of in the following categories:

- *Extremes of age:* Infants have a high body-surface-area-to-mass ratio, which puts them at risk for accelerated cooling.[24] In addition, their ability to seek shelter is often dependent on others. Elderly patients have lowered abilities to both vasoconstrict and generate metabolic heat (reduced lean body mass, impaired mobility, inadequate diet, and reduced shivering).[20,24,25]
- *Urban populations:* Urban populations are at risk of hypothermia, especially among patients with concurrent alcohol/drug use or psychiatric/socioeconomic barriers that preclude sheltering from cold.[23] Alcohol and illicit substances can impair judgment (such as to seek shelter or clothe appropriately for cold weather), cause cutaneous vasodilation (counteracting the intrinsic thermoregulatory response), and inhibit shivering.[22,24]
- *Low body mass index:* Hypothermia is more likely to affect those with low body fat percentages (decreased tissue insulation) and malnutrition (decreased available fuel for heat generation).[24]
- *Certain comorbidities:* There are many comorbidities that place patients at risk of hypothermia, including but not limited to the following:
  - Those that impair thermoregulation (via central nervous system failure, such as stroke or neoplasm, or via peripheral nervous system failure, such as diabetic peripheral neuropathy or spinal cord injury)[18,24,26]
  - Those that decrease heat production (seen in endocrine failure such as hypothyroidism or adrenal insufficiency, insufficient fuel such as hypoglycemia or malnutrition, or neuromuscular compromise such as debility)[18,24,26]
  - Those that increase heat loss (with dermatologic illness such as burns, infectious illness such as sepsis, and disease states like dementia that blunt the learned behavioral responses to cold)[18,24,26]
  - Those that necessitate using medications with alpha-blockade activity (phenothiazines, prazosin) or medications that can cause central thermoregulatory failure (barbiturates, tricyclic antidepressants, opioids, benzodiazepines)[20]

Populations who live in colder climates tend to have lower overall mortality, as they are accustomed to protecting themselves against the cold more effectively through means such as appropriate clothing and continuously moving while exposed to cold conditions.[27]

## PATHOPHYSIOLOGY OF HYPOTHERMIA
### Neurologic

Mild hypothermia can present with confusion, amnesia, dysarthria, and ataxia.[28] These findings transition to progressive decrease in level of consciousness throughout moderate hypothermia, resulting in a global loss of reflexes and coma by severe hypothermia. Pupillary dilation and loss of cerebral autoregulation occur below 26°C.[2] Electroencephalography becomes silent between 19 and 20°C.[2]

### Cardiovascular

With mild hypothermia, patients will experience initial tachycardia, hypertension, and an increase in cardiac output.[28] Patients will become increasingly bradycardic as core temperature falls below 34°C, and heart rates tend to be approximately 30 to 40 beats/min by 28°C and 10 beats/min by 20°C.[2,20,29] Dysrhythmias and other abnormal electrocardiographic (ECG) findings are common (discussed later).[30] As hypothermia progresses to moderate hypothermia, patients will initially display bradycardia, followed by decreased cardiac output.[2] Relative tachycardia in the moderately or severely hypothermic patient should prompt consideration of hypovolemia, hypoglycemia, or toxin ingestion/exposure.[30] By the time patients enter severe hypothermia, they display profound bradycardia and hypotension, and eventually loss of vital signs.

### Respiratory

Patients may initially display tachypnea and bronchorrhea in mild hyperthermia. However, as core temperature reduction progresses through moderate hypothermia, patients develop increasing bradypnea and loss of airway protection. Oxygen consumption and carbon monoxide production are decreased, both dropping approximately 50% by a core temperatures of 30°C.[20] Pulmonary edema and apnea will appear in severe hypothermia.[28]

### Metabolic/Endocrine

Shivering, initially present in mild hyperthermia, ceases between 30 and 33°C.[2]

Cellular oxygen consumption decreases by approximately 6% for every 1°C reduction in core temperature below normal.[31] This means that oxygen consumption is reduced by approximately 50% at 28°C, and by about 75% at 22°C.[31] For this reason, patients with severe hypothermia can have intact neurologic recovery even after prolonged cardiac arrest, so long as hypothermia sets in before asphyxia.[31]

Hyperglycemia is a common finding, as hypothermia inhibits insulin release and insulin uptake by membrane receptors at temperatures below 30°C.[2] However, insulin administration should be avoided, as it may cause rebound hypoglycemia during rewarming.[2] Alternatively, hypoglycemia is also commonly encountered, as it is a predisposing risk factor for hypothermia. Hypoglycemia should be corrected with oral glucose (as tolerated) or dextrose infusion.

### Renal

Mild and moderate hypothermia may be complicated by a phenomenon known as "cold diuresis," in which patients produce a large amount of dilute urine.[1] This is likely multifactorial and due to blunted tubular response to antidiuretic hormone, as well as peripheral vasoconstriction.[1] Severe hypothermia is associated with oliguria. Metabolic acidosis is common, and rhabdomyolysis may present upon rewarming, which can decompensate into renal failure.[1]

### Gastrointestinal

Gastrointestinal findings associated with hypothermia include ileus, pancreatitis, gastric stress ulcers (Wischnevsky ulcers), and decreased hepatic function leading to slow clearance of many CYP450 metabolized drugs and toxins.[1,16,20]

### Hematologic

Coagulopathies are commonly seen at temperatures below 33°C, as evidenced by prolonged prothrombin time/partial thromboplastin time and prolonged clot formation.[2] Platelet function decreases as well.[28] Coagulopathy strictly owing to hypothermia is not treated with clotting factor administration, but rather with rewarming.[2] Hemoconcentration also occurs as a result of hypothermia, with an increase in hematocrit of approximately 2% for every 1°C reduction in core body temperature.[28] Caution should be exercised when monitoring patients during rewarming, as disseminated intravascular coagulation may develop.[1]

### Musculoskeletal

Synovial fluid becomes more viscous at lower temperatures, and muscle/joint stiffness can become apparent.[20]

## DISCUSSION
### Approach to Prehospital Care and Initial Evaluation

#### Field assessment and core temperature measurement

Hypothermic patients differ from normothermic patients in that "No one is dead until warm and dead." This is because classic signs of death, including fixed and dilated pupils, apparent rigor mortis, and dependent lividity, cannot be interpreted in severely hypothermic patients.[32–35] However, on-site contraindications for resuscitation include obvious fatal injuries, including decapitation, open head injury with loss of brain matter, truncal transection, incineration, or a stiff chest wall that cannot be appropriately compressed.[34]

It is important to obtain a core temperature as soon as able for suspected hypothermic patients. The 2019 Wilderness Medical Society (WMS) Clinical Practice Guidelines recommend using an esophageal temperature probe whenever able in the patient with a secured airway, as this is the most accurate minimally invasive method of measuring core temperature.[34,36] For accurate readings, the probe must be inserted into the lower third of the esophagus (an average of 24 cm below the larynx in adult patients).[17,34] In the awake patient with an adequate cardiac output, an epitympanic thermometer can be used to obtain a core temperature.[34] The caveat is that the external auditory canal must be dry, free from impacted cerumen/snow, adequately sealed with the thermometer, and used with an isolating "cap" against environmental cold conditions.[34,37] This is not to be confused with an infrared tympanic thermometer, which should never be used to measure core temperature, as it is inaccurate.

Rectal and bladder temperatures are impractical to obtain in the field.[34] However, rectal (inserted to a depth of 15 cm) and bladder temperature probes may be used to monitor core temperatures as patients are rewarmed. Note that in both of these methods, the measured temperatures can lag behind core temperatures by as much as 1 hour.[16] Oral temperatures should only be used to rule out hypothermia, as liquid mercury/alcohol thermometers are generally unable to measure temperatures below 35.6°C.[17,34] Even with various modalities, obtaining accurate core temperatures in the prehospital arena is difficult, as emergency medical services and rescue teams are generally not equipped with esophageal temperature probes or epi-tympanic thermometers.[37]

In situations in which core temperature cannot be ascertained, the Revised Swiss System (**Fig. 1**) can be used to estimate the risk of cardiac arrest.[38] The Revised Swiss System was released by The Medical Commission of the International Commission of Alpine Rescue (ICAR-MEDCOM) in 2021. The Revised Swiss System uses level of consciousness as defined by the AVPU scale (Alert, Verbal, Painful, Unresponsive) to stratify patients, because literature demonstrates a linear relationship between decreased core temperature and decreased level of consciousness.[37,39]

Importantly, any somnolent or comatose hypothermic patient has a high risk of developing ventricular fibrillation.[31,40] Timely placement of defibrillation pads and careful handling of severely hypothermic patients are required.[32]

The Revised Swiss System replaced the original Swiss Staging Model developed by ICAR-MEDCOM in 2003 (**Fig. 2**) after the original Swiss Staging Model was found to only predict core temperature with about 60% accuracy based on physical examina-tion findings; shivering was found to be a poor predictor of hypothermia stage (given its high variability among individuals), and a series of case reports was published demonstrating measurable vital signs even below 24°C.[32,37,41]

The WMS developed their own staging system as well, which is less widely used and reported in the literature.[34,37]

### Extrication
Circumrescue collapse, otherwise known as rescue collapse, describes the phenom-enon of lightheadedness, collapse, syncope, or sudden death occurring in hypother-mic patients or victims of cold-water immersion in the period surrounding their rescue.[34] This is poorly understood but likely multifactorial, owing to mental relaxation and the resulting decrease in catecholamine output, decreased hydrostatic pressure allowing blood to pool in dependent areas, afterdrop, and mechanical stimulation of the irritable heart.[34,42] Therefore, hypothermic patients should be extricated in as much of a horizontal position as able (even from water or crevasse), limiting physical stimulation and keeping the patients mentally attentive and focused.[34] Once patients are extricated, they should be insulated within a vapor barrier to protect from further cooling.[34]

### Delayed/intermittent cardiopulmonary resuscitation
Palpating pulses or measuring blood pressure in a cold and stiff hypothermic patient can be difficult. Palpation for a pulse and observing for signs of life, using point-of-care ultrasound if available, should occur for a full 60 seconds before determining that there is no cardiac activity.[31,43] In addition, the presence of any organized cardiac rhythm

| Revised Swiss System for Staging Accidental Hypothermia | | |
|---|---|---|
| Stage | Clinical Findings | Risk of Cardiac Arrest |
| 1 | "Alert" from AVPU | Low |
| 2 | "Verbal" from AVPU | Moderate |
| 3 | "Painful" or "Unconscious" from AVPU AND vital signs present | High |
| 4 | "Unconscious" from AVPU AND no detectable vital signs | Hypothermic Cardiac Arrest |

**Fig. 1.** The revised Swiss system.

| Original Swiss Staging Model for Hypothermia | | |
|---|---|---|
| Stage | Clinical Findings | Estimated Core Temperature (°C) |
| HT I | Clear consciousness with shivering | 32–35 |
| HT II | Impaired consciousness without shivering | 28–32 |
| HT III | Unconsciousness | 24–28 |
| HT IV | Apparent death | 13.7–24 |
| HT V | Death due to irreversible hypothermia | < 13.7 |

**Fig. 2.** The original Swiss staging model. HT, hypothermia.

(excluding ventricular fibrillation) should be taken as a sign of life, and CPR should be avoided, as this could precipitate a nonperfusing rhythm, such as ventricular fibrillation.[2] Even a profoundly bradycardic rhythm with hypotension is usually enough to provide adequate perfusion in the hypothermic patient with a severely reduced metabolic rate.[2]

Attempting to maintain continuous CPR for profoundly hypothermic patients in cardiac arrest can be difficult, especially when extrication is required. Mechanical CPR devices should be used whenever able.[7,44] In addition, the WMS has endorsed the use of delayed and intermittent CPR in situations when necessary.[34] In practice, this means that CPR can be delayed for up to 10 minutes to allow rescuers time to move a victim to a safer location.[7] If core temperature is unknown or between 20 and 28°C, CPR should then be performed for at least 5 minutes at a time, with maximum 5-minute pauses between cycles. If core temperature is below 20°C, CPR should be performed for at least 5 minutes at a time, with maximum 10-minute pauses between cycles.[7]

Although there have been case reports of successfully transcutaneously pacing profoundly hypothermic patients with bradycardia and hypotension, transcutaneous pacing is neither routine nor recommended in the management of severe hypothermia, even if bradycardia and hypotension are present.[20,29]

### Defibrillation
Case reports exist regarding successful defibrillations of patients with core temperatures below 30°C, including a successful defibrillation at 18.2°C.[44–46] There are various recommended approaches to defibrillation in the hypothermic cardiac arrest patient, all of which are reasonable given on-going controversies.[16]

The 2021 European Resuscitation Council (ERC) Guidelines for Resuscitation recommend up to 3 defibrillation attempts for hypothermic patients with core temperatures below 30°C, and if unsuccessful, withholding further attempts until rewarmed to 30°C.[43]

Meanwhile, the 2019 WMS Clinical Practice Guidelines recommend only a single defibrillation attempt below 30°C, and if unsuccessful, withholding further attempts until rewarmed to 30°C.[34] Previous 2014 WMS guidelines suggested that multiple defibrillations below 30°C can be attempted while rewarming, but waiting for a core temperature increase of 1 to 2°C between successive attempts.[46,47]

### Vasoactive medications
Although some case reports have shown instances where vasoactive medications may have played a role in establishing return of spontaneous circulation (ROSC) below 30°C, this is not routine practice.[5] The 2020 American Heart Association Guidelines

recommend following standard advanced cardiac life support (ACLS) protocols, including the administration of vasoactive medications, for the treatment of hypothermic cardiac arrests.[48] However, the 2010 and 2021 ERC Guidelines for Resuscitation, as well as the 2019 WMS Clinical Practice Guidelines, recommend withholding vasoactive ACLS medications until the patient has been rewarmed to 30°C and then doubling standard dosing intervals while the core temperature is between 30 and 35°C.[31,34,43] Standard ACLS medication protocols may resume once the temperature has reached 35°C. These recommendations stem from the thought that hypothermic cardiac tissue is unresponsive to vasoactive medications, whereas potentially toxic levels of repeatedly dosed medications can accumulate in the setting of slowed metabolism from hypothermia.[31,34]

### Afterdrop
Afterdrop is the continued cooling of the core even after the process of rewarming has begun, owing to continued conductive heat loss (from the relatively warmer core to the relatively cooler periphery) and convective heat loss (owing to locally mediated vasodilation at the periphery).[49] The extent of afterdrop appears to be impacted by the rate of initial cooling, the rate of rewarming, and the extent of vasodilation achieved, although the scientific evidence is relatively sparse, and theories have been disputed.[50] The typical magnitude of afterdrop is only about 0.6°C, although afterdrop of up to 5 to 6°C has been reported in the literature and can still be clinically significant enough to precipitate cardiac arrest (especially at the threshold of moderate to severe hypothermia).[34,49]

### Destination determination
Although standardized guidelines to assist with destination determination do not exist in the United States, various European studies as well as the 2021 ERC Guidelines for Resuscitation recommend that hypothermic patients in cardiac arrest or at high risk of cardiac arrest (core temperature <30°C, systolic blood pressure <90 mm Hg, and/or ventricular arrhythmias) be transferred directly to a hospital with ECLS capabilities.[3,32,43,51]

### Approach to Further Emergency Department Evaluation

### Airway, Breathing, and Circulation Concerns
**Vital signs.** When assessing the vital signs of a hypothermic patient, hypothermia can significantly prolong the response time of finger pulse oximetry.[52] In addition, end-tidal capnography does not predict survival for hypothermic cardiac arrest patients.[53]

**Intubation.** Although there is a theoretic risk of precipitating ventricular fibrillation in the severely hypothermic patient, do not delay intubation if required.[20,28] The advantage of adequate oxygenation and protection against aspiration outweighs the risk of precipitating ventricular fibrillation by performing intubation.[31] The 2019 WMS Guidelines recommend decreased dosages of anesthetic and neuromuscular blockade agents in patients with core temperatures below 30°C, with extended intervals of dosing according to the degree of hypothermia.[34] Endotracheal tube cuff pressures should also be monitored during rewarming, as the warming air within the cuff may cause the cuff to expand, causing local pressure injury to the trachea.[1]

**Pacing.** Although not routinely recommended in the management of severely hypothermic patients with a perfusing rhythm, transcutaneous/transvenous pacing may be used to help facilitate hemodynamic status while using ECLS.[29]

### Electrocardiography
As patients develop worsening hypothermia below 35°C, their ECG may show Osborn waves particularly in the inferior and lateral precordial leads.[54] Otherwise known as "J

waves," "J deflections," or "Camel's humps," these prominent notches of the terminal QRS complex, followed by ST segment elevation, are due to an interventricular conduction delay associated with hypothermia (**Fig. 3**).[55] The presence or absence of Osborn waves does not appear to correlate with outcome, but their amplitude does seem to correlate with the degree of hypothermia.[56,57] However, they are a nonspecific ECG finding that can also be seen in other conditions, such as intracranial hemorrhage, myocardial ischemia, and hypercalcemia.[54]

With decreasing temperatures, initial sinus tachycardia in hypothermia gives way to sinus bradycardia, followed by atrial fibrillation.[31] Atrial fibrillation with slow ventricular response is common among hypothermic patients (occurring in 50%–60% of hypothermic patients) and is considered to be a benign dysrhythmia that resolves with rewarming (see **Fig. 3**).[54,58,59]

Other ECG findings associated with worsening hypothermia include junctional bradycardias, premature ventricular contractions, repolarization abnormalities (including ST depressions and ST elevations; see **Fig. 3**), and prolongation of the PR interval, QRS complex, and QT interval.[54,57]

Ventricular irritability increases and QRS complexes widen as temperature drops below 30°C, predisposing patients to developing ventricular fibrillation.[54,60] Dysrhythmias can progress to asystole, especially below 24°C.[60] There is some controversy surrounding whether asystole as the initial rhythm is a poor prognostic factor.[42]

### Laboratory Evaluation

Recommended laboratory testing includes the following[1,26]:

- *Blood glucose:* Although insulin is not indicated for hyperglycemia, glucose should be administered to the hypoglycemic hypothermic patient.[34]
- *Complete metabolic panel, including hepatic function panel:* Obtaining an early potassium level helps to guide further resuscitative efforts (a potassium level is one of the data points in the hypothermia outcome prediction after ECLS

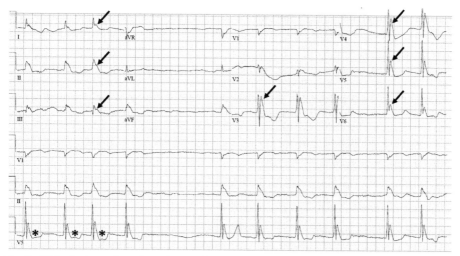

**Fig. 3.** ECG of a hypothermic patient with a core temperature of 26°C demonstrating atrial fibrillation with a slow ventricular response, J waves (*arrows*), and ST depressions (*asterisks*). (*Courtesy of* Dr Amal Mattu.)

(HOPE) and International accidental hypothermia extracorporeal life support (ICE) scores, described later, and termination of resuscitation is recommended in hypothermic cardiac arrest patients with an initial potassium level > 12 mmol/L).[34,61] Also evaluate for renal failure.

- *Complete blood count*: Evaluate for hemoconcentration, anemia, and thrombocytopenia.
- *Coagulation profile:* Evaluate for coagulopathies (although definitive treatment remains rewarming).
- *Arterial blood gas:* Note that reported values may be inaccurate in the patient, as arterial blood gas samples are usually warmed to 37°C before running the sample.
- *Creatine kinase level:* Evaluate for rhabdomyolysis.
- *Thyroid function tests:* Evaluate for hypothyroidism.
- *Lactic acid level:* Still used by some to guide resuscitative decisions involving ECLS and can also be trended as resuscitative measures are initiated.

### Radiographic Evaluation
The initial approach to assessing hypothermic patients for concurrent trauma is guided by clinical context. It can include the Advanced Trauma Life Support primary and secondary survey, an extended focused assessment of sonography in trauma (FAST), a chest radiograph, and a pelvic radiograph (if free intraabdominal fluid is found on the FAST examination).[62]

A computed tomography (CT) scan of the head should be considered in patients with suspected trauma, as findings may help guide the approach to heparinization in patients considered for or placed on ECLS.[63] However, early CT scans are limited in their ability to prognosticate neurologic outcomes.[64]

### Therapeutic Options

### Rewarming Techniques
There are a wide variety of rewarming techniques, many of which are commonly used in combination.[65,66] It is important that regardless of technique choices, core temperature be monitored throughout the entire rewarming process, with an end goal of 33 to 35°C.[67]

### Passive rewarming
Passive external rewarming is most suitable for previously healthy patients presenting with mild hypothermia. The aim is to prevent further heat loss and allow the patient's own metabolic heat production (generally by shivering) to raise their core temperature.[49] Vigorous shivering in a patient with adequate caloric availability can raise core temperature by approximately 3 to 4°C per hour.[34] Providing patients with blankets can allow additional rewarming rates of approximately 1 to 2°C per hour.[49]

### Active external rewarming
Convective rewarming should be accomplished using a forced-air device, such as one that is frequently available in postoperative care units. Forced-air rewarming rates can reach approximately 1.5 to 3°C per hour.[49,59]

### Active internal rewarming
Providing patients with warmed (42°C) humidified air via endotracheal tube can achieve an additional rewarming rate of approximately 0.5°C per hour.[28] Intravenous fluids should also be warmed to 40 to 42°C before administration. This does not contribute any meaningful rewarming but can prevent further heat loss.

Thoracic lavage can be performed using several different techniques: single or dual chest tube approach, unilateral or bilateral approach.[68] When performing thoracic lavage, keep in mind that left-sided chest tube insertion or lavage may precipitate ventricular fibrillation and cardiac arrest in the patient who presents with a perfusing rhythm.[68] Thoracic lavage can achieve additional rewarming rates of 0.5 to 3°C per hour. This is similar to peritoneal lavage, whereas bladder and gastric lavage have shown slower rewarming rates of 0.5 to 1°C per hour.[16,59,69] Irrigation of the stomach, bladder, and colon have limited utility given minimal area available for heat transfer.[1] However, bladder irrigation/dwell is often still performed, as it is relatively quick to deploy and uses minimal resources to maintain.

Intravascular rewarming catheters are central venous catheters with a closed-loop circuit through which temperature-controlled fluid (warmed by a bedside console) can be circulated.[70] Central venous catheterization (femoral approach preferred) is a relatively quick and routinely performed procedure by emergency physicians, and rewarming rates can achieve approximately 1.5 to 2.5°C per hour.[16,28,65]

Renal replacement therapy has been used as a rewarming modality, achieving rewarming rates of 2 to 3°C per hour.[69,71] It may be a viable option in hospitals that do not have access to extracorporeal membrane oxygenation (ECMO) circuits or specialized teams and provides the ability to correct and balance electrolyte and fluid status.[69,71]

The first successful use of cardiopulmonary bypass (CPB) was described as early as 1967.[23] It became standard therapy by 1987 to rewarm patients with severe accidental hypothermia and cardiac arrest, because CBP could achieve rewarming rates of up to 9°C per hour.[51,59]

With wider availability of ECMO, the use of CPB transitioned to the use of ECMO in the early 2000s, and studies have shown improved survival for patients rewarmed with ECMO over CBP.[12,72] ECMO has a few advantages over CPB: cannulation can be performed at bedside percutaneously and expeditiously, lower levels of anticoagulation are required, prolonged support for hours or days is possible, and the system can be transferred between hospitals if needed.[72,73] Although ECMO can provide rewarming rates of 4 to 10°C per hour, there is some evidence to suggest improved outcomes with slower rewarming rates, and a rewarming rate of 4 to 5°C per hour has been suggested as the optimal rewarming rate.[9,74,75] The use of venoarterial ECMO for resuscitative support is referred to as ECLS.

Liberal use of ECLS is costly, whereas restrictive use of ECLS can deny life-saving interventions to patients in need.[3] Two scores now exist to better predict outcomes and survival of hypothermic cardiac arrest patients rewarmed with ECLS, compared with using potassium levels alone: the HOPE score (more widely referenced in the literature) and the ICE score. The 2021 ERC Guidelines and other studies recommend the use of these scores in guiding patient selection for ECLS.[43]

The HOPE score takes into account the following 6 variables: age, sex, core temperature at admission, serum potassium level, mechanism of cooling, and CPR duration.[76] The score is based on a complex equation but can be easily calculated at www.hypothermiascore.org by entering the 6 parameters. When using a score cutoff of less than 0.1 as a criterion for poor prognosis, this score predicted that 27% of futile rewarming attempts using ECLS could have been prevented without one additional loss of life.[76] The study was externally validated in 2019.[77] However, the external validation suggested to exercise caution when applying the 0.1 cutoff to children.[77,78]

The ICE score is calculated based on gender, presence of asphyxiation, and serum potassium (**Fig. 4**).[3] Reported rates of survival with good neurologic outcomes following

| ICE Score | | |
|---|---|---|
| **Characteristic** | | **Points** |
| Gender | Male | 0 |
| | Female | -3 |
| Asphyxiation | No | 0 |
| | Yes | 5 |
| Serum Potassium (mmol/L) | < 5 | 0 |
| | 5-10 | 5 |
| | >10 | 10 |
| | Total Points: | (possible -3 to 15) |

**Fig. 4.** The ICE score.

hypothermic cardiac arrest are as follows: approximately 85% with an ICE score of −3, 60% with an ICE score of 0, 50% with an ICE score of 2, 30% with an ICE score of 5, 20% with an ICE score of 7, 10% with an ICE score of 10, and 0% with an ICE score of 12 to 15.[3,72] Per currently available literature, this score has not yet been externally validated.

Although the use of ECLS is mostly recommended for the severely hypothermic patient in or at risk for cardiac arrest, it should also be considered in patients who fail to improve with less invasive methods of rewarming, have comorbidities that limit tolerance of the low-flow state of hypothermia, or who develop life-threatening arrhythmias, hypotension, respiratory failure, or refractory acidosis.[79] The signs that a patient is failing to rewarm include a steady or decreasing core temperature, rising lactic acid level, decreasing level of consciousness, progressive hypotension, or the occurrence of ventricular dysrhythmias.[18]

ECLS is not recommended for patients with hypothermia greater than 30°C in cardiac arrest, as it is likely that the cardiac arrest is not primarily due to hypothermia.[42]

ECLS has also been used to successfully resuscitate and rewarm pediatric patients.[80] There is no guidance regarding the use of ECLS in pregnant patients, although there are reports of pregnant patients having been placed on ECMO for surgical procedures and acute respiratory distress syndrome.[63]

Complications of rewarming by ECLS include cerebral edema, renal failure, and a systemic inflammatory response.[15]

### Clinical Outcomes

When ECLS is used as a rewarming modality, survival rates of approximately 70% (range, 50%–100%) have been reported in the literature.[32,81,82] This is significantly higher when compared with survival rates of less than 40% for hypothermic cardiac arrests not treated with ECLS, which results in a number needed to treat 2 to 5 patients for ECLS rewarming of hypothermic cardiac arrests.[3,81,83] However, ECLS is not available at every hospital, and it is important to know what rewarming modalities are locally available, as successful resuscitation without ECLS is still possible.[84]

### Termination of Resuscitation

The indications to terminate resuscitative efforts in hypothermic cardiac arrest patients are a potassium level greater than 12 mmol/L (as recommended by the 2019 WMS Guidelines) and/or failure to achieve ROSC when rewarmed to 32 to 33°C.[16,34,85]

### Complications/concerns

As patients with moderate and severe hypothermia rewarm, consider their appropriate dispositions. Many will go on to require critical care because multiorgan failure is likely. Complications may include compartment syndrome, rhabdomyolysis, acute respiratory distress syndrome, acute tubular necrosis, disseminated intravascular coagulation, pancreatitis, heart failure, and even Wernicke encephalopathy.[1,26] This is by no means an exhaustive list of complications.

### Special Circumstances

#### Avalanche

Most avalanche deaths are due to hypoxia. Although hypothermia may protect avalanche victims from hypoxia during prolonged cardiac arrest, the hypothermic avalanche victim found in unwitnessed asystolic cardiac arrest has a particularly poor prognosis.[86] In addition, asystole at a hypothermic temperature greater than 24°C indicates likelihood of major concomitant pathologic condition, such as trauma or asphyxia.[86]

Avalanche victims are unlikely to survive when they are found in cardiac arrest with an obstructed airway on extrication and buried for ≥35 minutes, found in cardiac arrest with an obstructed airway on extrication and with an initial core temperature below 32°C, or found in cardiac arrest with an initial serum potassium greater than 8 mmol/L.[16,31]

The 2021 ECR Guidelines state to use prognostic scores, such as the HOPE score and/or ICE score, to guide resuscitative efforts for hypothermic arrest victims of avalanche.[43] However, if the HOPE score cannot be calculated, experts recommend that a combination of potassium less than 7 mmol/L and a core temperature below 30°C may indicate the need for ECLS.[14] The presence of an air pocket is associated with increased survival, whereas asystole is associated with a poor outcome in hypothermic cardiac arrests secondary to avalanche burial.[14]

Although the HOPE score has been shown to predict survival better than potassium alone, literature also suggests that a potassium level ≥7 or 8 mmol/L could be used to terminate resuscitative efforts in the hypothermic avalanche patient in arrest (compared with the classic ≥12 mmol/L in nonavalanche hypothermic arrest patients), even before full rewarming.[10,19,43,76] The 2021 ECR Guidelines also consider resuscitation futile in hypothermic avalanche patients with burial time greater than 60 minutes and evidence of airway obstruction.[14,43]

#### Drowning

Concomitant hypothermia in drowned patients appears to confer an improved prognosis, especially if the patient's history indicates an initial immersion in cold water (body exposed to cold water but still able to breathe).[59] If submersion during a drowning event occurs in icy (<5°C) water, and hypothermia develops rapidly before the onset of hypoxia from drowning, the hypothermia may confer protection against hypoxic neurologic insult, and survival without neurologic impairment is still possible.[16,31]

## SUMMARY

The prompt recognition, triage, and treatment of hypothermic patients are critical, as even those in hypothermic cardiac arrest with long downtimes can survive with excellent neurologic recovery. Mild hypothermia will present with a hallmark ramped-up metabolism (tachypnea, tachycardia, increased cardiac output, and shivering), whereas moderate hypothermia will present with slowed signs (bradypnea, bradycardia, and decreasing level of consciousness), and severe hypothermia may present with apparent death or cardiac arrest. Important deviations from standard ACLS include the approach to defibrillation and vasoactive medication administration. An accurate core temperature must be obtained and monitored throughout the process of rewarming. Survival rates of hypothermic cardiac arrest patients are remarkably improved when ECLS is used as a rewarming modality, and the HOPE score can be used to help guide the use of ECLS.

Although current literature and guidelines have been extensively reviewed in this article, there is still a relative paucity of studies on hypothermic human patients, and recommendations are usually based on animal studies and consensus opinions. The International Hypothermia Registry was created to increase the knowledge base of accidental hypothermia and to develop evidence-based guidelines.[19] Over the past decade, many of the entries are from mountainous regions in Europe, and thus, many of the cases involve primary hypothermia sustained during recreational activities. However, all are encouraged to contribute at https://hypothermia-registry.org/.[16,19]

## CLINICS CARE POINTS

- Classic signs of death, including fixed and dilated pupils, apparent rigor mortis, and dependent lividity, cannot be interpreted in severely hypothermic patients.
- Esophageal and epitympanic temperatures are the best minimally invasive modalities to measure accurate core temperature.
- The Revised Swiss Staging Model can be used to estimate risk of hypothermic cardiac arrest based on level of patient alertness according to the AVPU (Alert, Verbal, Painful, Unresponsive) scale.
- In the hypothermic cardiac arrest patient, perform only 1 to 3 defibrillations and withhold vasoactive advanced cardiac life support medications until the patient has been rewarmed to 30°C.
- Atrial fibrillation with slow ventricular response is common in hypothermic patients and will correct with rewarming.
- Although many rewarming methods exist, consider extracorporeal life support for hypothermic cardiac arrest patients—the HOPE score can help guide resuscitative efforts.
- Avalanche patients found in cardiac arrest on extrication have particularly poor outcomes.

## DISCLOSURE

The author has no financial disclosures.

## REFERENCES

1. Hanania NA, Zimmerman JL. Accidental hypothermia. Crit Care Clin 1999;15(2): 235–49.

2. Jurkovich GJ. Environmental cold-induced injury. Surg Clin North Am 2007;87(1): 247–67, viii.

3. Saczkowski RS, Brown DJA, Abu-Laban RB, et al. Prediction and risk stratification of survival in accidental hypothermia requiring extracorporeal life support: An individual patient data meta-analysis. Resuscitation 2018;127:51–7.

4. Vassal T, Benoit-Gonin B, Carrat F, et al. Severe accidental hypothermia treated in an ICU: prognosis and outcome. Chest 2001;120(6):1998–2003.

5. Wira CR, Becker JU, Martin G, et al. Anti-arrhythmic and vasopressor medications for the treatment of ventricular fibrillation in severe hypothermia: a systematic review of the literature. Resuscitation 2008;78(1):21–9.

6. Walpoth BH, Walpoth-Aslan BN, Mattle HP, et al. Outcome of survivors of accidental deep hypothermia and circulatory arrest treated with extracorporeal blood warming. N Engl J Med 1997;337(21):1500–5.

7. Gordon L, Paal P, Ellerton JA, et al. Delayed and intermittent CPR for severe accidental hypothermia. Resuscitation 2015;90:46–9.

8. Gilbert M, Busund R, Skagseth A, et al. Resuscitation from accidental hypothermia of 13.7 degrees C with circulatory arrest. Lancet 2000;355(9201):375–6.

9. Forti A, Brugnaro P, Rauch S, et al. Hypothermic Cardiac Arrest With Full Neurologic Recovery After Approximately Nine Hours of Cardiopulmonary Resuscitation: Management and Possible Complications. Ann Emerg Med 2019;73(1):52–7.

10. Brugger H, Bouzat P, Pasquier M, et al. Cut-off values of serum potassium and core temperature at hospital admission for extracorporeal rewarming of avalanche victims in cardiac arrest: A retrospective multi-centre study. Resuscitation 2019;139:222–9.

11. Debaty G, Moustapha I, Bouzat P, et al. Outcome after severe accidental hypothermia in the French Alps: A 10-year review. Resuscitation 2015;93:118–23.

12. Bjertnæs LJ, Hindberg K, Næsheim TO, et al. Rewarming From Hypothermic Cardiac Arrest Applying Extracorporeal Life Support: A Systematic Review and Meta-Analysis. Front Med 2021;8:641633.

13. Wanscher M, Agersnap L, Ravn J, et al. Outcome of accidental hypothermia with or without circulatory arrest: experience from the Danish Præstø Fjord boating accident. Resuscitation 2012;83(9):1078–84.

14. Pasquier M, Strapazzon G, Kottmann A, et al. On-site treatment of avalanche victims: Scoping review and 2023 recommendations of the international commission for mountain emergency medicine (ICAR MedCom). Resuscitation 2023;184: 109708.

15. Romlin BS, Winberg H, Janson M, et al. Excellent Outcome With Extracorporeal Membrane Oxygenation After Accidental Profound Hypothermia (13.8°C) and Drowning. Crit Care Med 2015;43(11):e521–5.

16. Paal P, Gordon L, Strapazzon G, et al. Accidental hypothermia-an update: The content of this review is endorsed by the International Commission for Mountain Emergency Medicine (ICAR MEDCOM). Scand J Trauma Resusc Emerg Med 2016;24(1):111.

17. Zafren K. Out-of-Hospital Evaluation and Treatment of Accidental Hypothermia. Emerg Med Clin North Am 2017;35(2):261–79.

18. Paal P, Pasquier M, Darocha T, et al. Accidental Hypothermia: 2021 Update. Int J Environ Res Public Health 2022;19(1):501.

19. Walpoth BH, Maeder MB, Courvoisier DS, et al. Hypothermic Cardiac Arrest - Retrospective cohort study from the International Hypothermia Registry. Resuscitation 2021;167:58–65.

20. Mallet ML. Pathophysiology of accidental hypothermia. QJM 2002;95(12): 775–85.
21. Tveita T, Sieck GC. Physiological Impact of Hypothermia: The Good, the Bad, and the Ugly. Physiology 2022;37(2):69–87.
22. Willmore R. Cardiac Arrest Secondary to Accidental Hypothermia: The Physiology Leading to Hypothermic Arrest. Air Med J 2020;39(2):133–6.
23. Vretenar DF, Urschel JD, Parrott JC, et al. Cardiopulmonary bypass resuscitation for accidental hypothermia. Ann Thorac Surg 1994;58(3):895–8.
24. Biem J, Koehncke N, Classen D, et al. Out of the cold: management of hypothermia and frostbite. CMAJ (Can Med Assoc J) 2003;168(3):305–11.
25. Stares J, Kosatsky T. Hypothermia as a cause of death in British Columbia, 1998-2012: a descriptive assessment. CMAJ Open 2015;3(4):E352–8.
26. Epstein E, Anna K. Accidental hypothermia. BMJ 2006;332(7543):706–9.
27. Näyhä S. Environmental temperature and mortality. Int J Circumpolar Health 2005;64(5):451–8.
28. Kempainen RR, Brunette DD. The evaluation and management of accidental hypothermia. Respir Care 2004;49(2):192–205.
29. Ho JD, Heegaard WG, Brunette DD. Successful transcutaneous pacing in 2 severely hypothermic patients. Ann Emerg Med 2007;49(5):678–81.
30. Danzl DF, Pozos RS. Accidental hypothermia. N Engl J Med 1994;331(26): 1756–60.
31. Soar J, Perkins GD, Abbas G, et al. European Resuscitation Council Guidelines for Resuscitation 2010 Section 8. Cardiac arrest in special circumstances: Electrolyte abnormalities, poisoning, drowning, accidental hypothermia, hyperthermia, asthma, anaphylaxis, cardiac surgery, trauma, pregnancy, electrocution. Resuscitation 2010;81(10):1400–33.
32. Pasquier M, Zurron N, Weith B, et al. Deep accidental hypothermia with core temperature below 24°C presenting with vital signs. High Alt Med Biol 2014;15(1): 58–63.
33. Hilmo J, Naesheim T, Gilbert M. "Nobody is dead until warm and dead": prolonged resuscitation is warranted in arrested hypothermic victims also in remote areas–a retrospective study from northern Norway. Resuscitation 2014;85(9): 1204–11.
34. Dow J, Giesbrecht GG, Danzl DF, et al. Wilderness Medical Society Clinical Practice Guidelines for the Out-of-Hospital Evaluation and Treatment of Accidental Hypothermia: 2019 Update. Wilderness Environ Med 2019;30(4S):S47–69.
35. Bunya N, Sawamoto K, Kakizaki R, et al. Successful resuscitation for cardiac arrest due to severe accidental hypothermia accompanied by mandibular rigidity: a case of cold stiffening mimicking rigor mortis. Int J Emerg Med 2018;11(1):46.
36. Pasquier M, Paal P, Kosinski S, et al. Esophageal Temperature Measurement. N Engl J Med 2020;383(16):e93.
37. Musi ME, Sheets A, Zafren K, et al. Clinical staging of accidental hypothermia: The Revised Swiss System: Recommendation of the International Commission for Mountain Emergency Medicine (ICAR MedCom). Resuscitation 2021;162: 182–7.
38. Deslarzes T, Rousson V, Yersin B, et al. An evaluation of the Swiss staging model for hypothermia using case reports from the literature. Scand J Trauma Resusc Emerg Med 2016;24:16.
39. Fukuda M, Nozawa M, Okada Y, et al. Clinical relevance of impaired consciousness in accidental hypothermia: a Japanese multicenter retrospective study. Acute Med Surg 2022;9(1):e730.

40. Barrow S, Ives G. Accidental hypothermia: direct evidence for consciousness as a marker of cardiac arrest risk in the acute assessment of cold patients. Scand J Trauma Resusc Emerg Med 2022;30(1):13.

41. Pasquier M, Carron PN, Rodrigues A, et al. An evaluation of the Swiss staging model for hypothermia using hospital cases and case reports from the literature. Scand J Trauma Resusc Emerg Med 2019;27(1):60.

42. Frei C, Darocha T, Debaty G, et al. Clinical characteristics and outcomes of witnessed hypothermic cardiac arrest: A systematic review on rescue collapse. Resuscitation 2019;137:41–8.

43. Lott C, Truhlář A, Alfonzo A, et al. European Resuscitation Council Guidelines 2021: Cardiac arrest in special circumstances. Resuscitation 2021;161:152–219.

44. Mair P, Gasteiger L, Mair B, et al. Successful Defibrillation of Four Hypothermic Patients with Witnessed Cardiac Arrest. High Alt Med Biol 2019;20(1):71–7.

45. Thomas R, Cahill CJ. Successful defibrillation in profound hypothermia (core body temperature 25.6 degrees C). Resuscitation 2000;47(3):317–20.

46. Kosiński S, Drzewiecka A, Pasquier M, et al. Successful Defibrillation at a Core Temperature of 18.2 Degrees Celsius. Wilderness Environ Med 2020;31(2):230–4.

47. Zafren K, Giesbrecht GG, Danzl DF, et al. Wilderness Medical Society practice guidelines for the out-of-hospital evaluation and treatment of accidental hypothermia. Wilderness Environ Med 2014;25(4):425–45.

48. Panchal AR, Bartos JA, Cabañas JG, et al. Part 3: Adult Basic and Advanced Life Support: 2020 American Heart Association Guidelines for Cardiopulmonary Resuscitation and Emergency Cardiovascular Care. Circulation 2020;142(16_suppl_2): S366–468.

49. Steele MT, Nelson MJ, Sessler DI, et al. Forced air speeds rewarming in accidental hypothermia. Ann Emerg Med 1996;27(4):479–84.

50. Mydske S, Thomassen Ø. Is prehospital use of active external warming dangerous for patients with accidental hypothermia: a systematic review. Scand J Trauma Resusc Emerg Med 2020;28(1):77.

51. Svendsen ØS, Grong K, Andersen KS, et al. Outcome After Rewarming From Accidental Hypothermia by Use of Extracorporeal Circulation. Ann Thorac Surg 2017;103(3):920–5.

52. MacLeod DB, Cortinez LI, Keifer JC, et al. The desaturation response time of finger pulse oximeters during mild hypothermia. Anaesthesia 2005;60(1):65–71.

53. Darocha T, Debaty G, Ageron FX, et al. Hypothermia is associated with a low ETCO2 and low pH-stat PaCO2 in refractory cardiac arrest. Resuscitation 2022;174:83–90.

54. Salinski EP, Worrilow CC. ST-segment elevation myocardial infarction vs. hypothermia-induced electrocardiographic changes: a case report and brief review of the literature. J Emerg Med 2014;46(4):e107–11.

55. Alsafwah S. Electrocardiographic changes in hypothermia. Heart Lung 2001; 30(2):161–3.

56. Graham CA, McNaughton GW, Wyatt JP. The electrocardiogram in hypothermia. Wilderness Environ Med 2001;12(4):232–5.

57. Doshi HH, Giudici MC. The EKG in hypothermia and hyperthermia. J Electrocardiol 2015;48(2):203–9.

58. Cocchi MN, Giberson B, Donnino MW. Rapid rewarming of hypothermic patient using arctic sun device. J Intensive Care Med 2012;27(2):128–30.

59. Brown DJA, Brugger H, Boyd J, et al. Accidental hypothermia. N Engl J Med 2012;367(20):1930–8.

60. Delaney KA, Vassallo SU, Larkin GL, et al. Rewarming rates in urban patients with hypothermia: prediction of underlying infection. Acad Emerg Med 2006;13(9):913–21.

61. Pasquier M, Blancher M, Buse S, et al. Intra-patient potassium variability after hypothermic cardiac arrest: a multicentre, prospective study. Scand J Trauma Resusc Emerg Med 2019;27(1):113.

62. Monika BM, Martin D, Balthasar E, et al. The Bernese Hypothermia Algorithm: a consensus paper on in-hospital decision-making and treatment of patients in hypothermic cardiac arrest at an alpine level 1 trauma centre. Injury 2011;42(5):539–43.

63. Jarosz A, Kosiński S, Darocha T, et al. Problems and Pitfalls of Qualification for Extracorporeal Rewarming in Severe Accidental Hypothermia. J Cardiothorac Vasc Anesth 2016;30(6):1693–7.

64. Ruttmann E, Dietl M, Kastenberger T, et al. Characteristics and outcome of patients with hypothermic out-of-hospital cardiac arrest: Experience from a European trauma center. Resuscitation 2017;120:57–62.

65. Klein LR, Huelster J, Adil U, et al. Endovascular rewarming in the emergency department for moderate to severe accidental hypothermia. Am J Emerg Med 2017;35(11):1624–9.

66. Prekker ME, Rischall M, Carlson M, et al. Extracorporeal membrane oxygenation versus conventional rewarming for severe hypothermia in an urban emergency department. Acad Emerg Med 2023;30(1):6–15.

67. Kjaergaard B, Bach P. Warming of patients with accidental hypothermia using warm water pleural lavage. Resuscitation 2006;68(2):203–7.

68. Plaisier BR. Thoracic lavage in accidental hypothermia with cardiac arrest–report of a case and review of the literature. Resuscitation 2005;66(1):99–104.

69. Mendrala K, Kosiński S, Podsiadło P, et al. The Efficacy of Renal Replacement Therapy for Rewarming of Patients in Severe Accidental Hypothermia-Systematic Review of the Literature. Int J Environ Res Public Health 2021;18(18):9638.

70. Laniewicz M, Lyn-Kew K, Silbergleit R. Rapid endovascular warming for profound hypothermia. Ann Emerg Med 2008;51(2):160–3.

71. Murakami T, Yoshida T, Kurokochi A, et al. Accidental Hypothermia Treated by Hemodialysis in the Acute Phase: Three Case Reports and a Review of the Literature. Intern Med 2019;58(18):2743–8.

72. Ledoux A, Saint Leger P. Therapeutic management of severe hypothermia with veno-arterial ECMO: where do we stand? Case report and review of the current literature. Scand J Trauma Resusc Emerg Med 2020;28(1):30.

73. Ruttmann E, Weissenbacher A, Ulmer H, et al. Prolonged extracorporeal membrane oxygenation-assisted support provides improved survival in hypothermic patients with cardiocirculatory arrest. J Thorac Cardiovasc Surg 2007;134(3):594–600.

74. Saczkowski R, Kuzak N, Grunau B, et al. Extracorporeal life support rewarming rate is associated with survival with good neurological outcome in accidental hypothermia. Eur J Cardio Thorac Surg 2021;59(3):593–600.

75. Austin MA, Maynes EJ, O'Malley TJ, et al. Outcomes of Extracorporeal Life Support Use in Accidental Hypothermia: A Systematic Review. Ann Thorac Surg 2020;110(6):1926–32.

76. Pasquier M, Hugli O, Paal P, et al. Hypothermia outcome prediction after extracorporeal life support for hypothermic cardiac arrest patients: The HOPE score. Resuscitation 2018;126:58–64.

77. Pasquier M, Rousson V, Darocha T, et al. Hypothermia outcome prediction after extracorporeal life support for hypothermic cardiac arrest patients: An external validation of the HOPE score. Resuscitation 2019;139:321–8.

78. Grin N, Rousson V, Darocha T, et al. Hypothermia Outcome Prediction after Extracorporeal Life Support for Hypothermic Cardiac Arrest Patients: Assessing the Performance of the HOPE Score in Case Reports from the Literature. Int J Environ Res Public Health 2021;18(22):11896.

79. Kosiński S, Darocha T, Jarosz A, et al. Clinical course and prognostic factors of patients in severe accidental hypothermia with circulatory instability rewarmed with veno-arterial ECMO - an observational case series study. Scand J Trauma Resusc Emerg Med 2017;25(1):46.

80. Gehrmann LP, Hafner JW, Montgomery DL, et al. Pediatric Extracorporeal Membrane Oxygenation: An Introduction for Emergency Medicine Physicians. J Emerg Med 2015;49(4):552–60.

81. Khorsandi M, Dougherty S, Young N, et al. Extracorporeal Life Support for Refractory Cardiac Arrest from Accidental Hypothermia: A 10-Year Experience in Edinburgh. J Emerg Med 2017;52(2):160–8.

82. Farstad M, Andersen KS, Koller ME, et al. Rewarming from accidental hypothermia by extracorporeal circulation. A retrospective study. Eur J Cardio Thorac Surg 2001;20(1):58–64.

83. Ohbe H, Isogai S, Jo T, et al. Extracorporeal membrane oxygenation improves outcomes of accidental hypothermia without vital signs: A nationwide observational study. Resuscitation 2019;144:27–32.

84. Kuhnke M, Albrecht R, Schefold JC, et al. Successful resuscitation from prolonged hypothermic cardiac arrest without extracorporeal life support: a case report. J Med Case Rep 2019;13(1):354.

85. Fister M, Knafelj R, Radsel P, et al. Cardiopulmonary Resuscitation with Extracorporeal Membrane Oxygenation in a Patient with Profound Accidental Hypothermia and Refractory Ventricular Fibrillation. Ther Hypothermia Temp Manag 2019;9(1):86–9.

86. Mair P, Brugger H, Mair B, et al. Is extracorporeal rewarming indicated in avalanche victims with unwitnessed hypothermic cardiorespiratory arrest? High Alt Med Biol 2014;15(4):500–3.

# Cold Injury

Jennifer Dow, MD, MHA, FAWM, DiMM[a,b,*]

## KEYWORDS

- Frostbite • Non-freezing cold injury • Iloprost • Thrombolytics

## KEY POINTS

- Cold injury can be prevented by use of appropriate clothing, seeking shelter, or avoiding freezing environments.
- Early recognition of a cold injury and the initiation of rapid rewarming can minimize tissue damage.
- Management with thrombolytic therapy and/or Iloprost is time dependent and has been shown to improve tissue salvage.
- All cold related injuries can have long-term sequelae, if not recognized and treated appropriately.

## INTRODUCTION

The sequelae of cold injury can have profound and debilitating consequences in terms of functional loss and economic instability. Injury leading to amputation garners extensive medical costs, including acute care and long-term management. Those whose injury does not progress to amputation may still experience chronic neuropathic pain, arthritis, cold sensitivity, and/or chronic ulcers. Early recognition and treatment will mitigate the long-term impacts of cold injury.

Cold injury encompasses hypothermia, freezing, and non-freezing injuries. Hypothermia is discussed in depth elsewhere in this volume. Freezing injury is frostbite. Non-freezing cold injury (NFCI) is commonly referred to as trench foot. This chapter focuses on frostbite, with a brief overview of other cold related conditions.

## HISTORY AND EPIDEMIOLOGY OF COLD INJURY

Cold weather injury is historically an occupational hazard – predominantly attributed to laborers and military personnel. Military losses were attributed to cold as early as the fourth century BCE, with references to frostbite by Hippocrates, Aristotle, and Galen.[1] Dominque Jean Larrey, Napoleon Bonaparte's surgeon, is credited with the first clinical descriptions of cold injury.[2] Mountaineers and other winter sports enthusiasts

[a] Department of Emergency Medicine, Alaska Regional Hospital, Anchorage, AK, USA;
[b] National Park Service, Alaska Region
* PO Box 1229, Girdwood, AK 99587.
E-mail address: jenndow@mac.com

Emerg Med Clin N Am 42 (2024) 513–525
https://doi.org/10.1016/j.emc.2024.02.012
0733-8627/24/© 2024 Elsevier Inc. All rights reserved.
emed.theclinics.com

endure extreme cold to pursue their passions and are not exempt from sustaining cold injuries. Whether secondary to safety – as seen by those escaping military bombardment or a storm – or pushing for a goal, the inability or unwillingness to treat early injury contributes to deeper injury and more extensive tissue trauma.

Avoiding cold exposure is a simple preventative measure but may be impractical for many professions and a challenge for those facing housing insecurity. If cold exposure cannot be avoided, preventative measures including appropriate equipment and clothing, education, and frequent self-assessment are valuable. Early recognition of a cold injury is critical to mitigating tissue loss or progressive injury. Recognition may be impaired by intoxicants, hypoxia, hypoglycemia, and other chronic conditions affecting sensation. Insulated clothing, including gloves, should be worn to protect from the cold, wind, and moisture. Further preventative measures include avoiding constricting clothing or jewelry, wearing well-fitting footwear, using extreme caution to minimize exposure when removing gloves to perform tasks, and instituting a buddy check system to ensure team members are aware of each other's status. Team members can monitor each other for frostnip. Frostnip, while not associated with cellular damage like frostbite, is a condition that occurs in freezing conditions. It is associated with vasoconstriction of superficial vessels underlying exposed skin and frost, or ice crystals, forming on the surface. It resolves rapidly upon rewarming without sequalae. If frostnip is observed, it does indicate that conditions are extreme enough to cause a freezing cold injury, and precautions should be taken.

The incidence of cold injury is challenging to define. Studies may include hypothermia, may exclude minor injuries such as frostnip, or may only include severe frostbite. Frostbite is the most common cold injury reported by the US Armed Forces,[3,4] and some studies have described up to 36% of mountaineers reporting some degree of frostbite.[5] The hands and feet are the most commonly affected areas.[6–8]

## FROSTBITE
### Pathophysiology

Frostbite is a cold injury secondary to tissue exposure to temperatures below its freezing point, approximately $-0.5°C$.[9] There are four pathologic phases: prefreeze, freeze-thaw, vascular stasis, and late ischemic. Direct cellular injury occurs during the prefreeze and freeze-thaw phases. Prefreeze is characterized by tissue cooling without ice crystal formation. Vasoconstriction during this phase may cause ischemia, manifesting as hyperesthesia or paresthesia. Intracellular and extracellular ice crystals form during the freeze-thaw phase, causing cell wall lysis, cellular electrolyte shifts, lipid and protein derangement, and cellular death.[10] The thawing stage of this phase may trigger an inflammatory response, ischemia, and reperfusion injury. During vascular stasis, intravascular sludging occurs, leading to the late ischemic phase. A cascade of inflammatory response, vasoconstriction, reperfusion injury, embolic showers, and larger vessel thrombosis marks this phase. Microvascular destruction contributes to cellular death.[11,12] Refreezing after an initial injury leads to intracellular ice formation and the further release of destructive mediators, causing additional tissue damage.

### Classification

Frostbite injury has a component of tissue ischemia and is similar to the heart or brain; rapid identification and initiation of therapy improves tissue salvage and recovery.[13,14] Time is tissue. Like burns, frostbite is classified by degree based on the acute physical findings present once the tissue has thawed.[15] The four-tier classification system may be challenging in the field after rewarming and prior to imaging. A simplified classification field classification system identifies superficial and deep injury.[16] (**Table 1**)

Patients may have a frostbitten extremity with multiple degrees of injury – for example, third-degree injury to the tips of the fingers and second-degree injury to more proximal areas. Cauchy proposed a grading scale for frostbite injury based on cyanosis present after rewarming with a correlation to amputation risk. No cyanosis and no amputation risk characterizes a grade 1 injury. Grade 2 has a moderate risk of amputation with cyanosis of the distal phalanx. Grade 3 demonstrates cyanosis to the metacarpal-phalangeal or metatarsal-phalangeal (MP) joint with a high risk of amputation. Grade 4 has a 100% risk of amputation and is characterized by cyanosis proximal to the MP joint.[15,17] This classification system, and more specifically, the amputation risk, is based on both the appearance of the injury after immediate rewarming and advanced imaging performed on day 2 (**Fig. 1**).

### Management and Treatment

Historically, frostbite has been managed conservatively, with the common saying, "freeze in January, amputate in July" summarizing treatment. Deep frostbite leads to dry gangrene, with mummification of the damaged tissue. This obvious line of demarcation provided the guide for amputation (**Fig. 2**). Advances in imaging and the availability of new treatments have made tissue salvage a real possibility. Success is predicated upon minimizing initial injury by rapid warming (if possible), preventing re-freeze of thawed issue of tissue, and timely imaging. If the patient is a candidate; thrombolytic or prostaglandin inhibitor therapy can be initiated (**Fig. 3**).

### Field management

The field management of frostbite includes a complete assessment, prevention of further injury, and treatment, including warming, injury protection, pain management, and evacuation considerations.

The initial field assessment of frostbite does not differ from any other injury. Completing the primary survey using the C-ABCDE approach is followed by immediate treatment of threats to life (C: catastrophic hemorrhage, A: airway, B: breathing, C: circulation, D: disability, E: exposure). Hypothermia needs to be managed or prevented prior to active frostbite treatment. Once frostbite is identified, prevent further exposure to the cold and remove constricting jewelry or clothing. Do not rub or

**Table 1**
**Classification and description of depth of frostbite injury**

|  | Characteristics | Field Description |
|---|---|---|
| First degree | • Mild edema and erythema<br>• Numbness of tissue<br>• Area of injury white or yellow and firm<br>• Absence of blisters or blebs | Superficial<br>• Minimal tissue loss anticipated |
| Second degree | • Superficial skin blebs with clear or milk fluid<br>• Blebs with surrounding edema and erythema |  |
| Third degree | • Hemorrhagic blisters – (indicates deep dermal involvement and extension into the vascular plexus and reticular dermis) | Deep<br>• Significant tissue loss anticipated |
| Fourth degree | • Extension of injury into subcutaneous tissue, potential for necrosis of muscle and bone |  |

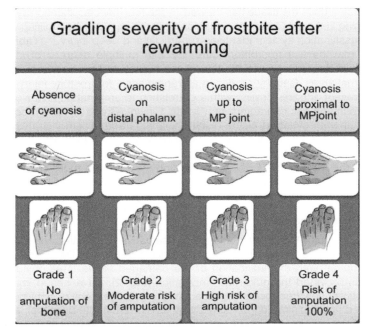

**Fig. 1.** Grading and severity of frostbite after rewarming. (*From*: Cauchy E, Davis CB, Pasquier M, Meyer EF, Hackett PH. A New Proposal for Management of Severe Frostbite in the Austere Environment. Wilderness Environ Med. 2016 Mar;27(1):92-9.)

massage the skin, as this causes additional injury. Wrap the area with a dry protective dressing, such as bulky gauze, and protect against mechanical damage with a splint if necessary. If in an urban area, transport the patient to the nearest medical facility.[16]

Austere or wilderness settings follow the same guidelines, but initiating rewarming in the field may be necessary. Only initiate rewarming if there is no chance of refreezing, which causes additional reperfusion injury.[17–19] If the injury is to the feet, consider whether walking is necessary to establish safety. If the boots are removed and spontaneous thaw begins, it is unlikely that the injured person will be able to wear their boots again due to swelling.

Frostbitten tissue will spontaneously thaw when removed from the freezing environment, and this should not be prevented. Do not continuously expose the injury to freezing temperatures; this will worsen the frostbite and contribute to hypothermia. Slow warming measures may speed tissue thaw, such as placing the frostbitten part in an axilla or in a sleeping bag with insulated hot water bottles. Do not apply dry heat to the injury. Rapid rewarming has been championed and is thought to improve outcomes,[20] especially if established care is greater than 2 hours away. Rapid rewarming may be realistic in a field medical clinic or basecamp. To prevent burns, heat the water to no greater than 38-39°C.[16] Circulating the water will help maintain a more consistent temperature, and alert those monitoring treatment that the water is cooling and needs to be exchanged. Anticipate a minimum of 30 minutes to achieve thaw, which will be evident when the injured tissue becomes more pliable and appears red or purple.

### Field treatment
**Blisters.** Blisters form as the tissue thaws. Clear blisters are believed to contain prostaglandins and thromboxanes and may damage the underlying tissue. Hemorrhagic

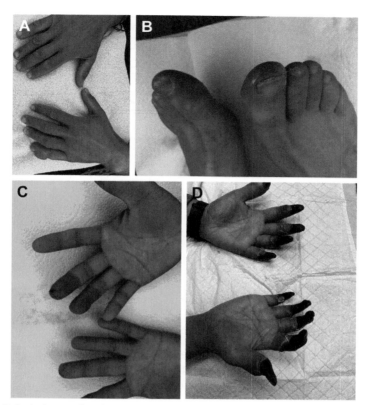

**Fig. 2.** (*A*) 2nd degree frostbite with clear blebs, (*B*) 3rd degree frostbite of the toes: Hemorrhagic blebs present – grade 2, (*C*) 3rd degree frostbite of the hand on a dark skinned individual; Grade 2 to 3, (*D*) 4th degree frostbite demonstrating dry gangrene and demarcation. (Photo Credit: A, B, C: Melis Coady, Executive Director, Alaska Avalanche School.)

blisters indicate deep tissue injury and involve the vascular plexus. Clear blisters may be aspirated in the field if they are large or interfere with movement. Hemorrhagic blisters should not be aspirated in the field. Blisters may rupture spontaneously; care should be taken to prevent additional tissue damage. If available, apply aloe vera and a sterile dressing to the injury, even if the blisters are intact. Aloe vera is a thromboxane inhibitor and minimizes local vasoconstriction, potentially decreasing tissue loss.[21,22]

**Pain management.** Pain management must be considered and balanced against the need for the patient to be alert. Nonsteroidal anti-inflammatory drugs (NSAIDs) decrease the production of prostaglandins and thromboxanes; mediators contributing to vasoconstriction and progressive ischemia.[23,24] Administer ibuprofen at 12 mg/kg divided over two daily doses. (The maximum recommended dose of ibuprofen, in an otherwise healthy individual, is 3200 mg/24 hrs.) Opioids, whether oral or parenteral, may be considered and should be slowly titrated to response, minimizing sedation. Other methods for pain control, such as nerve blocks or sympathetic blockade, should be reserved for the hospital setting.

**Evacuation and special considerations.** Evacuate all patients with frostbite from the field. Ideally, the patient will not travel in the cold, but, if necessary, ensure that all

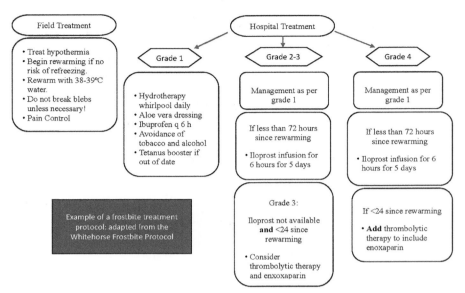

**Fig. 3.** Example of a frostbite treatment protocol, adapted from Whitehorse Frostbite Treatment Protocol.

skin is protected from additional exposure. This is especially critical if the patient's mental status is altered. Careful monitoring during the rescue process prevents additional cold injury and the refreeze of thawing skin. Prevention and treatment of hypothermia take precedence over frostbite treatment.

The depth and extent of the cold injury influence the destination hospital. Some locales will only have community medical centers or a limited capacity to treat frostbite. If there is a choice of healthcare facilities, factors influencing the decision include the clinical grade of injury, the length of time since tissue thaw, the presence of other trauma or medical comorbidities, and the availability of diagnostic and specialty therapeutic modalities. As will be further discussed, there are time limits for initiating aggressive pharmacologic therapy.

**Oxygen.** While frostbite does have an ischemic component, supplemental oxygen is not indicated unless the patient is otherwise hypoxic, which may be secondary to altitude or underlying disease processes. Maintaining an oxygen saturation greater than 90% is likely beneficial.[17] Some centers advocate hyperbaric oxygen therapy early in frostbite care. Based on these protocols, the use of portable hyperbaric chambers in the field is postulated to improve oxygen delivery to damaged tissues. There is currently no support for or against using portable hyperbaric chambers to treat frostbite in the field.

**Pharmacologic therapies.** The use of thrombolytic agents and prostaglandin inhibitors in the field is limited to case reports. These agents are discussed in depth in the following sections. The patient and medical provider must carefully balance the administration of these agents against the lack of imaging and physiologic monitoring. It is the author's opinion that this may be considered if the degree of injury is great, the time to access the treatment facility will exceed the time parameters for treatment, and a careful and thorough informed consent is completed.

### Hospital management

Not unlike field management, a thorough patient assessment using the C-ABCDE mnemonic guides treatment. Care for hypothermia, unstable illness, and trauma takes precedence over frostbite management.[16] Once stabilized, rapid rewarming of frost-bitten tissue can be initiated using circulating 38-39°C water.

### Patient history

Determining the appropriate therapy for frostbite requires knowledge of the following.

- Length of exposure and environmental conditions preceding injury
- Length of time from injury identification to tissue warming (thaw)
- Length of time since tissue warming (warm ischemia)
  - less than 24 h or greater than 24 h, less than 72 hours
- Any freeze-thaw-refreeze pattern or history of walking on frozen feet
- Field treatment measures

In addition to the details of the cold injury, a complete history, to determine the presence or absence of predisposing conditions or risk factors will help guide and anticipate potential obstacles to therapy.

- Use of intoxicants or illicit drugs
- Use of nicotine (eg, cigarettes, chewing tobacco, gum)
- History of peripheral vascular disease including Reynaud's phenomenon
- Altered peripheral sensation (eg, neuropathy, central nervous system pathology, spinal injury)
- History of prior cold injury
- Housing and food security and the ability to access care.

**Imaging.** The determination of treatment modality is guided by the severity of tissue injury and imaging results. Frostbite is caused by vascular thrombosis resulting in tissue ischemia. Angiography demonstrates the perfusion status of the injured tissue. Results are utilized to guide thrombolytic therapy in the acute phase of treatment.[25,26] Repeat angiography can be performed after thrombolysis to assess the treatment response. Multiphase bone scintigraphy – or a SPECT/CT – is a valuable adjunct to predicting injury extent and level of amputation.[27] Routine radiography will not guide frostbite treatment but can identify associated fractures or soft tissue foreign bodies that require management

**Wound care.** While routine debridement of blisters is not recommended in the field, it is appropriate in the hospital setting. Topical agents, such as aloe vera, are applied to inhibit additional thromboxane activity. Secondary to the concern of damaging the underlying vascular bed, hemorrhagic blisters are traditionally not debrided. There is little supporting evidence for either pathway.[21,28] Apply protective, non-constricting dressings to open wounds.

### Pharmacotherapy

**Pain management and anti-inflammatories.** Ibuprofen (12 mg/kg divided BID) is recommended both for pain relief and for its anti-inflammatory properties; specifically for thromboxane and prostaglandin inhibition. As in the field, opioids can be used for moderate to severe pain.

**Infection control.** Prophylactic antibiotic use is not recommended for frostbite treatment. While not initially infection prone, secondary infection can occur. Antibiotic choice should be determined by local susceptibilities and patterns.[16] Frostbite is not a tetanus prone injury; immunoglobulin is not necessary, and booster vaccination should be administered according to the regular schedule.

**Thrombolytic therapy.** Frostbite is an ischemic injury, and as with a stroke or myocardial infarction, restoring circulation limits tissue damage. Patients with a grade 3 or 4 injury, presenting within 24 hours of tissue thaw, are candidates for thrombolytic therapy – potentially reversing the ischemic injury. Successful treatment protocols currently include the systemic administration of both alteplase and tenecteplase.[29–31] (**Table 2**) Systemic intravenous therapy is not inferior to intra-arterial directed therapy and makes this therapy available at institutions without interventional radiology or catheterization lab capacity.[13,32] Fibrinolysis does have a procoagulant effect, thus anticoagulants, either unfractionated heparin (UFH) or low-molecular-weight heparin (LMWH) is co-administered. LMWH is preferred secondary to it predictable anticoagulant effect.[16,33] Before administration, the patient must be screened for general exclusion criteria, including severe hypertension, recent stroke or trauma, bleeding disorder, pregnancy, and inability to consent. Frostbite specific exclusion criteria include repeated freeze-thaw-refreeze cycles and greater than 24 hours since rewarming. Thrombolytic therapy has been administered in the field in cases of severe frostbite with a high risk of amputation.[17]

**Iloprost.** Iloprost is a synthetic analog of prostaglandin $I_2$, a potent vasodilator and inhibitor of platelet aggregation. Its use in frostbite treatment was first reported in 1984 in Austria.[34] An extensive investigation by Cauchy, followed by encouraging case reports has made Iloprost a mainstay of treatment for severe frostbite.[14,33] Use of Iloprost for severe frostbite has demonstrated a reduction in amputations compared to historic controls.[33,35] Approved in February of 2024 for use from frostbite in the US by the FDA, its use is established in Canada, Europe, and other countries. It can be administered up to 72 hours after tissue thaw with fewer significant side-effects as compared to thrombolysis. It should be considered for patients with grade 2 to 4 injuries.[14] Administered as a continuous infusion over 6 hours, for 5 to 6 consecutive days, patients are often admitted to an inpatient service (**Table 3**). Outpatient infusion centers with simple hemodynamic monitoring capacity are another option if the patient does not otherwise require admission. Adverse reactions to Iloprost are dose related, with the most common reactions being flushing and headaches. These reactions, as well as the more significant reaction of hypotension, can be avoided by careful dose titration. All reactions resolve quickly after the cessation of the infusion.[36]

**Surgical intervention.** Except for intervention via fasciotomy for compartment syndromes, immediate surgical intervention is not generally needed for frostbite injuries. Early amputation is indicated in instances of wet gangrene, liquefaction necrosis, or sepsis. Late amputation can be guided by SPECT/CT imaging, perfusion studies, or the extent of mummification.

**Hyperbaric oxygen therapy.** Hyperbaric oxygen therapy (HBOT) is established as an adjunct for wound healing through its actions of hyperoxygenation of hypoxic tissue.

| Table 2 Indications and dosing recommendations for thrombolytic therapy | | |
|---|---|---|
| **Indications** | **Alteplase (Activase)** | **Tenecteplase (TNKase)** |
| • No refreeze injury <br> • <24 h since thaw <br> • Grade 3 or 4 injury | • 0.15 mg/kg IV bolus over 15 min <br>   • followed by <br> • 0.15 mg/kg/hr infusion <br>   for 6 h – total dose <100 mg. | • 25 mg – 0.5 mg/kg up to 50 mg single bolus |

| Table 3 | |
|---|---|
| **Iloprost infusion strategy, based upon the Yukon/Whitehorse Frostbite treatment protocol** | |
| Indications<br>• Grade 2–4 frostbite injury<br>• <72 h since tissue thaw<br>Contraindications<br>• Pregnancy/lactation<br>• Severe coronary artery disease or unstable angina<br>• Acute or chronic severe congestive heart failure<br>• Conditions with increased risk of hemorrhage | • 50mcg Iloprost Diluted into 250 mL D5W: Concentration of 0.2mcg/ml<br>• Infusion Imitated at 10 mL/hr<br>• Increase Infusion rate by 10 mL/hr Every 30 min up to 50 mL/hr<br>• Continue Infusion of at Least 50mcg (250 mL) and for a Minimum of 6 h – Starting a second bag if Necessary<br>• Adverse Reaction: Decrease rate by 10 mL/hr and Reassess in 30 min – Side Effects Will Rapidly Resolve if Dose Related<br>Day 3, 4, 5<br>• if the patient Tolerates the Infusion, may start at the Maximum rate |

https://yukon.ca/en/whitehorse-frostbite-protocol.

Inflammatory processes that accompany infection or edema associated with chronic wounds can restrict blood flow. HBOT can increase oxygenation up to 5 times in infected tissue.[37] HBOT has been utilized in cases of delayed frostbite, but studies investigating immediate treatment have not demonstrated conclusive improvement in tissue salvage.[38] Importantly, it did not lead to worse outcomes. Current studies suggest that a combination of HBOT and Iloprost may improve outcomes.[39]

### Long-term impact
A challenge in identifying the long-term sequelae in frostbite patients is follow-up. Patients may receive initial care a distance from their home, in another country, principality, state, or municipal region. While a health center with an established frostbite treatment protocol may actively assess for associated sequelae, an institution unfamiliar with the injury may not attribute a condition to frostbite. Tissue loss is the most obvious long-term impact of frostbite injuries. Difficulties with ambulation or loss of dexterity may contribute to job loss, the inability to participate in nonvocational activities (hobbies, volunteerism, etc.), and may negatively impact mental health. Cold injuries have less obvious complications. Patients have reported impaired circulation, leading to cold hypersensitivity and intolerance. Also identified are chronic neuropathies including dysesthesia, hyperhidrosis, and pain.[9] Chronic wounds and ulcerations have been reported, both in patients with access to health care and those with poor access.

**Socioeconomic considerations.** All prolonged episodes of medical care have a considerable financial impact. Severe frostbite requires hospitalization, followed by scheduled treatments for wound care. Beyond the cost of health care, the patients who do not live near a capable facility may have to relocate for the duration of treatment. Patients who sustain frostbite in an urban environment tend to have a plethora of risk factors that negatively impact both access to health care and the sequelae of injury. Risk factors include economic instability, homelessness, substance abuse, and medical comorbidities including diabetes and peripheral vascular disease.[40] Unfortunately, these patients may require readmission for chronic wound care.[41]

## COLD ASSOCIATED CONDITIONS
### Nonfreezing Cold Injury

While not associated with cellular damage due to freezing, NFCI can also cause long term disability. Cold, but non-freezing, conditions and exposure to moisture are precipitants to injury. NFCI is commonly known as trench foot, but it can occur in the hands and other areas with prolonged exposure to cold, moist conditions. It is also called an immersion foot or a cold-immersion injury. NFCI can be prevented by not allowing tissue to remain moist and keeping the feet dry. In combat situations, soldiers were often unable to remove their boots. Trench foot has had a devastating impact on military operations throughout history. Prolonged exposure to a cold, wet environment contributes to skin breakdown. Further injury is caused by prolonged vasoconstriction, causing direct injury to vasculature.[42] Further damage and maceration of the tissue occur with walking. Treatment, like frostbite, is to rewarm the tissue and keep it dry. Trench foot has three distinct phases after exposure to cold. The early stage, or prehyperemic phase is characterized by waxy, yellow, or white, but has no blisters. The hyperemic phase occurs after several hours of rewarming and is characterized by edema, pain, and erythematous tissue. The pain associated with this phase can be extreme and may last for weeks. The final phase may not occur in minor cases and has no obvious physical signs. Characterized by hyperhidrosis, persistent aches, and anesthesia, this phase may last for weeks to years.[43] Amitriptyline or gabapentin may be used for chronic symptoms.

### Chilblains

Chilblains, or pernio, is an idiopathic condition associated with cold exposure. An inflammatory condition manifests as painful lesions, most commonly in the distal extremities. It may be mistaken for vasculitis. Characteristics of chilblains include exposure to cold weather, familial clusters, and spontaneous resolution as the season warms.[44]

### Cold-induced Urticaria

Cold-induced urticaria is urticaria, or hives, triggered by exposure to cold. Typically, the urticaria manifests after cold exposure, upon return to the warmth. Most cases resolve within an hour. It is believed to be immunologically mediated and may involve the formation of auto allergens. Symptoms can range from an isolated skin response to anaphylaxis. Symptoms are mitigated by avoidance of the cold. Specific treatment regimens are under investigation, and patients with severe symptoms should be referred to an allergist or immunologist.[45] The patient presenting with anaphylaxis is treated with standard protocols.

### SUMMARY

Most cold injuries can be prevented by wearing appropriate clothing and limiting exposure to cold and freezing temperatures. When injury does occur; rapid recognition, prevention of further cold exposure, and early intervention with rapid rewarming and pharmacologic intervention will prevent tissue loss and long-term morbidity. After the initial treatment phase, patients with significant injuries require prolonged wound care, specialized imaging, and possibly amputation. Understanding the pathophysiology, treatment options, and extended care regimens of these injury patterns will mitigate potential long-term sequalae and improve patient outcomes.

### CLINICS CARE POINTS

- Early recognition and treatment of cold injury is critical for tissue salvage.
- Rapid initiation of rewarming with warm water will minimize tissue damage.

- HIgh grade freezing cold injury can be managed with thrombolytic and/or iloprost, but these therapies are time dependent.

## DISCLOSURE

No financial conflicts or disclosures.

## REFERENCES

1. Lee JWI. A Greek army on the march : soldiers and survival in Xenophon's Anabasis. xii: Cambridge University Press; 2007. p. 323.
2. Larrey DJ. Memoirs of military surgery: and campaigns of the French armies on the Rhine. In: Hall RWt, editor. Corsica, Catalonia, Egypt, and Syria: at Boulogn, Umm, and Austerlitz: in Saxony, Prussian Poland, Spain, and Austria (Vol 2). Baltimore MD: Joseph Cushing; 1814.
3. Connor RR. Update: cold weather injuries, active and reserve components, U.S. Armed Forces. MSMR 2014;21(10):14–9.
4. Heil KM, Oakley EH, Wood AM. British Military freezing cold injuries: a 13-year review. J R Army Med Corps 2016;162(6):413–8.
5. Harirchi I, Arvin A, Vash JH, et al. Frostbite: incidence and predisposing factors in mountaineers. Br J Sports Med 2005;39(12):898–901, discussion 901.
6. Imray C, Grieve A, Dhillon S, et al. Cold damage to the extremities: frostbite and non-freezing cold injuries. Postgrad Med J 2009;85(1007):481–8.
7. Juopperi K, Hassi J, Ervasti O, et al. Incidence of frostbite and ambient temperature in Finland, 1986-1995. A national study based on hospital admissions. Int J Circumpolar Health 2002;61(4):352–62.
8. Kyosola K. Clinical experiences in the management of cold injuries: a study of 110 cases. J Trauma 1974;14(1):32–6.
9. Regli IB, Strapazzon G, Falla M, et al. Long-Term Sequelae of Frostbite-A Scoping Review. Int J Environ Res Public Health 2021;(18):18.
10. Mazur P. Causes of Injury in Frozen and Thawed Cells. Fed Proc 1965;24: S175–82.
11. Murphy JV, Banwell PE, Roberts AH, et al. Frostbite: pathogenesis and treatment. J Trauman 2000;48(1):171–8.
12. Kulka JP. Microcirculatory Impairment as a Factor in Inflammatory Tissue Damage. Ann N Y Acad Sci 1964;116:1018–44.
13. Nygaard RM, Lacey AM, Lemere A, et al. Time Matters in Severe Frostbite: Assessment of Limb/Digit Salvage on the Individual Patient Level. J Burn Care Res 2017;38(1):53–9.
14. Cauchy E, Cheguillaume B, Chetaille E. A controlled trial of a prostacyclin and rt-PA in the treatment of severe frostbite. N Engl J Med 2011;364(2):189–90.
15. Cauchy E, Chetaille E, Marchand V, et al. Retrospective study of 70 cases of severe frostbite lesions: a proposed new classification scheme. Wilderness Environ Med. Winter 2001;12(4):248–55.
16. McIntosh SE, Freer L, Grissom CK, et al. Wilderness Medical Society Clinical Practice Guidelines for the Prevention and Treatment of Frostbite: 2019 Update. Wilderness Environ Med 2019;30(4S):S19–32.
17. Cauchy E, Davis CB, Pasquier M, et al. A New Proposal for Management of Severe Frostbite in the Austere Environment. Wilderness Environ Med 2016; 27(1):92–9.

18. Mills WJ Jr. Summary of treatment of the cold injured patient. Frostbite. Alaska Med 1983;25(2):33–8.
19. Mills WJ, Frostbite Jr. A discussion of the problem and a review of an Alaskan experience. Alaska Med 1973;15(2):27–47.
20. Mills WJ Jr, Douglas JD, Gottmann AW. Clinical experiences in treatment and rehabilitation of frostbite in Alaska. Tech Rep Arct Aeromed Lab US 1960; 59-24:1–9.
21. McCauley RL, Heggers JP, Robson MC. Frostbite. Methods to minimize tissue loss. Postgrad Med 1990;88(8):67–8, 73-68.
22. Hekmatpou D, Mehrabi F, Rahzani K, et al. The Effect of Aloe Vera Clinical Trials on Prevention and Healing of Skin Wound: A Systematic Review. Iran J Med Sci 2019;44(1):1–9.
23. Robson MC, DelBeccaro EJ, Heggers JP, et al. Increasing dermal perfusion after burning by decreasing thromboxane production. J Trauma 1980;20(9): 722–5.
24. Rainsford KD. Ibuprofen: pharmacology, efficacy and safety. Inflammopharmacology 2009;17(6):275–342.
25. Gao Y, Wang F, Zhou W, et al. Research progress in the pathogenic mechanisms and imaging of severe frostbite. Eur J Radiol 2021;137:109605.
26. Zaramo TZ, Green JK, Janis JE. Practical Review of the Current Management of Frostbite Injuries. Plast Reconstr Surg Glob Open 2022;10(10):e4618.
27. Manganaro MS, Millet JD, Brown RK, et al. The utility of bone scintigraphy with SPECT/CT in the evaluation and management of frostbite injuries. Br J Radiol 2019;92(1094):20180545.
28. Robson MC, Heggers JP. Evaluation of hand frostbite blister fluid as a clue to pathogenesis. J Hand Surg Am 1981;6(1):43–7.
29. Nygaard RM, Whitley AB, Fey RM, et al. The Hennepin Score: Quantification of Frostbite Management Efficacy. J Burn Care Res 2016;37(4):e317–22.
30. Lacey AM, Rogers C, Endorf FW, et al. An Institutional Protocol for the Treatment of Severe Frostbite Injury-A 6-Year Retrospective Analysis. J Burn Care Res 2021; 42(4):817–20.
31. Gonzaga T, Jenabzadeh K, Anderson CP, et al. Use of Intra-arterial Thrombolytic Therapy for Acute Treatment of Frostbite in 62 Patients with Review of Thrombolytic Therapy in Frostbite. J Burn Care Res 2016;37(4):e323–34.
32. Drinane J, Kotamarti VS, O'Connor C, et al. Thrombolytic Salvage of Threatened Frostbitten Extremities and Digits: A Systematic Review. J Burn Care Res 2019; 40(5):541–9.
33. Gauthier J, Morris-Janzen D, Poole A. Iloprost for the treatment of frostbite: a scoping review. Int J Circumpolar Health 2023;82(1):2189552.
34. Groechenig E. Treatment of frostbite with iloprost. Lancet 1994;344(8930): 1152–3.
35. Poole A, Gauthier J, MacLennan M. Management of severe frostbite with iloprost, alteplase and heparin: a Yukon case series. CMAJ Open 2021;9(2): E585–91.
36. Grant SM, Goa KL. Iloprost. A review of its pharmacodynamic and pharmacokinetic properties, and therapeutic potential in peripheral vascular disease, myocardial ischaemia and extracorporeal circulation procedures. Drugs 1992; 43(6):889–924.
37. Zamboni WA, Browder LK, Martinez J. Hyperbaric oxygen and wound healing. Clin Plast Surg 2003;30(1):67–75.

38. Ghumman A, St Denis-Katz H, Ashton R, et al. Treatment of Frostbite With Hyperbaric Oxygen Therapy: A Single Center's Experience of 22 Cases. Wounds 2019; 31(12):322–5.

39. Magnan MA, Gayet-Ageron A, Louge P, et al. Hyperbaric Oxygen Therapy with Iloprost Improves Digit Salvage in Severe Frostbite Compared to Iloprost Alone. Medicina (Kaunas) 2021;57(11).

40. Endorf FW, Nygaard RM. Socioeconomic and Comorbid Factors Associated With Frostbite Injury in the United States. J Burn Care Res 2022;43(3):646–51.

41. Endorf FW, Nygaard RM. High Cost and Resource Utilization of Frostbite Readmissions in the United States. J Burn Care Res 2021;42(5):857–64.

42. Zafren K. Nonfreezing Cold Injury (Trench Foot). Int J Environ Res Public Health 2021;(19):18.

43. Imray CH, Richards P, Greeves J, et al. Nonfreezing cold-induced injuries. J R Army Med Corps 2011;157(1):79–84.

44. Pratt M, Mahmood F, Kirchhof MG. Pharmacologic Treatment of Idiopathic Chilblains (Pernio): A Systematic Review. J Cutan Med Surg 2021;25(5): 530–42.

45. Maltseva N, Borzova E, Fomina D, et al. Cold urticaria - What we know and what we do not know. Allergy 2021;76(4):1077–94.

# Altitude-Related Illness

Jessica Gehner, MD*

## KEYWORDS

- Altitude-related illness • AMS • HACE • HAPE

## KEY POINTS

- Proper acclimatization is crucial in avoiding altitude-related illness. Acclimatization is optimized by a slow, graded ascent profile and prophylaxis with medications such as acetazolamide.
- The diagnosis of altitude-related illness most commonly occurs in resource-limited environments. Acute mountain sickness is diagnosed based on history, while more severe manifestations of altitude illness such as high-altitude cerebral edema (HACE) and high-altitude pulmonary edema (HAPE) have abnormal physical exam findings.
- The definitive treatment for all altitude-related illnesses is descent. Supplemental oxygen and pharmacologic treatment are temporizing measures until the patient can be evacuated to a lower altitude.

## INTRODUCTION

*So, if you cannot understand that there is something in man that responds to the challenge of this mountain and goes out to meet it, that the struggle is the struggle of life itself upward and forever upward, then you won't see why we go. What we get from this adventure is just sheer joy. And joy is, after all, the end of life.*
—*George Mallory*

Climbers, mountaineers, and trekkers are often asked why they intentionally place themselves in such dangerous and harsh environments, just to stand upon a summit. "Because it's there" is the resounding answer. Yet, even the most experienced and well-trained athletes are not immune to the effects of high altitude. This text reviews the physiologic response to high altitude, as well as the spectrum of altitude-related illnesses, how to treat them, and when decent is necessary.

## BACKGROUND AND DEFINITIONS

One does not have to be summiting Everest to be at risk for altitude-related illness. Elevations above 1500m (4,921 ft) are considered high altitude, above 3500m

Wilderness Medicine Fellowship, Department of Emergency Medicine, Virginia Tech Carilion School of Medicine, Roanoke, VA, USA
* 4759 Mountain View Church Road, Blue Ridge, VA 24064.
*E-mail address:* Gehnerj@gmail.com

Emerg Med Clin N Am 42 (2024) 527–539
https://doi.org/10.1016/j.emc.2024.02.013
0733-8627/24/© 2024 Elsevier Inc. All rights reserved.

emed.theclinics.com

(11,483 ft) are considered very high altitude, and those greater than 5500m (18,045 ft) are considered extreme altitude. While still possible, it is extremely rare to see an altitude-related illness below 2500m (8,200 ft).[1] (**Fig. 1**)

As altitude increases, barometric pressure decreases, also decreasing the partial pressure of inhaled oxygen. The result is hypobaric hypoxia, which drives the physiologic changes seen in acclimatization, the process of our bodies becoming accustomed to a low-oxygen environment. When the body does not properly acclimatize, conditions such as acute mountain sickness (AMS), high-altitude cerebral edema (HACE), and high-altitude pulmonary edema (HAPE) may occur. AMS and HACE can be thought of as a spectrum of disease, with HACE being the most severe manifestation.

### Acclimatization

Acclimatization occurs in two phases: acute and chronic. Within hours of arrival at high altitude, the hypoxic ventilatory response (HVR) increases the respiratory rate. This improves oxygenation by decreasing the partial pressure of carbon dioxide in the alveoli, but it also causes a respiratory alkalosis. The kidneys respond to the increased pH by secreting bicarbonate in the urine, causing a compensatory metabolic acidosis and diuresis. This diuresis causes hemoconcentration, thereby increasing hematocrit. The increase in hematocrit is due to decreased water content in the blood during the acute phase of acclimatization. Adequate diuresis is associated with proper acclimatization.[1] Acetazolamide, oftentimes taken as an altitude illness prophylactic medication, facilitates this process. The pH-sensitive respiratory centers in the brain then respond to the more acidic environment with an increased respiratory rate, thus improving oxygenation.

After 3 to 4 weeks at high altitude, increased erythropoietin production results in increased red blood cell (RBC) mass, further increasing the hematocrit. Full acclimatization usually takes 4 to 6 weeks, but varies greatly based on multiple factors: rate of ascent, geographic location, and physiologic differences in populations.[2] This is the rationale behind climbers living at a high-altitude base camp for weeks prior to attempting high summits such as Mt. Everest.

### PATHOPHYSIOLOGY

When proper acclimatization does not occur, patients may develop one or more altitude-related illness: AMS, HACE, or HAPE. Each of these disease processes is ultimately the result of hypobaric hypoxia, relative hypoventilation, increased sympathetic drive, and fluid redistribution. The pathophysiology of AMS is not fully understood, with several hypotheses still being studied to further delineate this subjective and nebulous disease process. Some experts discuss the *"leaky-vessel theory,"* in which inflammation from hypoxia increases endothelin and cyclooxygenase

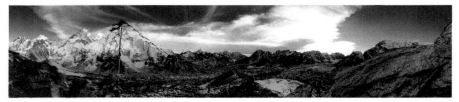

**Fig. 1.** Mt. Everest and Khumbu Glacier as seen from Kalapathar (Photo courtesy of Dr. Jessie Gehner, used with permission.)

and causes fluid to leak from blood vessels into the interstitium.[3] In a more severe form, this edema can result in HACE or HAPE. This is one reason non-steroidal anti-inflammatory drugs (NSAIDs) have been explored as a possible prophylactic and/or therapeutic option.[1]

Relative hypoventilation, as well as commonly experienced sleep apnea that develops in people visiting high altitude, contributes to the symptoms of altitude illness. Chemoreceptors in the respiratory centers of the brain are pH-sensitive. These chemoreceptors trigger a decreased respiratory rate in response to a high pH, and an increased respiratory rate in response to low pH. If acclimatization is inadequate or alkalosis is too extreme, the respiratory rate can decrease even to the point of apnea while asleep, causing not only lower peripheral oxygen saturation ($SpO_2$) but also very poor sleep at high altitude.

## EPIDEMIOLOGY

The incidence and severity of AMS depend on the rate of ascent, altitude attained (especially sleeping altitude), duration of altitude exposure, level of exertion, recent altitude exposure, and genetic susceptibility.[4] One of the most predictive factors is a previous history of AMS. The incidence of AMS ranges from 5% to 68% depending on the rate of ascent or gain in altitude. Significantly less common, the incidence of high-altitude cerebral edema is approximately 1% and the incidence of high-altitude pulmonary edema is approximately 2%.[5]

The altitude of residence also plays a role in the incidence of AMS. Those living at greater than 900m had an 8% incidence of AMS, compared to a 27% incidence among those living at sea level.[6] Age may be a protective factor for AMS; one study shows age greater than 60 years had half the incidence when compared to younger patients.[7] One hypothesis for this finding is that cerebral atrophy provides additional room in the skull to accommodate swelling. Children and young adults seem to be equally susceptible to AMS, while women may have the same or slightly higher incidence of AMS compared to their male counterparts.[7,8] Obesity is associated with an increased risk of developing AMS.[6] However, physical fitness is not a predictor of susceptibility to AMS. Elite athletes are often willing to push through extreme discomfort, and may ultimately become significantly more ill from altitude illness prior to alerting others of their distress.

## PREVENTION OF ALTITUDE-RELATED ILLNESS

Travel to high altitude locations often involves extensive training, planning, expensive gear, and a significant time commitment. Countless trekkers and mountaineers have had to abort their trips due to altitude-related illness. Others have proceeded despite concerning symptoms and/or dangerous conditions and have lost their lives. While many Emergency Medicine physicians may never work in a clinical setting where altitude-related illness is commonly treated (**Fig. 2**), all Emergency Medicine physicians can counsel patients on the proper prevention of altitude-related illness.

### Graded Ascent

*"Climb high, sleep low."* Sleeping elevation is the most important consideration when planning a high-altitude expedition.[9] In order to prevent AMS, the Wilderness Medical Society (WMS) Clinical Practice Guidelines recommend a maximum daily gain in sleeping the elevation of less than 500 m/day.[10] An acclimatization day, in which there is no gain in sleeping elevation, should be taken for every 1000m gain in altitude. If routes and logistics require a gain in the elevation of greater than 500m in a single

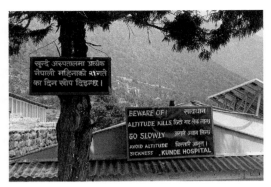

**Fig. 2.** Kunde Hospital, Nepal. (Photo courtesy of Dr. Jessie Gehner, used with permission.)

day, an extra acclimatization day should be taken to simulate a more gradual ascent.[10] While rest and refueling are important, taking a short hike on those days is common practice and may aid in acclimatization.

### Pharmacologic Prophylaxis

For those with a higher likelihood of developing AMS (i.e. those using a steep ascent profile or those with a history of AMS), pharmacologic prophylaxis should be considered. The first-line medication in both the prevention and treatment of AMS is acetazolamide. Prophylaxis should begin 24 hours prior to ascent. Current recommendations are for oral doses of 125 mg twice daily, though lower doses have recently been shown to be effective.[11] More data is needed to validate these results and change the current recommendations.

For those who cannot take acetazolamide, such as those with a known allergy to acetazolamide or other sulfa drugs, dexamethasone (2 mg orally every 6 hours) can also be used as prophylaxis. Using steroids as prophylaxis can result in adrenal insufficiency if taken for more than 10 days without a subsequent taper. It is also theorized that the adjuvant treatment of HACE with dexamethasone may be less effective if a patient is already taking corticosteroids.[10]

Several studies have evaluated the use of NSAIDs such as ibuprofen for the prevention of AMS. Trekkers taking 600 mg of ibuprofen three times daily had overall higher oxygen saturations than the control group.[3] Ibuprofen can be used for AMS prevention in persons who do not wish to take acetazolamide or dexamethasone, or have allergies or intolerance to these medications.[10]

Numerous natural remedies, including ginger tea, ginkgo biloba, and coca leaves, have been strongly recommended for centuries by locals living at high altitude to prevent altitude-related illness and improve acclimatization. However, studies are extremely limited on these substances and there are no formal recommendations for their use.

For patients with a history of HAPE, or for those who may be at higher risk, nifedipine (30 mg extended-release orally every 12 hours) is recommended as prophylaxis. Other therapeutic medications such as sildenafil, tadalafil, and salmeterol, have been evaluated for prophylactic use but are not recommended for the prevention of HAPE.[10]

### Adequate Hydration

A person exerting themselves at high altitude has many reasons to be dehydrated. Fluid losses due to increased respiration, sweating, and/or diuretic use (if on acetazolamide) all contribute to dehydration. This is often compounded by poor oral intake due to nausea and/or a low thirst drive in cold conditions. Therefore, many trekking guides encourage their clients to drink copious amounts of water at high altitude, which can conversely result in fluid overload and hyponatremia. The WMS consensus guidelines recommend drinking to thirst and watching urine coloration.[10] Addition of an electrolyte mix can also help maintain overall nutrition when oral intake is poor.

## DIAGNOSIS OF ALTITUDE-RELATED ILLNESS

The diagnosis of altitude-related illness is often made in an austere and resource-limited environment (as with most wilderness medicine-related conditions). For this reason, a thorough history and physical exam may be the only diagnostic modality available. While it is important to keep a broad differential diagnosis, persons at high altitude who experience signs and symptoms consistent with altitude-related illness should be presumed to have altitude-related illness, and preparations for descent (if necessary) should be made immediately.

### Diagnosis of Acute Mountain Sickness

The diagnosis of AMS is subjective, without any specific findings on physical examination, laboratory evaluation, or radiography. AMS should be considered in those patients who develop headache at high altitude, which is often accompanied by other symptoms including nausea, anorexia, fatigue, dizziness, and/or difficulty sleeping. Symptom onset occurs 6 to 12 hours after arrival at high altitude.

The Lake Louise AMS Score is the sum of the severity ratings across four categories of symptoms: headache, gastrointestinal symptoms, fatigue/weakness, and dizziness/lightheadedness (**Fig. 3**). The AMS score should be calculated only after 6 hours after arrival to high altitude, to avoid confusing AMS with confounding symptoms from travel or responses to acute hypoxia. Other conditions on the differential diagnosis include dehydration, migraine headache, hyponatremia, or viral illness.

### Diagnosis of High-Altitude Cerebral Edema

The diagnosis of HACE should be made in any patient who has symptoms of severe AMS, along with a new neurologic deficit, ataxia, visual change, altered mental status, seizures, or in cases of impending cerebral herniation, a comatose state.[1] The classic patient with HACE may appear to be intoxicated, dysarthric, unable to walk in a straight line, vomiting, and/or altered.

The use of portable point-of-care ultrasound (POCUS) is becoming more common in austere environments, and ocular ultrasound may reveal an increased diameter of the optic nerve sheath.[13] Nerve sheath diameters of greater than 0.55 cm are indicative of elevated intracranial pressure (ICP) (**Fig. 4**). In the rare cases where magnetic resonance imaging (MRI) scans were obtained on patients with HACE, the findings were consistent with vasogenic edema. Other conditions that should be on the differential include intracranial hemorrhage, ischemic stroke, seizure disorder, atypical migraine, intoxication, and other metabolic disturbances.

### Diagnosis of High-Altitude Pulmonary Edema

The diagnosis of high-altitude pulmonary edema should be made in the person at high altitude who demonstrates at least two of the following four symptoms (chest tightness or pain, cough, dyspnea at rest, or decreased exercise tolerance), along with at least two of the following four signs (central cyanosis, rales/wheezes, tachycardia,

## 2018 Lake Louise Acute Mountain Sickness Score

| | 0 | 1 | 2 | 3 |
|---|---|---|---|---|
| Headache | None at all | A mild headache | Moderate headache | Severe headache, incapacitating |
| Gastrointestinal Symptoms | Good appetite | Poor appetite or nausea | Moderate nausea or vomiting | Severe nausea and vomiting, incapacitating |
| Fatigue and/or Weakness | Not tired or weak | Mild fatigue/weakness | Moderate fatigue/weakness | Severe fatigue/ weakness, incapacitating |
| Dizziness/ lightheadedness | No dizziness/ light-headedness | Mild dizziness/ light-headedness | Moderate dizziness/ light-headedness | Severe dizziness/ light-headedness, incapacitating |
| AMS Clinical Function Score: Overall, if you had AMS symptoms, how did they affect your activities? | Not at all | Symptoms present, but did not force any change in activity or itinerary | My symptoms forced me to stop the ascent or to go down on my own power | Had to be evacuated to a lower altitude |
| *Score Interpretation: AMS present if headache score of at least one point, and a total score of at least three points.* | *3-5 points Mild AMS* | *6-9 points Moderate AMS* | *10-12 points Severe AMS* | |

**Fig. 3.** The Lake Louise Acute Mountain Sickness scoring system and interpretation. (Used with permission from the International Society of Mountain Medicine.[12])

or tachypnea).[14] The onset of HAPE usually occurs 2 to 4 days after arrival at high altitude.

If available, a chest x-ray (CXR) may show patchy alveolar infiltrates with a normal-sized mediastinum/heart. An ultrasound may show B-lines consistent with pulmonary edema (**Fig. 5**). Electrocardiography (ECG) may show signs of right axis deviation and/ or ischemia. Labs are of limited utility. Patients with HAPE are very quickly responsive to supplemental oxygen.

The classic HAPE patient will be extremely dyspneic, complain of orthopnea with crackles on auscultation, and may have a cough productive of pink, frothy sputum. Other conditions that should be on the differential diagnosis include pulmonary embolism, cardiomyopathy, pneumonia, or congestive heart failure.

## TREATMENT OF ALTITUDE-RELATED ILLNESS

The definitive treatment for all altitude-related illness is descent. The treatments discussed below are only temporizing measures until a safe descent can be made. Remote locations, communication difficulties, dangerous weather, and rough terrain may make a timely evacuation impossible. Most symptoms typically improve or resolve after a descent of 300-1000m, but the required decrease in altitude varies among individuals.[10]

### Treatment of Acute Mountain Sickness

The symptoms of mild to moderate AMS may be treated in the backcountry without mandating descent; however, a patient with AMS should not continue to ascend until symptoms improve. One strategy is taking an extra acclimatization day while starting

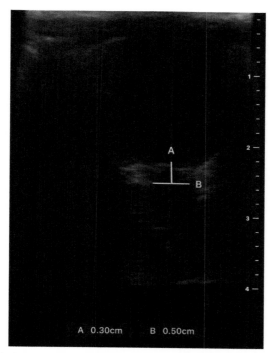

**Fig. 4.** Ultrasound showing measurements of optic nerve sheath diameter. Ultrasound demonstrating that the measurement of the optic nerve sheath diameter should be taken at a distance of 0.3 cm behind the eye. (*Courtesy of* Dr. Jessie Gehner, used with permission.)

the treatment dose of acetazolamide (250 mg orally twice a day), providing other supportive care medications (NSAIDs, antiemetics), and ensuring adequate hydration. Supplemental oxygen can be utilized if available. If the patient's symptoms improve, they may consider continuing their trip at high altitude while continuing the treatment dose of acetazolamide.

Severe AMS mandates descent. Supplemental oxygen should be initiated, and acetazolamide and other supportive care medications should be administered. Due to the nausea and vomiting that are often present in severe AMS, antiemetics can be useful (ie, ondansetron orally disintegrating tablets and promethazine rectal suppositories).[10] The patient should be monitored closely for any neurologic changes, and should not be allowed to descend independently in case they progress from severe AMS to HACE. On prolonged treks or travel to very high altitude, AMS can still occur upon descent. Acetazolamide may be initiated at the treatment dose even while descending.

### Treatment of High-Altitude Cerebral Edema

HACE can rapidly progress to herniation and death, so immediate descent is indicated for any neurologic abnormality at high altitude. Supplemental oxygen should be administered and if possible, the patient should be placed in a portable hyperbaric chamber (commonly known as a "Gamow bag") while awaiting descent. A portable hyperbaric chamber simulates a decrease in altitude by up to thousands of feet while awaiting evacuation and descent.[15] However, portable hyperbaric chambers are

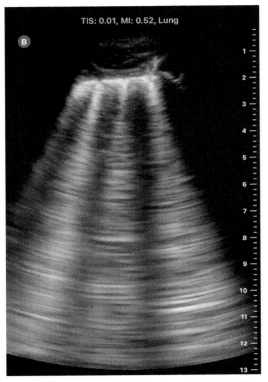

TIS: 0.01, MI: 0.52, Lung

**Fig. 5.** Ultrasound showing B lines as in HAPE. (*Courtesy of* Dr. Jon Noguiera (Virginia Tech Carilion Ultrasound Fellowship), used with permission.)

fraught with limitations/difficulties, including the need for the constant pumping of a foot pedal by an attendant and the inability to closely monitor a critical patient.[15]

Dexamethasone should be administered to the patient with HACE: an initial 8 mg dose, followed by 4 mg every 6 hours, which can be given orally, subcutaneously or intravenously.[10] Therapeutically dosed acetazolamide (250 mg twice daily) should also be considered, as should NSAIDs and antiemetics to assist with symptom management.[10] Patients with HACE may be altered and uncooperative, making treatment interventions extremely difficult. As with severe AMS, these patients should be monitored closely and not left alone.

### Treatment of High-Altitude Pulmonary Edema

As with other altitude-related illness, the definitive treatment for HAPE is rapid descent. Supplemental oxygen and portable hyperbaric chambers can be utilized while awaiting evacuation. High-altitude pulmonary edema may appear similar to cardiogenic pulmonary edema on examination and radiography, but the treatments are unique. Diuretics such as furosemide are not recommended.

The goals in the treatment of HAPE are to improve oxygenation and reduce pulmonary vascular resistance. The first-line therapy is nifedipine (30 mg extended-release orally every 12 hours). Other therapies to reduce pulmonary vascular resistance include phosphodiesterase inhibitors such as tadalafil or sildenafil.[10] Vasodilators should be used with caution in patients with baseline low blood pressure, and are contraindicated in patients using nitroglycerin. While sometimes used in treatment, inhaled beta agonists have not been shown to be effective but are not likely harmful.[10]

### Treatment of Concurrent High-Altitude Cerebral Edema and High-Altitude Pulmonary Edema

Once again, rapid descent is mandatory and both supplemental oxygen and a portable hyperbaric chamber can be used as therapeutic temporizing measures until a definitive descent can take place. Dexamethasone should be added to the above treatment regimen for HAPE. It may be difficult in the backcountry to discern whether neurologic dysfunction is due to hypoxic encephalopathy or HACE, so it is important to treat both entities if the patient meets the criteria. While phosphodiesterase inhibitors and calcium channel blockers are not contraindicated in the treatment of HACE, patients should be monitored closely for hypotension. A decrease in cerebral perfusion pressure may worsen cerebral ischemia if it is present.

## OTHER ALTITUDE-RELATED CONDITIONS
### Retinal/Vitreous Hemorrhage

Hypoxia at high altitude brings about retinal neovascular changes. Increased blood pressure during strenuous work at altitude can increase the pressure in retinal blood vessels, resulting in capillary leaks and subsequent high-altitude retinal hemorrhage.[16] These findings can be seen on ophthalmoscopy and sometimes on ultrasound. Patients should be counseled to avoid exertion if vision changes are present and should have close ophthalmologic follow-up.

### High Altitude Cough

Sometimes called the *"Khumbu cough,"* this nonproductive, persistent, paroxysmal cough is common and quite bothersome to many high-altitude travelers. The cough can be so severe that it causes rib fractures.[17] Though the exact etiology is not clearly understood, the previously held belief that it was due solely to the inspiration of cold, dry air was refuted by observations and experiments in long-duration hypobaric chamber studies. High-altitude cough is likely a symptom of several possible perturbations in the cough reflex arc that may exist independently or together. These include loss of water from the respiratory tract, respiratory tract infections, or sub-clinical HAPE.[17] Silica dust has also been implicated as a possible cause of the *"Khumbu cough,"* as many trekkers inhale this sparkling dust while on their journey. Wearing a moist facial covering so that particulate matter is filtered and inspired air is warmed/moistened may prevent or decrease this troublesome symptom.

### Chronic Mountain Sickness

CMS is seen in patients with long-term residence at altitudes greater than 3,000m (10,000 ft) above sea level. It is insidious in onset, presenting with increasing weakness, shortness of breath, fatigue, somnolence, and slowed mental functioning. It can progress to complete incapacitation. CMS is characterized by severe symptomatic erythrocytosis (Hgb $\geq$19 g/dL for women and Hgb $\geq$21 g/dL for men) and accentuated hypoxemia, frequently associated with pulmonary hypertension. In advanced cases, the condition may evolve into cor pulmonale and congestive heart failure.[18] Patients with suspected CMS should be evaluated at a facility where cardiology and pulmonology can diagnose and manage sequelae (heart failure, pulmonary hypertension, or thrombosis).

## CASE REPORT: 34-YEAR-OLD FEMALE WITH HEADACHE
### Presentation

- *History of Present Illness*: 34-year-old female presents with headache, anorexia, vomiting, lightheadedness, and fatigue. She is on day 9 of a trek to Everest Base Camp at 5125m (16,814 ft). The ascent profile has been gradual, taking acclimatization days at 3840m (12,598 ft) and 4410m (14,470 ft). She complains of a worsening headache for the past 24 hours, anorexia, fatigue, and dizziness. She denies any weakness or numbness but does have paresthesias in her hands and feet. She reports some visual disturbance (floaters/blurriness) but denies vomiting, diarrhea, or chest pain. She reports mild shortness of breath (SOB), which has been present since arrival at high altitude. When it is suggested to this patient that she may have AMS, she insists that this is a migraine headache.
- *Past Medical History*: Migraine headaches, anorexia nervosa.
- Social History: Endurance athlete. The maximum altitude reached on previous treks was 15,000 ft without significant symptoms.
- *Medications*: 125 mg oral acetazolamide twice daily for AMS prophylaxis that was initiated 24 hours before the start of her trek.
- Allergies: none
  - Physical Exam:
  - Vital Signs: Heart rate 125beats/min, SPO2 85% on room air, respiratory rate 25, blood pressure (not available), temperature (not available)
  - General: Alert, oriented, appears fatigued
  - HEENT: Mucous membranes are dry, no other abnormalities
  - Cardiac: Radial pulse 2+ bilaterally, regular
  - Respiratory: Mild tachypnea, no audible wheezing or crackles
  - Skin: Pale, cool, dry, no cyanosis
  - Neurologic: No focal deficits

### Patient's Course

The patient is started on the therapeutic dosing of acetazolamide (250 mg twice daily), ondansetron (4 mg orally disintegrating tablets as needed), and ibuprofen (600 mg three times daily). She is encouraged to increase her oral fluid intake, although she is reluctant to do so due to feeling unwell. Her team is scheduled to leave for Everest Base Camp (EBC) in the morning.

The patient's symptoms worsen upon awakening the following morning, though she remains without focal neurologic symptoms. Despite medications, her headache worsens. It is recommended that the patient descend and not proceed to EBC. She says that this is her regular migraine headache, and she is not turning back.

One hour into the trek, the patient becomes more fatigued and ataxic. She begins slurring her speech. The headache continues to worsen. She is given dexamethasone 8 mg orally but immediately vomits. Fortunately, another team has injectable dexamethasone, and she is subsequently given 8 mg intramuscularly.

The patient is able to ambulate, so she is assisted down to 4940m (16,000 ft), where she is evacuated by helicopter to Kathmandu. By the time she arrives at the receiving facility, her symptoms have almost completely resolved.

### Discussion

Since this patient had a history of migraine headaches, she was reluctant to descend, attributing her symptoms to migraines rather than AMS. This was complicated by her desire to reach her destination, for which she had extensively trained, planned, and funded.

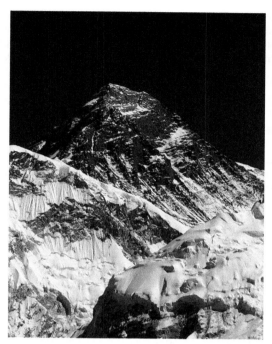

**Fig. 6.** Mt. Everest (Sagarmatha or Chomolungma), Nepal. (Photo courtesy of Dr. Jessie Gehner, used with permission.)

The patient started out with moderate AMS. She was treated appropriately. However, since she did not descend, she progressed to severe AMS by the next morning. Once neurologic signs became present (ataxia, slurred speech), the patient met the diagnostic criteria for HACE.

She could not tolerate oral dexamethasone due to her nausea and vomiting, so it was potentially lifesaving that she received it intramuscularly. Her teammates took advantage of her ambulatory status and assisted her to a lower altitude immediately. It would have been a much more prolonged extrication if she were no longer ambulatory, which would have delayed her definitive descent to a lower altitude and may have resulted in a worsened outcome. Air evacuation was thankfully available, but this is not always an option when visibility is limited.

While it is important to keep a broad differential diagnosis, her symptoms should not have been attributed to a complex migraine at high altitude. The quick resolution of her symptoms upon arrival to Kathmandu at 1,340m (4,396 ft) suggests that the patient had HACE.

## SUMMARY

Travel to high altitude can be one of the most beautiful and breathtaking experiences of a person's life (**Fig. 6**). It also can be the most dangerous. Diagnostic and therapeutic options are extremely limited in most cases, and altitude-related illness should be assumed until proven otherwise. Patients should be counseled prior to high altitude travel, so that they are educated about high altitude illness, prophylactic and therapeutic pharmacologic options, and most importantly, when to descend. For travelers who have planned a rapid ascent or have a history of altitude-related illness, pharmacologic prophylaxis should be considered. Most of all, the mountains should be respected, not only for their grandeur, but also for their awesome power to destroy. The prudent mountain enthusiast must know when to push on and when to turn back.

*Getting to the top is optional. Getting down is mandatory.*

*—anonymous*

## CLINICS CARE POINTS

- If altitude illness is suspected, the definitive treatment is DESCENT. Pharmacologic agents and supplemental oxygen are only temporizing measures until descent is accomplished.
- Concerning symptoms should be considered altitude-related until proven otherwise, and diagnostics should not delay descent. However, small portable point-of-care ultrasound (POCUS) is becoming more common as a diagnostic tool in the backcountry and can help the practitioner diagnose conditions including high-altitude cerebral edema (HACE) and high-altitude pulmonary edema (HAPE).
- Patients with mild symptoms of acute mountain sickness (AMS) should not continue to ascend until symptoms have improved.
- Oxygen saturation does not always correlate with the severity of altitude-related illness; consider the entire clinical picture, including the patient's functional status.
- Graded ascent (gaining no more than 500 m/night in sleeping elevation) is recommended to prevent altitude-related illness. Acetazolamide is the first-line medication for both the treatment and prevention of AMS.

## DISCLOSURE

The author has nothing to disclose.

## REFERENCES

1. Auerbach PS, Cushing TA, Stuart Harris N. Auerbach's wilderness medicine. Philadelphia, PA: Elsevier; 2017.
2. Waeber B, Kayser B, Dumont L, et al. Impact of Study Design on Reported Incidences of Acute Mountain Sickness: A Systematic Review. High Alt Med Biol 2015;16(3):204–15.
3. Kanaan NC, Peterson AL, Pun M, et al. Prophylactic Acetaminophen or Ibuprofen Result in Equivalent Acute Mountain Sickness Incidence at High Altitude: A Prospective Randomized Trial. Wilderness Environ Med 2017;28(2):72–8.
4. Bloch KE, Latshang TD, Turk AJ, et al. Nocturnal Periodic Breathing during Acclimatization at Very High Altitude at Mount Muztagh Ata (7,546 m). Am J Respir Crit Care Med 2010;182(4):562–8.
5. Basnyat B, Subedi D, Sleggs J, et al. Disoriented and ataxic pilgrims: an epidemiological study of acute mountain sickness and high-altitude cerebral edema at a sacred lake at 4300 m in the Nepal Himalayas. Wilderness Environ Med 2000; 11(2):89–93.
6. Honigman B, Theis MK, Koziol-McLain J, et al. Acute mountain sickness in a general tourist population at moderate altitudes. Ann Intern Med 1993;118:587–92.

7. Schneider M, Bernasch D, Weymann J, et al. Acute mountain sickness: Influence of susceptibility, preexposure, and ascent rate. Med Sci Sports Exerc 2002;34: 1886–91.
8. Wu T. Children on the Tibetan plateau. ISSM Newslett 1994;4:5–7.
9. San T, Polat S, Cingi C, et al. Effects of high altitude on sleep and respiratory system and their adaptations. Sci World J 2013;2013:241569.
10. Luks AM, Auerbach PS, Freer L, et al. Wilderness Medical Society Practice Guidelines for the Prevention and Treatment of Acute Altitude Illness: 2019 Update. Wilderness Environ Med 2019;30(4).
11. McIntosh SE, Hemphill M, McDevitt MC, et al. Reduced Acetazolamide Dosing in Countering Altitude Illness: A Comparison of 62.5 vs 125 mg (the RADICAL Trial). Wilderness Environ Med 2019;30(1):12–21.
12. Roach RC, Hackett PH, Oelz O, et al. The 2018 Lake Louise Acute Mountain Sickness Score. High Alt Med Biol 2018;19(1):4–6.
13. Kanaan NC, Lipman GS, Constance BB, et al. Optic Nerve Sheath Diameter Increase on Ascent to High Altitude: Correlation With Acute Mountain Sickness. J Ultrasound Med 2015;34(9):1677–82.
14. Jensen JD, Vincent AL. High altitude pulmonary edema. PubMed. Available at: 2021 https://www.ncbi.nlm.nih.gov/books/NBK430819/. [Accessed 2 December 2021].
15. Taber RL. Protocols for the use of a portable hyperbaric chamber for the treatment of high altitude disorders. J Wilderness Med 1990;1(3):181–92.
16. Wiedman M, Tabin GC. High-altitude retinopathy and altitude illness. Ophthalmology 1999;106(10):1924–7.
17. Mason NP. Altitude-related cough. Cough 2013;9(1):23.
18. Villafuerte FC, Corante N. Chronic Mountain Sickness: Clinical Aspects, Etiology, Management, and Treatment. High Alt Med Biol 2016;17(2):61–9.

# Drowning

Christopher A. Davis, MD[a],*, Stephanie Lareau, MD[b]

## KEYWORDS

- Drowning • Submersion • Immersion • ARDS

## KEY POINTS

- Drowning is defined as "the process of experiencing respiratory impairment from submersion/immersion in liquid." There can be 3 outcomes: death, survival with morbidity, or survival with no morbidity.
- The drowning process is primarily driven by hypoxia, and can be interrupted by delivering oxygen and ventilation (which should occur as soon as feasible).
- Upon rescue from the water, rescuers should initiate resuscitation using an "Airway, Breathing, Circulation" approach, as opposed to "Circulation, Airway, Breathing" or chest compression-only cardiopulmonary resuscitation.
- Patients who remain stable and asymptomatic or only minimally symptomatic can be safely discharged from the emergency department after an observation period of 4 to 6 hours without any diagnostic imaging or laboratory studies.
- Drowning is responsible for significant morbidity and mortality, especially among children. Prevention strategies should focus on adult supervision of children around water, physical barriers, and life jacket use.

## INTRODUCTION

Drowning is a significant global public health concern, representing the third leading cause of unintentional death worldwide. Despite substantial efforts to prevent drowning, the complex interplay of contributing factors and the rapidity with which life-threatening events unfold necessitate an ongoing exploration of strategies to improve emergency care and mitigate the substantial associated morbidity.[1] Drowning incidents encompass a broad spectrum of scenarios ranging from accidents occurring in bathtubs or backyard swimming pools to natural bodies of water. This review aims to provide a comprehensive synthesis of the current state of knowledge surrounding drowning, equipping health care professionals with the required understanding and tools to improve patient outcomes.

Prior to 2002, there were over 33 different identified definitions of drowning, leading to widespread confusion and inconsistent reporting. In 2002, the World Congress on

a Wake Forest University School of Medicine, 1 Medical Center Boulevard, Winston-Salem, NC 27157, USA; b Virginia Tech Carilion School of Medicine, Roanoke, VA, USA
* Corresponding author.
E-mail address: christda@wakehealth.edu

Emerg Med Clin N Am 42 (2024) 541–550
https://doi.org/10.1016/j.emc.2024.02.014
0733-8627/24/© 2024 Elsevier Inc. All rights reserved.
emed.theclinics.com

Drowning offered a definition that has become recognized by the World Health Organization (WHO), defining drowning as "the process of experiencing respiratory impairment from submersion or immersion in liquid."[2] Depending on the outcome, drowning can be further classified as drowning with morbidity, drowning with mortality, or drowning with neither morbidity nor mortality. The severity of non-fatal drowning can be divided into (1) mild: breathing, involuntary distressed coughing, and fully alert, (2) moderate: difficulty breathing and disoriented but conscious, or (3) severe: not breathing and unconscious.[3]

Drowning can be further classified as undetermined intent, intentional (in the case of suicide), unintentional (when it occurs by accident), or natural disaster. Terms such as "near drowning," "dry drowning," and "delayed drowning" should be avoided, as they are dated and do not align with the current understanding of the pathogenesis of drowning.

## EPIDEMIOLOGY

There were an average of 4083 fatal unintentional drownings annually in the United States between 2012 and 2021.[4] The CDC reports that drowning is the leading single cause of death in children 1 to 4 years of age, and it remains the second leading cause of unintentional injury or death among children 5 to 14 year old.[4] Risk factors include male sex, alcohol use, low income, rural residence, risky behavior, and lack of supervision.[5-9] Autism and epilepsy have both been shown to increase risk of drowning in children.[10] In the elderly, certain conditions including dementia, sarcopenia, cardiac conditions, and epilepsy increase the risk of drowning.[10]

Although the incidence of drowning is higher among males, the WHO reports females account for about one-third of drownings. The incidence of female drowning increases with age. When studied in 5 high-income countries, females now partake in risky activities at similar rates to males, including alcohol consumption and swimming in unsafe locations. However, it is thought that their risk assessment differs, which may account for the decreased rate of drowning. Females are more likely to drown due to falls or unanticipated entry into water than their male counterparts.[11]

## PATHOPHYSIOLOGY

Drowning occurs when there is respiratory impairment due to submersion or immersion in liquid. Drowning deaths all follow the same common pathway of hypoxia leading to cardiac arrest. Drowning occurs on a spectrum, and patients presenting with drowning may have symptoms that range from a mild cough to severe respiratory distress and respiratory failure.

The drowning process begins when the airway is immersed or submersed in a liquid medium. The initial reflex is to hold one's breath. However, as carbon dioxide accumulates, the hypercapnic respiratory drive overcomes the desire to hold one's breath, which causes an involuntary gasp resulting in the aspiration of water (and sometimes laryngospasm). This process ultimately leads to profound hypoxemia and eventual cardiac arrest.[12]

Surfactant is destroyed when water reaches the alveolar bed, causing a disturbance in the alveolar-capillary membrane. Fluid then shifts into the alveolar space, leading to pulmonary edema and poor gas exchange. Over time, this leads to increased left-to-right shunting and decreased lung compliance, ultimately leading to acute respiratory distress syndrome (ARDS).[13] Without interruption, the process of drowning results in profound hypoxia, which decompensates into cardiac arrest. As this process unfolds, the heart initially responds with tachycardia, then bradycardia, followed by pulseless electrical activity, and ultimately asystole. Although uncommon, ventricular fibrillation (VF) or ventricular tachycardia in a drowned patient may indicate that the patient suffered cardiac arrest from an underlying cardiac event and not the drowning process. This subset of patients can benefit from early defibrillation.

The brain is very sensitive to periods of hypoxia, and irreversible neurologic injury can occur in 4 to 10 minutes. Full neurologic recovery is rare after 10 minutes of anoxia in normothermic conditions.[14]

Pre-existing or chronic illness also plays a large role in drowning. Studies have shown up to 2.8% of motor vehicle accidents that lead to drowning can be attributed to underlying chronic illness, and underlying chronic conditions were found to be the reason for drowning in up to 24.6% of elderly drowned patients.[15] Chronic illnesses across multiple organ systems are implicated in drownings. The most common chronic illness contributing to drowning is epilepsy, but cardiac arrhythmias are also implicated in many drownings. One study performed cardiac channel molecular autopsies on unexplained drowning victims in the United States and found that 22% of drowning deaths had evidence of arrhythmia.[16] A similar study in Australia found a similar rate of 21.7%.[17] This suggests that many unexplained drownings may occur due to fatal arrythmias. Additionally, psychotic disorders and mood disorders were the most implicated psychiatric illnesses related to drowning deaths.

Canine studies from the 1960s raised questions about the potential differential effects of saltwater, freshwater, and chlorinated water on drowning physiology. Early studies found that instilling greater than 11 mL/kg of various fluids into the lungs of dogs could cause hemodilution and electrolyte abnormalities.[18] However, subsequent extensive research involving human drowning victims has failed to show any conclusive evidence demonstrating clinically significant electrolyte or hematologic abnormalities among the various aspirated fluid types/compositions. The small volumes of liquid aspirated by human victims, typically less than 4 mL/kg, generally fall within a range that does not seem to induce the same level of physiologic disturbance observed in animal experiments. Consequently, the distinctions between saltwater, freshwater, and chlorinated water drowning in terms of their physiologic impact are likely of minimal relevance to clinical practice.

## PRE-HOSPITAL CARE

Tragically, bystanders or rescuers without water rescue training are at increased risk of becoming victims when trying to perform a rescue of a victim from water. It is advised that only people with appropriate training and equipment enter the water to attempt the rescue of a drowning victim. Those without appropriate training should attempt to assist the victim only by reaching out to them with a long rigid object (such as a paddle or pole) or by throwing a rope (or another object that will float).[19] A study in Turkey demonstrated 114 fatalities among rescuers in a 3-year period, demonstrating that there is a significant risk to untrained would-be rescuers.[20]

As death from drowning occurs due to hypoxia, early attempts to reverse that process with rescue breaths have shown to improve outcomes in certain situations. Trained rescuers can attempt in-water resuscitation (IWR), which consists of providing ventilations while still in the water. Studies have shown that IWR performed by trained lifeguards is feasible even in open water without floatation devices, while other studies have shown that IWR is ineffective, exhausting, and inefficient when performed by laypersons.[21–23] Organizations including the American Red Cross, International Lifesaving Federation, and United States Lifesaving Association recommend IWR by trained rescuers when a patient is rescued from shallow water or from deep water when a flotation device is present. Chest compressions are ineffective in the water and should be delayed until the patient is on a hard surface.[19] Guidelines also generally recommend removing or unbuckling life jackets prior to performing chest compressions, as the foam padding has been shown to decrease the efficacy of compressions.

Initial prehospital resuscitation should focus on airway, breathing, and circulation (A-B-C) as opposed to C-A-B or compressions-only resuscitation.[19,24] Since cardiac arrest in drowning is due to profound hypoxia, it is important to address airway and breathing first by administering oxygen and providing positive pressure ventilation. Many organizations, such as the European Resuscitation Council, recommend starting resuscitation with 5 rescue breaths.[24] Efforts to try to remove water from the airway, such as abdominal thrusts or positioning the patient head-down, should be avoided as they delay oxygenation and potentially increase the risk of aspiration.[3] Guidelines recommend administering oxygen at the highest concentration available, and recommend positive pressure ventilation over passive oxygen administration for patients in respiratory distress or cardiac arrest.[19] Recent studies have demonstrated the safety and efficacy of using noninvasive positive pressure ventilation (NIPPV) in drowned patients, with a single study showing improved neurologic outcomes when compared to mechanical ventilation.[25] Patients with moderate to severe drowning often present with copious frothy and foamy secretions due to noncardiogenic pulmonary edema from the washout of pulmonary surfactant and subsequent alveolar endothelial injury and vascular leak. Attempts to suction and clear the foam are futile and will delay delivery of rescue breaths, mask ventilation, or other means of oxygen delivery. Therefore, the current recommendations are to provide oxygen and ventilations despite the presence of foamy secretions in the airway.[19] If aspiration of foreign bodies during a drowning event (or from subsequent vomiting) is suspected, the airway should be carefully evaluated. One study showed 54% of the cases of drowned patients on a surf-beach had foreign bodies such as sand or seaweed in their airways.[26]

During the drowning process, victims often swallow a large volume of water, and rescue breaths often will insufflate the stomach with air. This leads to a high likelihood of vomiting among drowned patients. Vomiting has been reported in up to 86% of drowned patients who receive cardiopulmonary resuscitation.[26] Therefore, patients who are unconscious but breathing should be placed in the lateral decubitus or recovery position to prevent aspiration. Likewise, the potential for emesis and aspiration should be considered when deciding on airway management and strategies. Due to the high risk of vomiting, ensure that drowned patients are alert enough to protect their airways if considering NIPPV.

Automated external defibrillators (AEDs) are integral in cardiac arrest management, as VF can be a common presenting rhythm in cardiac arrest due to acute coronary syndromes. However, VF is rare in drowned patients, so AEDs may play a more limited role.[27,28] The use of an AED has been proven safe in a wet environment.[29–32] However, efforts should be made to dry the patient's chest to promote pad adhesion, and rescuers should avoid contacting the pads during defibrillation.

Patients who have drowned are oftentimes treated as trauma patients with cervical spine immobilization and trauma center activation. However, a retrospective review of drowned patients over a 12-year period showed only a 4.3% rate of traumatic injuries, none of which required operative intervention.[10] If a patient has a witnessed traumatic event or obvious external signs of trauma, they should be treated as a trauma patient. However, drowned patients without clear history or physical evidence of trauma do not require trauma care, and providing trauma care may actually limit or delay rapid airway management and oxygenation. Furthermore, the routine use of cervical collars for spinal immobilization is not recommended, as the incidence of cervical spine injury in drowning patients is low and usually associated with specific scenarios such as diving from cliffs.[19,33,34]

## IN-HOSPITAL CARE

Emergency clinicians often find the care of patients in cardiac arrest or profound hypoxia straightforward, as much of emergency medicine training focuses on the resuscitation of critically ill patients. Nonetheless, drowned patients will present on a spectrum of severity.

In a drowned patient who arrives to the emergency department without a severe cough, respiratory complaints, vital sign abnormalities, or physical examination abnormalities, studies have shown that discharge home is safe if they remain stable over a 4 to 6 hour observation period. Further imaging or work up is not indicated, assuming that the patient does not need further evaluation for an underlying condition that led to drowning. Some studies show these patients do not even need to be transported to a hospital if they have a reliable person to watch them.[19,35–39] A study of on-scene decision-making among lifeguards reviewed 1831 cases of drowned patients with normal clinical examinations (aside from mild cough) after the drowning event, and found a 0% mortality rate without further intervention.[40]

A subset of patients will have a normal mental status with mild respiratory symptoms and require supplemental oxygen. Oxygen requirements can range from 1 to 2 L of oxygen via nasal cannula, to significantly higher oxygen demands in a patient demonstrating increased work of breathing and respiratory failure. A trial of NIPPV is reasonable in a drowned patient with a normal mental status. NIPPV provides increased airway pressure, which can decrease respiratory effort and decrease atelectasis. One small retrospective study demonstrated non-inferiority of NIPPV with regards to correction of hypoxemia and acidosis when compared to endotracheal intubation. It also showed benefits of NIPPV, including decreased hospital length of stay and decreased infection rates.[25]

In patients who are critically ill after drowning, and are profoundly hypoxic and/or unable to manage their own airway, the focus should be on airway management. It can be very challenging to manage the drowned patient's airway due to large amounts of foamy secretions from pulmonary edema and vomitus. The traditional attempts to clear secretions with suction are oftentimes unsuccessful, as secretions are copious and cannot be fully cleared. As cardiac arrest in drowning is secondary to hypoxia, additional time spent trying to clear the airway increases the degree and time of hypoxia. Current recommendations are to use the suction-assisted laryngoscopy and airway decontamination (SALAD) technique for managing the drowned airway. In this method, a large bore suction catheter, such as the SSCOR DuCanto catheter, is placed near the left side of the airway or esophagus while intubation is performed. In some situations, this catheter can be used to pass through the vocal cords. Then, the suction tubing is unplugged, allowing a gum elastic bougie to be placed into the airway. Next, the suction catheter is removed leaving the gum elastic bougie in place and the endotracheal tube can be placed over the bougie using seldinger technique.

One study showed that the use of some supraglottic airways was unsuccessful in drowning resuscitations, as they do not allow the high positive pressures needed for adequate oxygenation and ventilation. The high pressures were noted to overcome the seal, decreasing oxygen delivery, and increasing the risk of aspiration. Lung compliance in drowned experimental animal models is decreased by 66% when compared to non-drowned animal models. The decreased compliance after drowning requires higher than typical pressures for oxygenation and ventilation.[41] Compliance is believed to be decreased due to widespread closing of terminal airways and increased resistance from fluid and foam.[41]

Knowing that profound hypoxia in the drowned patient leads to morbidity and can decompensate into cardiac arrest, it is vital to recognize when orotracheal intubation efforts are unsuccessful and quickly move to rescue strategies such as the bedside surgical airway.

Once the airway is secured via endotracheal intubation or surgical airway, lung protective ventilation strategies should be employed. One recommendation is the ARDS Net protocol, which is a lung protective strategy employing low-volume ventilation, typically 4 to 8 mL/kg of ideal body weight. Another key point in the ARDS Net protocol is maintaining plateau pressures of less than 30 cm $H_2O$, allowing for permissive hypercapnia; however, hypercapnia should be avoided to prevent further neurologic sequelae in drowned patients. After determining the desired positive end-expiratory pressure (PEEP) to maintain adequate oxygenation, attempts to wean PEEP should also be delayed for at least 48 hours to allow for generation of new surfactant.[3]

To maintain adequate tissue perfusion, initial resuscitation with crystalloid fluids is recommended. There is no evidence that ingestion or aspiration of freshwater or saltwater has any clinically significant impact on electrolyte concentrations or fluid status, as once thought. Drowned patients frequently have evidence of pulmonary edema; this is noncardiogenic pulmonary edema, and results from the inflammatory cascade triggered by lung injury secondary to hypoxia, loss of surfactant, and atelectasis. Therefore, diuresis is not recommended in drowned patients, as patients are generally not hypervolemic.[19]

Corticosteroids, such as methylprednisolone and dexamethasone, have been used in various lung conditions to modulate inflammation and reduce tissue damage. Their potential role in mitigating the inflammatory response and lung injury in drowning patients has garnered attention in recent years. While some studies have shown benefit to giving steroids in cases of hypoxia secondary to pneumonia, studies of steroid use in drowned patients have failed to show any benefit and steroids are therefore not recommended.[19,42]

Empiric antibiotics are not necessary or recommended, as most pools, oceans, and rivers do not have the bacterial colony count needed to rapidly cause pneumonia. Pneumonitis is common in drowned patients, and has a similar radiographic appearance to pneumonia, leading to frequent misdiagnosis.[3] When pneumonia does occur, it is generally diagnosed 48 to 72 hours after the drowning event based on high fevers, increasing leukocytosis, and new infiltrates on radiography. In ICU patients with ventilator-associated pneumonia, culture data and hospital pathogens should be considered when selecting antibiotics.[3] Empiric antibiotics should only be considered when drowning events occur in water sources with known high bacterial counts, such as sewage systems.[3]

While numerous studies have examined the prognostic factors influencing survival to hospital discharge of patients who suffer drowning, fewer have examined the criteria for observation or discharge.[36,37,40] The Wilderness Medical Society has provided recommendations for observation based on best available evidence: "Any patient who is asymptomatic (other than a mild cough) and displays normal lung auscultation may be considered for release from the scene. Ideally, another individual should be with them for the next 4 to 6 [hours] to monitor for symptom development, or the patient should be advised to seek medical assistance if symptoms develop."[19]

The duration of submersion is 1 factor that can help predict the probability of neurologically intact survival to discharge. Data for normothermic drownings show that patients with a duration of submersion of less than 5 minutes have only a 10% chance of death or severe neurologic impairment. Submersion of 5 to 10 minutes drastically increases the probability of death or severe neurologic impairment to 56%. In submersion greater than 25 minutes, the chance of death or severe neurologic impairment is 99.9%.[3]

## PREVENTION

It is estimated that greater than 90% of drownings are preventable.[3] Drownings usually occur when victims underestimate the danger or overestimate their competency in the water. Drownings can also occur when young children who are unable to effectively swim gain access to pools or other bodies of water. It is state law in many localities that pools must be protected by a closed physical barrier, such as a fence. Lack of appropriate, attentive adult supervision is a factor in pediatric drownings. Dirty or murky water and unprotected drain pipes at the bottoms of pools are also factors that increase the chance of drowning events.[9]

Life jacket or personal flotation device use is helpful in preventing drownings. A study by the US Coast Guard evaluated 1597 recreational boaters and found that wearing a life jacket could potentially prevent 1 out of every 2 drowning deaths. It has been shown that 76% of boating-related fatalities occur from drowning, and 85% of those fatalities are in individuals not wearing life jackets.[6,43,44]

Drowning is the leading cause of death among those engaged in recreational aquatic activity, and 30% to 70% of those individuals who suffer a fatal drowning have a detectable blood alcohol level. A blood alcohol level of 0.10 g/dL holds a 10-fold increase in the risk of recreational boating death when compared to people who have not been drinking.[45] An encouraging statistical is that some studies have shown a decline in alcohol-associated drowning deaths since the 1980s.[45]

While the presence of lifeguards is common at public swimming pools, their presence is uncommon around natural bodies of water. The United States Lifesaving Association data from 2021 demonstrated greater than 7 million prevention actions, such as verbal warnings, and greater than 50,000 water rescues in a population of 260 million beachgoers. Significantly more deaths (80) were reported at beaches without lifeguards than at beaches with lifeguards, from which only 30 fatal drownings were reported.[46]

Significant data associating swimming lessons with drowning prevention do not exist. However, expert opinion from the American Academy of Pediatrics suggests that children should take swimming lessons.[19] Experts from the Wilderness Medical Society (WMS) recommend "All persons who participate in activities conducted in or around water should have, at a minimum, enough experience and physical capability to maintain their head above water, tread water, and make forward progress for a distance of 25 m (82 ft)."[19]

## SUMMARY

Drowning is a significant yet preventable cause of death, especially in the pediatric population. "Drowning" is the term used to describe respiratory impairment from immersion or submersion in a liquid medium, and can occur with or without morbidity or mortality. Although evidence is sparse, the key in caring for the drowned patient is rapid reversal of hypoxia, which is the ultimate etiology of cardiac arrest. Therefore, focus on airway and breathing ahead of circulation for drowning resuscitations. There is no evidence to support the use of empiric steroids or antibiotics. On the other hand, positive pressure ventilation using lung protective strategies has shown benefit. The rapidly improved and well-appearing drowned patient with normal lung sounds and no hypoxia on scene is unlikely to suffer any sequelae from drowning. This can help guide field care and decisions for evacuation.

## CLINICS CARE POINTS

- Drowning remains a leading cause of accidental death worldwide, and is responsible for considerable morbidity. Supervision of children around water, wearing life jackets, and not abusing alcohol can dramatically decrease the likelihood of drowning.
- The cornerstone of the treatment of drowning is rapidly addressing hypoxia. Lifeguards, Emergency Medical Services (EMS) personnel, and others who are responsible for others around water should be trained in delivering rescue breaths. Recommendations are to provide rescue breaths first prior to chest compressions in drowning patients.
- Asymptomatic patients can be safely discharged from the ED after a 4 to 6 hour observation period without any diagnostic studies beyond a physical examination.
- Patients with severe lung injury from drowning may be treated with high-flow oxygen, NIPPV, or mechanical ventilation using a lung protective ventilatory strategy.

## DISCLOSURE

Dr C.A. Davis receives funding from the National Institutes of Health, United States. Dr S. Lareau has no financial conflicts of interest to disclose.

## REFERENCES

1. World Health Organization. Drowning fact sheet. Available at: https://www.who.int/news-room/fact-sheets/detail/drowning.
2. van Beeck EF, Branche CM, Szpilman D, et al. A new definition of drowning: towards documentation and prevention of a global public health problem. Bull World Health Organ 2005;83(11):853–6.
3. Szpilman D, Morgan PJ. Management for the Drowning Patient. Chest 2021; 159(4):1473–83.
4. Centers for Disease Control and Prevention NCfIPaC. Web-based Injury Statistics Query and Reporting System (WISQARS). Available at: https://www.cdc.gov/injury/wisqars/index.html.
5. Borse NNGJ, Dellinger AM, Rudd RA, et al. DC childhood injury report: patterns of unintentional Injuries among 0–19 year olds in the United States, 2000–2006. Atlanta: Centers for Disease Control and Prevention; 2008.
6. Cummings P, Mueller BA, Quan L. Association between wearing a personal floatation device and death by drowning among recreational boaters: a matched cohort analysis of United States Coast Guard data. Inj Prev 2011;17(3):156–9.
7. Peden MMK, Sharma K. The injury chart book: a graphical overview of the global burden of injuries. Geneva: World Health Organization; 2002.
8. Linnan MAL, Cuong PV, Anhm LV. Special series on child injury: child mortality and injury in Asia: survey results and evidence. Florence, Italy: NICEF Innocenti Research Center; 2007.
9. Modell JH. Prevention of needless deaths from drowning. South Med J 2010; 103(7):650–3.
10. Hunn ES, Helmer SD, Reyes J, et al. Patterns of injuries in drowning patients - do these patients need a trauma team? Kans J Med 2020;13:165–78.

11. Roberts K, Thom O, Devine S, et al. A scoping review of female drowning: an underexplored issue in five high-income countries. BMC Publ Health 2021; 21(1):1072.

12. Szpilman DSA, Graves S. Section 7.11: classification systems. In: Bierens J, editor. Handbook on drowning: prevention, rescue, treatment. Berlin, Germany: Springer-Verlag; 2005. p. 427–32.

13. Matthew JRC, Hofmeyr R, Hofmeyr R. Update on drowning. S Afr Med J 2017; 107(7):562–5.

14. Topjian AA, Berg RA, Bierens JJ, et al. Brain resuscitation in the drowning victim. Neurocrit Care 2012;17(3):441–67.

15. Peden AE, Taylor DH, Franklin RC. Pre-existing medical conditions: a systematic literature review of a silent contributor to adult drowning. Int J Environ Res Public Health 2022;19(14).

16. Tester DJ, Medeiros-Domingo A, Will ML, et al. Unexplained drownings and the cardiac channelopathies: a molecular autopsy series. Mayo Clin Proc 2011; 86(10):941–7.

17. Lippmann J, Walker D, Lawrence C, et al. Provisional report on diving-related fatalities in Australian waters 2006. Diving Hyperb Med 2011;41(2):70–84.

18. Modell JH, Davis JH. Electrolyte changes in human drowning victims. Anesthesiology 1969;30(4):414–20.

19. Davis CA, Schmidt AC, Sempsrott JR, et al. Wilderness Medical Society Clinical Practice Guidelines for the Treatment and Prevention of Drowning: 2024 Update. Wilderness Environ Med 2024;35(1_suppl):94S–111S.

20. Turgut A, Turgut T. A study on rescuer drowning and multiple drowning incidents. J Safety Res 2012;43(2):129–32.

21. Perkins GD. In-water resuscitation: a pilot evaluation. Resuscitation 2005;65(3): 321–4.

22. Szpilman D, Soares M. In-water resuscitation–is it worthwhile? Resuscitation 2004;63(1):25–31.

23. Winkler BE, Eff AM, Ehrmann U, et al. Effectiveness and safety of in-water resuscitation performed by lifeguards and laypersons: a crossover manikin study. Prehosp Emerg Care 2013;17(3):409–15.

24. Lott C, Truhlar A, Alfonzo A, et al. European Resuscitation Council Guidelines 2021: Cardiac arrest in special circumstances. Resuscitation 2021;161:152–219.

25. Michelet P, Bouzana F, Charmensat O, et al. Acute respiratory failure after drowning: a retrospective multicenter survey. Eur J Emerg Med 2017;24(4): 295–300.

26. Manolios N, Mackie I. Drowning and near-drowning on Australian beaches patrolled by life-savers: a 10-year study, 1973-1983. Med J Aust 1988;148(4): 170–1, 165–7.

27. Quan L, Cummings P. Characteristics of drowning by different age groups. Inj Prev 2003;9(2):163–8.

28. Bierens JJ, Knape JT, Gelissen HP. Drowning. Curr Opin Crit Care 2002;8(6): 578–86.

29. Lyster T, Jorgenson D, Morgan C. The safe use of automated external defibrillators in a wet environment. Prehosp Emerg Care 2003;7(3):307–11.

30. Klock-Frezot JC, Ohley WJ, Schock RB, et al. Successful defibrillation in water: a preliminary study. Conf Proc IEEE Eng Med Biol Soc 2006;2006:4028–30.

31. Schratter A, Weihs W, Holzer M, et al. External cardiac defibrillation during wet-surface cooling in pigs. Am J Emerg Med 2007;25(4):420–4.

32. Bierens J, Bray J, Abelairas-Gomez C, et al. A systematic review of interventions for resuscitation following drowning. Resusc Plus 2023;14:100406.
33. Watson RS, Cummings P, Quan L, et al. Cervical spine injuries among submersion victims. J Trauma 2001;51(4):658–62.
34. Hawkins SC, Williams J, Bennett BL, et al. Wilderness Medical Society Clinical Practice Guidelines for Spinal Cord Protection. Wilderness Environ Med 2019; 30(4S):S87–99.
35. Causey AL, Tilelli JA, Swanson ME. Predicting discharge in uncomplicated near-drowning. Am J Emerg Med 2000;18(1):9–11.
36. Shenoi RP, Allahabadi S, Rubalcava DM, et al. The Pediatric Submersion Score Predicts Children at Low Risk for Injury Following Submersions. Acad Emerg Med 2017;24(12):1491–500.
37. Brennan CE, Hong TKF, Wang VJ. Predictors of safe discharge for pediatric drowning patients in the emergency department. Am J Emerg Med 2018;36(9): 1619–23.
38. Cantu RM, Pruitt CM, Samuy N, et al. Predictors of emergency department discharge following pediatric drowning. Am J Emerg Med 2018;36(3):446–9.
39. Cohen N, Capua T, Lahat S, et al. Predictors for hospital admission of asymptomatic to moderately symptomatic children after drowning. Eur J Pediatr 2019; 178(9):1379–84.
40. Szpilman D. Near-drowning and drowning classification: a proposal to stratify mortality based on the analysis of 1,831 cases. Chest 1997;112(3):660–5.
41. Baker PA, Webber JB. Failure to ventilate with supraglottic airways after drowning. Anaesth Intensive Care 2011;39(4):675–7.
42. Orlowski JP, Szpilman D. Drowning. Rescue, resuscitation, and reanimation. Pediatr Clin North Am 2001;48(3):627–46.
43. Bugeja L, Cassell E, Brodie LR, et al. Effectiveness of the 2005 compulsory personal flotation device (PFD) wearing regulations in reducing drowning deaths among recreational boaters in Victoria, Australia. Inj Prev 2014;20(6):387–92.
44. O'Connor PJ, O'Connor N. Causes and prevention of boating fatalities. Accid Anal Prev 2005;37(4):689–98.
45. Driscoll TR, Harrison JA, Steenkamp M. Review of the role of alcohol in drowning associated with recreational aquatic activity. Inj Prev 2004;10(2):107–13.
46. US Lifesaving Association. National lifesaving statistics. 2021. Available at: https://www.usla.org/page/STATISTICS.

# Underwater and Scuba Diving Accidents

David Lambert, MD*, Mark Binkley, MD, Zachary Gaskill, DO

## KEYWORDS

- Immersion pulmonary disease • Dive physics • Nitrogen narcosis
- Decompression sickness • Arterial gas embolism • Hyperbaric oxygen therapy
- Dive history

## KEY POINTS

- Environmental factors (temperature, marine life, and breathing gas) can affect diving performance and lead to injuries.
- Barotrauma is a major risk factor for the development of ear pain, sinus pain, dental pain, pneumothorax and air-gas embolism.
- Arterial gas embolism (AGE) occurs when gas, typically from pulmonary over inflation (barotrauma), enters the arterial circulation leading to sudden injury (heart and CNS).
- Decompression sickness (DCS) typically presents between 1 and 6 hours after surfacing from prolonged underwater activities.
- Treatment of AGE and DCS typically requires hyperbaric oxygen therapy.
- Transporting injured divers requires special considerations.

## INTRODUCTION

There are 4 major components to the evaluation and management of an injured scuba diver, or any individual who is exposed to greater than sea-level atmospheric pressures for extended periods. Categorically, this includes the following: (1) taking a thorough dive history; (2) considering the major fundamental risks inherent to underwater activities and the pathophysiology of immersion pulmonary edema (IPE) and decompression illness; (3) completing a detailed physical examination with emphasis on skin, lymphatic, musculoskeletal, pulmonary, and neurologic findings; and (4) providing supportive care, knowing when to consult a dive medicine expert and transportation considerations. A working knowledge of these 4 tenants enables the emergency physician to systematically evaluate an injured diver in the acute setting, create a

Division of Undersea and Hyperbaric Medicine, University of Pennsylvania, 3610 Hamilton Walk, 1 John Morgan Building, Philadelphia, PA 19104, USA
* Corresponding author. Department of Emergency Medicine, Hospital of the University of Pennsylvania, 3400 Spruce Street, Philadelphia, PA 19104
E-mail address: david.lambert@pennmedicine.upenn.edu

Emerg Med Clin N Am 42 (2024) 551–563
https://doi.org/10.1016/j.emc.2024.02.015     emed.theclinics.com
0733-8627/24/© 2024 Elsevier Inc. All rights reserved.

differential diagnosis and provide, when necessary, the proper (and safe) evacuation to more definitive care in the event of a serious injury that requires an undersea medical expert. Conversely, it may also prevent unnecessary transfer and/or intervention (**Table 1**).[1]

Open-circuit recreational scuba diving is the most popular and most common form of diving encountered by the emergency provider in the United States and Canada.[2] There are many other forms of diving that involve various degrees of risk, such as technical diving using a closed-circuit rebreather apparatus and specialized military or commercial diving using surface-supplied breathing gas. Open circuit means exhaled gas is released, unlike closed circuit where air is scrubbed to remove $CO_2$ and recycled. In open-circuit recreational scuba diving, divers carry a tank of gas with them, whereas in surface supplied breathing, air is forced down an umbilical to them from the surface. Regardless of the type of underwater activity, the mechanisms leading to injury are similar; therefore, the management is the same. Overall, diving remains a safe activity with only 1.8 deaths per million recreational dives.[3]

When it comes to diving, experience matters, as there are many divers with limited training and certification, including resort diving certification, which does not meet industry standards. The inexperienced divers often have a poor understanding of the risks of diving, limited familiarity with their diving gear, and a lack of understanding of emergency procedures that lead to a compounding of errors. In addition to these human factors, many accidents are associated with pre-existing comorbidities such as diabetes, cardiopulmonary diseases (eg, asthma and chronic obstructive pulmonary disease), and poor physical conditioning. The most recent recommendation for recreational scuba divers is that they should be able to meet a moderate energy expenditure with a 7 metabolic equivalent (MET) capacity for uncomplicated recreational dives.[4]

## ENVIRONMENTAL FACTORS
### Temperature

Both the water temperature and environmental temperature can affect a diver's ability to maintain an ideal body temperature. Cold water can lead to hypothermia, even when wearing proper diving gear (wet or dry suit).[5] Nitrogen narcosis, a change in consciousness brought on by breathing compressed gas, reduces perception of cold and inhibits central temperature regulation and heat generation.[6] Susceptibility to hypothermia is increased in divers with dehydration, low body mass index, and alcohol and/or tobacco use.[7] Hyperthermia is rarely caused by immersion in water, but if the water temperature is 86°F or warmer, divers are at risk of overheating.[8] Both

| Table 1 | |
|---|---|
| **General overview of scuba diver evaluation and management** | |
| Risk Factors and Pathophysiology | Past Medical History, Environmental Exposure, Immersion Pulmonary Edema, Decompression Illness (DCS/AGE) |
| Dive history | Diving experience, prior injuries, and recent dive-related events |
| Physical examination | Skin, lymphatic, musculoskeletal, pulmonary, and neurologic findings |
| Disposition and referral | IV fluids, supplemental oxygen, dive medical expert consultation, and transportation considerations |

*Abbreviations*: AGE, arterial gas embolism; DCS, decompression sickness; IV, intravenous.

extremes may present with altered mental status, confusion, and poor motor skills leading to an increasing risk for loss of consciousness and subsequent drowning.[9]

### Immersion

Immersion into the water column leads to fluid shifts within the pulmonary and circulatory system. Immersion in water has a compressive effect on the circulatory system where the increased ambient pressure increases blood flow to the heart and leads to diuresis (immersion diuresis) and subsequent hypovolemia.[10]

Usually this is tolerated well, but sometimes prior to diuresis the fluid shift can lead to cardio-respiratory distress with chest pain, dyspnea, coughing, hemoptysis, and syncope. This phenomenon is known as IPE. Risk factors include cold water immersion, excessive hydration, increased breathing resistance, increased exertion, and pulmonary hypertension.[11] IPE has been seen in scuba divers, swimmers, and snorkelers. During immersion in water, the increased fluid shift may cause an increased volume returning to the heart, leading to an increased pulmonary capillary wedge pressure.[12] This in turn leads to leakage of fluid into the alveolar spaces and pulmonary edema.[13] This phenomenon is one reason that patients with a history of cardiomyopathy and congestive heart failure are advised against swimming or diving.[14] Treatment of patients with IPE involves removal from the water to reverse the hydrostatic pressures and supplemental oxygen or positive pressure ventilation.[15] IPE may respond to β2-adrenergic agonist or diuretic therapy.[16] Patients with IPE are at high risk of recurrence (up to 40%) so should be warned to take precautions prior to any future underwater activities.[17]

Conductive heat exchange occurs with any diver exposed to the water environment even when wearing a wetsuit.[18] Most cases result in heat loss as water temperature is typically less than body temperature. In rare circumstances, where ambient water temperature exceeds body temperature, heat is transferred to the diver. Strategic rewarming of patients after removal from the in-water environment is a priority to prevent chilling and hypothermia.

### Contaminated Breathing Gas

Compressed air, as well as various gas mixtures, is used selectively based on its inherent properties to address a proposed constraint such as depth, duration, or operational logistics. While careful dive planning and gas analysis may mitigate risk while filling scuba cylinders, the risk of contamination persists. One of the most common contaminants is carbon monoxide, which is introduced in small amounts from environmental sources such as compressors, generators, or other pollution near a filling station.[19] This risk exists not only for scuba divers, but for commercial divers who are receiving their breathing gas via a surface supplied breathing apparatus.[20] The small amount of carbon monoxide is amplified at depth as the partial pressure increases according to Henry's gas law. Contaminated breathing gas and carbon monoxide poisoning should be suspected if a diver reports symptoms starting concomitant with reaching the bottom of their dive or upon the start of their ascent, as the concentration of gaseous molecules is most concentrated at depth. Other breathing gases that have been reported include excessive carbon dioxide, volatile hydrocarbons, oils, and dust (see **Table 2**).

### Dive profile factors

There are 2 principal gas laws to keep in mind when caring for scuba divers: Boyle's law and Henry's law. They account for the changes in pressure, volume, and the amount of gas dissolved in the body when diving. Understanding them is vital to understanding diving accidents.

**Table 2**
**Dive injury factors and presentation[15,21–25]**

| Dive Injury Related Factors | Effects | Clinical Signs/Symptoms |
|---|---|---|
| Environmental factors | | |
| Temperature | Ambient and/or water temperature | Hypothermia/hyperthermia and severe dehydration |
| Contaminated breathing gas | Scuba cylinder or surface supplied air | SOB, cough, AMS, headache, and LOC |
| Immersion effects | Pulmonary edema | SOB, cough, and respiratory arrest |
| Dive profile factors | | |
| Barotrauma | Ears | Ear pain and bleeding |
| | Sinuses | Sinus congestion and bleeding |
| | Dental | Toothache |
| | Eyes/mask | Subconjunctival hemorrhages |
| | Pulmonary | SOB/CP, hypoxia, tension PTX, and AGE |
| Breath gas effects | Oxygen toxicity | Seizure |
| | Carbon dioxide | LOC and cardiac dysfunction |
| | Nitrogen narcosis | Giddiness, AMS, and confusion |
| DCS | Musculoskeletal | Joint ache/pain (typically shoulder, elbow, hip, and knees) |
| | Cutaneous | Erythematous poorly demarcated truncal/proximal rash |
| | Lymphatic | Isolated lymphatic swelling (typically truncal/upper chest) |
| | Spinal cord | Motor neuron deficits and bladder dysfunction |
| | Inner ear | Vertigo, ataxia, HL, and tinnitus |
| | CNS | AMS, confusion, VF deficits, and Ataxia |
| | Pulmonary | Dyspnea, cough, and CP |
| | Constitutional | Generalized weakness/fatigue/malaise |

*Abbreviations:* AMS, altered mental status; CP, chest pain; HL, hearing loss; LOC, loss of consciousness; PTX, pneumothorax; SOB, shortness of breath; VF, visual field.
Based on data from sources and the experience of the authors.

### Barotrauma (Boyle's Law) and Air-Gas Embolism

As a diver descends in the water column, the ambient pressure surrounding their body increases. As ambient pressure changes (increase with descent, decrease with ascent) gas-filled pockets will naturally change volume in relation to depth and pressure increases according to Boyle's law, which states that pressure and volume are inversely related, $P1V1 = P2V2$.[26] Injuries related to pressure–volume changes are termed barotrauma and they can occur in the lungs, middle ears, sinuses, and other air-filled pockets, such as within teeth, gastrointestinal tract, and even in the dive mask.[27–34] During descent, divers use Valsalva maneuvers to inject air into their middle ear to equalize against the increasing pressures and prevent injury, commonly termed a "squeeze." Conversely, upon ascent, divers open their jaws, swallow, and utilize other maneuvers to allow expanding middle ear air to escape via the Eustachian tube to prevent a "reverse squeeze." Signs and symptoms of the various forms of barotrauma are described in **Table 3**.

Clinically, middle ear barotrauma may cause sudden onset pain, bleeding, and tympanic membrane rupture. This may lead to vertigo and vomiting that may ultimately lead to drowning. Inner ear barotrauma (IEBT) presents in a similar manner but is often associated with a diver being unable to equalize and/or forcibly performing a Valsalva maneuver, causing trauma to the inner ear membranes, the round and oval windows. IEBT is difficult to diagnose without direct visualization, and therefore, the onset and presenting signs and symptoms in the dive history are vital to creating an accurate differential diagnosis in the emergency department (ED). Symptoms of IEBT need to be distinguished from inner ear decompression sickness (DCS) as recompression of a patient with isolated barotrauma may exacerbate rather than improve symptoms.[35]

The most clinically significant barotrauma is pulmonary barotrauma (PBT), which can have life-threatening consequences. For every 33 feet of seawater (fsw) depth, there is an increase of 1 atm absolute (ATA) of pressure. For example, a diver at a depth of 33 fsw will experience an absolute pressure of 2 ATA, double the pressure at the surface. If that same diver does not exhale during ascent, the volume of air in his lungs at 33 ft will expand to twice its volume upon reaching the surface leading to PBT. The expanding gas, if trapped, leads to pneumothorax, pneumomediastinum, or enters the pulmonary circulation leading to Arterial air-Gas Embolization (AGE) with near-immediate consequences. PBT symptoms typically manifest immediately upon ascent when a diver approaches the surface and almost always less than 10 minutes after surfacing.[21] PBT may occur from depths as shallow as 5 to 10 ft since the greatest change, relative to ambient pressure, occurs near the surface. Divers who hold their breath when ascending from depth are at risk of lung overexpansion and subsequent injury regardless of depth unless the breath was taken at the surface and no other inhalation occurred at depth. For this reason, the incidence is rare in breath-hold divers unless they take a breath from another source of air while they are underwater (no longer a breath-hold diver).

Ultimately, beyond the risk of developing a pneumothorax while scuba diving, the greatest risk to PBT is the introduction of air directly into the arterial circulation and

**Table 3**
**Contaminated breathing gas symptoms**

| Contaminant | Symptoms |
|---|---|
| Carbon monoxide | Headache, dizziness, weakness, nausea/vomiting, shortness of breath, altered mental status, confusion, and syncope |
| Carbon dioxide | Hyperventilation, dizziness, confusion, and syncope |
| Volatile hydrocarbons | Fatigue, headache, confusion, impaired judgment, numbness, cardiac arrhythmias, and syncope |
| Oil (condensed) | Headache, nausea, and impaired respiratory function |
| Dust (particles) | Impaired respiratory function |

*Adapted from* Divers Alert Network Website: Safety and Prevention - Diver Safety - Breathing Gas Contamination (https://dan.org/safety-preventipon/diver-safety/)

subsequent downstream consequences with air going to directly to vital organs and causing sudden and severe stroke-like symptoms, including death (**Tables 4** and **5**).[5]

### Breathing Gas Effects and Decompression Sickness

Henry's law states that the amount of a gas dissolved in the body is directly proportional to the partial pressure of that gas.[26] As a diver descends into the water column, the partial pressure of the inhaled gas increases correspondingly, which means more of whatever gas mixture the diver is breathing will be absorbed. Most recreational divers breathe regular compressed air, which is approximately 21% oxygen and 79% nitrogen—at sea level. Divers breathing compressed air will absorb increasing amounts of nitrogen the deeper and longer they dive. DCS occurs when a diver surfaces after being underwater for either too long of a time and/or too deep of a depth. Nitrogen, absorbed while at depth, will come out of solution and form bubbles. If a diver ascends too quickly, it may accelerate the process of nitrogen gas coming out of solution, overwhelming what the body can handle. This leads to excessive amounts of nitrogen bubbles in the body causing possible downstream sequelae involving multiple organ systems: neurologic, pulmonary, cardiac, musculoskeletal, lymphatic, and skin. This can be referred to as the "bends."

The vast majority of the time (approximately 90%), the onset of DCS typically occurs between 1 and 12 hours after surfacing from a dive.[21] Historically, DCS was described by symptom severity as Type 1 (mild) and Type 2 (severe); however, more commonly it is simply described by the organ system affected. The key to the evaluation of an injured diver is taking an accurate dive history. The dive profile (depth and duration), number of dives per day, surface intervals (time between dives), type of breathing gas, experience level, timing of onset of symptoms, problems during the dive, and predive events are helpful details to obtain. It often helps to talk with your EMS personnel as they may have collateral history from dive instructors, fellow divers, family members, and other

**Table 4**
**Signs and symptoms of barotrauma**

| | | |
|---|---|---|
| Ears | Middle ear bleeding, TM rupture, and round/oval window rupture | Severe unilateral headache, vertigo, disorientation, and nausea/vomiting |
| Lungs | Ruptured alveoli, pneumothorax, and pneumomediastinum | Chest pain, shortness of breath, and air-gas embolism AGE |
| Sinuses | Bleeding, congestion, and pneumocephalus (rare) | Pain, pressure, and headache |
| Eyes (mask squeeze) | Periorbital congestion/hyperemia and subconjunctival hemorrhages | Pain |
| Dental | Cary/cavity/crown with trapped air pocket | Severe dental pain and dental fracture (rare) |
| Skin | Poor fitting wetsuit or with dry suit air pockets | Linear marks and bruises, typically painless |
| Gastrointestinal | Stomach and intestinal expansion | Eructation, vomiting, flatus, bloating, colicky pain, and stomach rupture (rare) |

*Abbreviation:* TM, tympanic membrane.

**Table 5**
**Clinical presentation of arterial air-gas embolism in divers age—always less than 10 minutes upon surfacing and rapid in onset**[21–25,36]

| Loss of Consciousness | Altered Mental Status/Seizure |
|---|---|
| Dizziness/presyncope | Paralysis/paresthesia |
| Cardiac dysrhythmia/ischemia/shock | Paralysis/paresthesia |
| Bowel/bladder dysfunction | Vision changes |
| Headache | Cranial nerve deficits |

witnesses. Always ask for any available dive computer information. Determining the type of injury a patient sustained often requires this detailed history and physical examination. For example, a weight belt worn around the waist may compress the lateral femoral cutaneous nerve causing tingling, numbness, and pain in the thigh. This may easily be confused with and treated as DCS if not determined from a thorough history and physical.

As nitrogen gas accumulates during ascent, the majority of the nitrogen gas is filtered by the lungs. However, when there is an overwhelming amount of gas bubbles, they may coalesce and obstruct musculature, joint spaces, lymphatic regions and central nervous system (CNS) leading to characteristic signs and symptoms (**Table 6**). In severe cases, the lungs, which filter the nitrogen bubbles returning to the heart, may become overwhelmed allowing gas bubbles to escape in the arterial system. This is another way in which a patient may develop an AGE with similar consequences as noted previously in relation to PBT. Additionally, in patients who have pre-existing heart defects such as a patent foramen ovale (PFO), nitrogen gasses may shunt from the right heart to the left heart leading to an AGE. Obtaining this information in a past medical history may be helpful for the diagnosis and treatment, if available.

## HISTORY AND EXAMINATION OF THE INJURED DIVER
### Diving History

Keeping in mind the risk factors previously discussed, a detailed history with a focus on both remote and recent diving events is more vital to developing a working differential diagnosis and care plan than most diagnostic testing.[21] Knowing a diver's lifetime experience, level of certifications, type of diving, and prior decompression illness events helps put the current presentation in better context as experience matters when it comes to diving, and an experienced technical diver or commercial diver will most often be able to provide very detailed history of events. In the event that a diver is incapacitated, they will likely have a dive buddy or have been diving with a dive instructor who can also provide detailed history. An inexperienced or novice diver is more likely to violate many of the basic tenets of diving and therefore, the clinician may want to consider events such as running out of air, panic, omitted decompression stop, or rapid ascent. Ultimately, all divers can suffer from decompression illness, and a thorough examination is warranted in everyone, but having as much historical information as possible helps not only in the emergency department but also when speaking to a dive medical expert in consultation.

### Physical Examination

As mentioned in **Table 7**, certain physical findings can be indicative of DCS, which is nearly always a clinical diagnosis. The examination of any diver should include a general physical examination with emphasis on particular organ systems looking for evidence of barotrauma or DCS. This would include eye, ears, sinuses, neck, pulmonary,

| Table 6 Taking a dive history | |
|---|---|
| **Lifetime Diving** | |
| Level and date of diving certifications | |
| Certifying agency | |
| Total lifetime dives | |
| History of prior decompression illness | |
| **Current dive history** | |
| Location of diving | Saltwater and freshwater |
| Type of diving activity | Recreational, commercial, military, rescue/public service, and scientific |
| Temperature | Ambient, water (°F) |
| Suit type | Wet, dry, style, and thickness |
| Number of dives/day | |
| Dive profiles over preceding 48 h | Maximum depth per dive, dive durations, ascent rates, and surface interval times |
| Breathing gas | Standard air, enriched air (aka "Nitrox"), mixed gas, surface supplied |
| Location of scuba tank service/fill | |
| Any strenuous events during dive | Unexpected physical exertion, trauma, missed decompression stops, dive computer warnings, or violations |
| Buddy diver | Any symptoms or complaints |
| Collateral reports | EMS, dive instructors, family, and other observers (eg, boat captain) |

skin, neurologic, musculoskeletal, and psychiatric. On the Head, Ears, Eyes, Nose, Throat (HEENT) examination, one would look for evidence of barotrauma to the ears, eyes, or sinuses. Neck examination would look for crepitus secondary to a pneumomediastinum from a pneumothorax. Pulmonary examination may show evidence of pneumothorax or pulmonary edema. Subcutaneous emphysema from "skin bends" or cutis marmorata, an itchy or painful area of skin that is a red-bluish discolored area of the skin, is easily missed if a patient is not disrobed and fully examined. Musculoskeletal examination of painful joints after diving that appear normal but pain relieved with compression with a blood pressure cuff is consistent with a diagnosis of DCS. A full neurologic examination is vital in helping rule-in or rule-out DCS, which may mimic findings of stroke. Strength, weakness, sensory, motor, cranial nerves, reflexes, cerebellar, proprioception, and gait testing must be performed. For example, signs such as mild urinary retention, ataxia, and hyperesthesia are possible findings easily missed by a cursory neurologic examination. Evaluation of tandem gait both forward and backward and well as both a Romberg and Sharpened Romberg are high-yield tests for picking up subtle findings of truncal instability. Sharpened Romberg is performed in a manner similar to the Romberg, but in this test, the patient places their feet in tandem, with one foot in front of the other heel to toe. They then cross their arms across their chest and place open palms on opposite shoulder. They then hold their chin level to the ground. The test is performed with eyes open first, and then with eyes closed. **Table 7** outlines the major organ systems, signs, and symptoms affected in DCS.

**Table 7**
Decompression sickness—signs and symptoms[2,21,22,36]

| | | |
|---|---|---|
| Musculoskeletal ("bends") | Major joints (elbows, shoulder, knees, hip, and ankle), Large muscle groups (legs and arms) | Localized, deep, constant, not affected by movement, nontender, may range from mild (aka "niggle") to excruciating |
| Cutaneous ("skin bends") | Skin especially around head, neck, and upper torso most common | Mottled/marbled appearance and itching |
| Pulmonary ("chokes") | Lungs | Substernal pleuritic chest pain, dyspnea, dry cough, choking, cardiopulmonary arrest, AGE formation secondary to massive bubble formation that overwhelms normal pulmonary filtration and/or PFO in the heart |
| Neurologic | Brain  Spinal cord | Confusion, altered mental status, headache, visual complaints (spots, double or blurred vision), extreme fatigue, seizure, vertigo, nausea, vomiting, syncope, and loss of consciousness  Weakness, numbness, tingling and/or paralysis, and urinary or bowel incontinence |
| Lymphatic | Peripheral lymphatics | Peripheral edema and swelling, typically localized to one region |

*Adapted from* various sources and author clinical experience.

### Diagnostic Testing

The majority of dive-related injuries are diagnosed clinically with minimal required testing. It may be helpful to consider basic blood work such as complete blood count, basic metabolic panel, and urinalysis for the evaluation for other causes of the patient's presentation. If not clinically apparent on initial physical examination, sometimes these tests will alert the provider to possible electrolyte imbalances or signs of dehydration that can be readily treated while awaiting more definitive care, such as transfer for hyperbaric oxygen therapy (HBOT). If available, it is helpful to check a postvoid residual as urinary retention findings can be a subtle clue to spinal cord DCS. Other testing may include biomarkers such as a troponin to evaluate for possible cardiac injury in the event of an AGE in the coronary arteries leading to myocardial ischemia. All patients should receive a chest radiograph to rule-out the presence of pneumothorax, an absolute contraindication to HBOT.

The remainder of testing performed in the emergency department most often will be in the pursuit of alternative diagnoses, including CT brain when patients present with stroke-like symptoms. It should be noted that the absence of air-gas emboli on CT or MRI radiographs does not rule out the presence of an AGE.[21]

### Treatment and Disposition

Decompression illness is a rare event with an estimated incidence of 3 cases per 10,000 dives.[37] Once decompression illness is identified, the definitive treatment is HBOT. Treatment can be arranged, typically by transfer to a center with 24/7 HBOT availability. To locate such facilities, physicians are encouraged to call the Divers Alert Network Call Center Hotline, which is available 24/7 to assist with the assessment, triage, and possible treatment of all injured divers. They are staffed by on-call diver medical technicians as well as diving physicians. They have a 24 hour hotline number (919) 684-9111, and the staff will help provide closest hyperbaric facility location information in the event it is deemed necessary.

While preparing for and awaiting transfer to an HBO capable facility, there are other adjunctive measures that can be and should be taken by the emergency physician. As mentioned previously, many injured divers are dehydrated and may benefit from rehydration. Supine positioning is the recommended position for most patients when AGE remains on the differential. Trendelenburg positioning is not recommended by the authors to reduce air-emboli migration as it introduces the transportation challenges as well as potentially lead to cerebral edema if maintained for too long.[38] Lastly, the mainstay of treatment of all injured divers is supplemental oxygen via nonrebreather.[21] This is not for hypoxia but rather to aid the elimination of excess nitrogen gas molecules in the body that will continue to off-gas for many hours after completion of a dive. This is commonly referred to as their residual nitrogen time.

For a patient who needs transfer to for HBOT, this may involve the use of aircraft and/or ground transportation over mountainous (ie, high elevation) terrain, which introduces the risk of exacerbating symptoms of DCS. When requesting transportation aircraft, it is important to request fixed-wing aircraft with the ability to either fly at sea-level cabin pressure via either a minimum safe altitude flight or a pressurized cabin pressure that matches sea level. Commercial aircrafts that are traditionally pressurized to a cabin altitude pressure equivalent of 8000 ft are not recommended due to the increased risk of exacerbating the effects of DCS. A literature review found DCS symptoms worsened in patients when elevation exceeded 500 ft above ground level.[39] The vibratory actions of flight, especially rotary-wing aircraft, have been theorized to introduce the added risk of increased nitrogen bubble formation. For this reason, it is recommended to package and locate a patient within the aircraft to minimize vibrations.[40] It is incumbent on the emergency physician to confirm with the receiving facility any other adjunctive measures to be taken prior to transport such as intravenous (IV) access, airway cuff balloons being replaced with water or saline to mitigate any reduction in pressure with changes in altitude pressure. Lastly, it is vital that the medical records, imaging, and any diving computers are included with the patient transport to aid with reassessments.

### SUMMARY

In summary, the evaluation and care of an injured scuba diver requires an understanding of the different types of underwater activities that may be deemed scuba diving. Such activities may range from the complex (eg, commercial or technical diving) all the way up to basic recreational scuba or snorkeling. From this comes an understanding of the physiologic effects of breathing compressed air underwater and the pathophysiology of diving. Once a diver presents himself or herself to the ED, the most important component of the evaluation and management of the patient is taking a detailed history, as this information may be critically important when considering possible referral and/or transfer to a dive medicine clinic with hyperbaric oxygen capabilities. Next, a thorough physical examination should be completed as early as possible with a focus on specific areas at risk for injury and etiology, such as a detailed cardiopulmonary, skin, and neurologic examination. Serial reassessments and supportive care are as equally important as consultation with a dive medicine expert, especially one with hyperbaric capabilities. Lastly, stabilization and suitability for transport via air–ground assets demand consideration of risk–benefit analysis.

## CLINICS CARE POINTS

- Taking a thorough dive history should include information about environment, equipment and dive plan, or profile. Additionally, access to dive computer, dive logs, and diving companion history are valuable assets.
- Chronologic presentation of symptoms and evolution of symptoms are needed for an accurate diagnosis of a dive injury.
- AGE should be included in the differential diagnosis when symptoms (loss of consciousness, altered mental status, or neuro deficit) begin within 10 minutes of surfacing.
- IPE is a process that can occur from any depth of immersion in water and should be considered in patients with shortness of breath after swimming.
- Detailed full body musculoskeletal, skin, cardiopulmonary, and detailed neurologic examinations are crucial in diagnosing the varied presentations of decompression sickness.
- Imaging can help corroborate DCS diagnosis, but the diagnosis is largely based on history and physical examination.
- Supportive care and repeat physical examinations are useful when consulting with dive medicine physicians and can be done concurrently while arranging transfer.

## DISCLOSURE

None declared.

## REFERENCES

1. Xu W, Liu W, Huang G, et al. Decompression illness: clinical aspects of 5278 consecutive cases treated in a single hyperbaric unit. PLoS One 2012;7(11): e50079.
2. Available at:. In: Denoble PJ, editor. DAN annual diving report 2019 edition: a report on 2017 diving fatalities, injuries and incidents. Durham, NC: Divers Alert Network; 2019. p. 113 https://www.ncbi.nlm.nih.gov/books/NBK562527/?report=classic.
3. Buzzcott P, Schiller D, Crain J, et al. Epidemiology of morbidity and mortality in US and Canadian recreational scuba diving. Publ Health 2018;155:62–8.
4. Buzzcott P, Pollock NW, Rosenberg M. Exercise intensity inferred from air consumption during recreational scuba diving. Available at: Diving Hyperb Med 2014;44(2):74–8 https://pubmed.ncbi.nlm.nih.gov/24986724/.
5. Pendergast DR, Mollendorf J. Exercising divers' thermal protection as a function of water temperature. Available at: Undersea Hyperb Med 2011;38(2):127–36 https://pubmed.ncbi.nlm.nih.gov/21510272/.

6. Rocco M, Pelaia P, Di Benedetto P, et al. ROAD Project Investigators. Inert gas narcosis in scuba diving, different gases different reactions. Eur J Appl Physiol 2019;119(1):247–55.
7. Tipton M, Mekjavic I, Golden F. Chapter 13: hypothermia." Bove and Davis' diving medicine. 4th edition. Philadelphia, PA: Alfred Bove. Saunders; 2004. p. 261–73 (ISBN-9780721694245).
8. Dinsmore D, Bozanic J. Diving physiology: types of heat stress" NOAA diving manual. 5th edition. Palm Beach, FL: Best Publishing; 2013. 4:40.
9. Dinsmore D, Bozanic J. Diving physiology: effects of cold" NOAA diving manual. 5th edition. Palm Beach, FL: Best Publishing; 2013. 4:37.
10. Epstein M. Water immersion and the kidney: implications for volume regulation. Available at: Undersea Biomed Res 1984;11(2):113–21 https://pubmed.ncbi.nlm.nih.gov/6567431/.
11. Kumar M, Thompson PD. A literature review of immersion pulmonary edema. Physician Sportsmed 2019;47(2):148–51.
12. Giauzzi P, Tavazzi L, Meyer K, et al. Recommendations for exercise training in chronic heart failure patients. Eur Heart J 2001;22:125–35.
13. Bosco G, Rizzato A, Moon RE, et al. Environmental Physiology and Diving Medicine. Front Psychol 2018;9:72.
14. Wilmshurst PT. Immersion pulmonary oedema: a cardiological perspective. Diving Hyperb Med 2019;49(1):30–40.
15. Seiler C, Kristiansson L, Klingberg C, et al. Swimming-Induced Pulmonary Edema: Evaluation of Prehospital Treatment with CPAP or Positive Expiratory Pressure Device. Chest 2022;162(2):410–20.
16. Moon R, Martina S, Peacher D, et al. Swimming-Induced Pulmonary Edema Pathophysiology and Risk Reduction With Sildenafil. Circulation 2016;133(10):988–96.
17. Smith R, Ormerod JOM, Sabharwal N, et al. Swimming-induced pulmonary edema: current perspectives. Open Access J Sports Med 2018;9:131–7.
18. Aguilella-Arzo M, Alcaraz A, Aguilella V. Heat loss and hypothermia in free diving: Estimation of survival time under water. Am J Phys 2003;71:333.
19. Hampson NB. Carbon monoxide poisoning while scuba diving a rare event? UHM 2020;47(3). 487-450.
20. Lippmann J. Fatalities involving divers using surface-supplied breathing apparatus in Australia, 1965 to 2019. Diving Hyperb Med 2021;51(1):53–62.
21. Mitchell SJ, Bennett MB, Mood RE. Decompression Sickness and Arterial Gas Embolism. N Engl J Med 2022;386:1254–64.
22. Greene KM: Causes of death in submarine escape training casualties: Analysis of cases c and review of the literature. Admiralty Marine Technology Establishment Report No. AMTE (E) R 78-402, 1978.
23. Harker CP, Neuman TS, Olson LK, et al: The roentgenographic findings associated with air embolism in sport scuba divers. J Emerg Med 1993;11:443–9.
24. Pearson RR, Goad RF. Delayed cerebral edema complicating cerebral air embolism: Case histories. Available at: Undersea Biomed Res 1982;9(4):283–96 https://pubmed.ncbi.nlm.nih.gov/7168093/.
25. Kizer KW. Dysbaric cerebral air embolism in Hawaii. Ann Emerg Med 1987 May; 16(5):535–41.
26. Melamed Y, Shupak A, Bitterman H. Medical problems associated with underwater diving. N Engl J Med 1992;326(10):30–5.
27. Pearson RR. Diagnosis and treatment of gas embolism. In: Schilling CW, Carlston CB, Mathias RA, editors. The physician's guide to diving medicine. New York: Plenum Press; 1984.

28. Weissman D, Green RS, Roberts PT. Frontal sinus barotrauma. Laryngoscope 1972;82(2):160–2.
29. Becker GD, Parell GJ. Otolaryngologic aspects of scuba diving. Otolaryngol Head Neck Surg 1979;87(5):569–72.
30. Burman F. Compressed gas (air) supply system. Available at:. Belgrade, Serbia: Presented at the Ninth European Committee for Hyperbaric Medicine (ECHM) Consensus Conference; 2012 https://www.uhms.org/images/Safety-Articles/Compressed_Gas_Supply_System.pdf.
31. Gas Association Compressed. CGA G-7.1-2011. Commodity specification for air. Available at:. 6th edition. Chantilly, Virginia: Compressed Gas Association; 2011 https://portal.cganet.com/Publication/Details.aspx?id=G-7.1.
32. Available at:Health and safety executive. Diver's breathing air standard and the frequency of examination and tests. DVis9(Rev1). Suffolk: HSE Books; 2008 https://scubaengineer.com/documents/hse_divers_breathing_air_standard_frequency_of_tests.pdf.
33. Millar IL, Mouldey PG. Compressed breathing air: the potential for evil from within. Available at: Diving and Hyperbaric Medicine 2008;3(3):145–51 https://pubmed.ncbi.nlm.nih.gov/22692708/.
34. Available at:US navy diving manual revision 6. SS521-AG-PRO-010. Washington, DC: Naval Sea Systems Command; 2008 https://www.navsea.navy.mil/Portals/103/Documents/SUPSALV/Diving/Dive%20Manual%20Rev%206%20with%20Chg%20A.pdf.
35. Rozycki SW, Brown MJ, Camacho M. Inner ear barotrauma in dievers: an evidence-based tool for evaluation and treatment. Diving Hyperb Med 2018;48(3):186–93.
36.. Bove AA, Davis JC. Diving medicine. 4th edition. Philadelphia, PA: Saunders; 2004 (ISBN: 9780721694245).
37. Pollock NW, Buteau D. Update in Decompression Illness. Emerg Med Clin North Am 2017;35(2):301–19.
38. Cooper JS, Hanson KC. Decompression sickness. [Updated 2022 Sep 2]. In: StatPearls [Internet]. Available at:. Treasure Island (FL): StatPearls Publishing; 2023 https://www.ncbi.nlm.nih.gov/books/NBK537264/.
39. MacDonald RD, O'Donnell C, Allan GM, et al. Interfacility transport of patients with decompression illness: literature review and consensus statement. Available at:. In: Database of abstracts of reviews of effects (DARE): quality-assessed reviews [Internet]. York (UK): Centre for Reviews and Dissemination (UK); 1995; 2006 https://www.ncbi.nlm.nih.gov/books/NBK72658/.
40. Stephenson J. Pathophysiology, treatment and aeromedical retrieval of SCUBA - related DCI. Journal of Military and Veterans' Health 2009;17(3):10–9.

# Desert Medicine

Geoffrey Comp, DO, FACEP, FAWM[a,b,c],*, Andrea Ferrari, MD[a],
Savannah Seigneur, DO[a,c]

## KEYWORDS

- Desert medicine • Desert climate • Wilderness medicine • Hyperthermia
- Bites and stings • Dehydration

## KEY POINTS

- Variations in temperature, humidity, and topography in desert climates predispose patients to medical conditions that practitioners in both rural and urban deserts must recognize and manage.
- Heat emergencies represent a variety of disorders ranging from minor to severe when the environmental and metabolic heat burden outpaces an individual's thermoregulatory mechanisms for heat transfer and the core temperature rises.
- Hydration needs vary significantly with activity level, environmental conditions (temperature and humidity), as well as individual factors such as acclimatization, sweat production, and sweat electrolyte content.
- The desert landscape is home to a tremendous variety of animal species, ranging from the harmless desert spiny lizard to the infamously venomous rattlesnake. Mammals such as the coyote and javelina occasionally collide with humans, while creatures like the bark scorpion and the Gila monster pose a smaller but impactful threat.

 Video content accompanies this article at http://www.emed.theclinics.com.

## INTRODUCTION

Deserts are defined by their arid nature, characterized by little rainfall, and often featuring vast stretches of sandy terrain with sparse vegetation. The resulting variations in temperature, humidity, and topography predispose patients to medical conditions that practitioners in both rural and urban deserts must recognize and manage. This article will equip medical practitioners with the essential knowledge and tools to navigate these complexities. It will focus on specific environmental considerations and challenges encountered while providing care in these desert locations and

[a] Valleywise Health Medical Center; [b] University of Arizona College of Medicine-Phoenix;
[c] Creighton University School of Medicine-Phoenix
* Corresponding author. Valleywise Health Hosptial - Department of Emergency Medicine, C/O Geoffrey Comp, 2601 E. Roosevelt Street, Phoenix, AZ 85008.
E-mail address: geoffbc@gmail.com

Emerg Med Clin N Am 42 (2024) 565–580
https://doi.org/10.1016/j.emc.2024.02.016
0733-8627/24/© 2024 Elsevier Inc. All rights reserved.

emed.theclinics.com

conditions associated with extreme heat and solar radiation, as well as native animal encounters.

## PATIENT CARE CONSIDERATIONS
### Assessment, Management, and Evacuation

When providing medical care in extreme heat and arid conditions, it is of particular importance to also consider the patient's core temperature and hydration status. While assessing and evacuating a patient, it is important to ensure that the management plan continues to monitor and prevent the development of hyperthermia and dehydration, as these can complicate any medical condition.

### Temperature Management

There are 2 important areas to protect the patient from the heat: the ground and the sky. The ground surface is the hottest place in the desert. When air temperatures range from 32 to 47°C, the surface temperature of rock at noon ranges from 37 to 59°C, and at 6 PM it can still be as hot as 32 to 43°C.[1] Patients should be immediately insulated or separated from the ground with material such as an insulation pad, towel, blanket, backpack, car seat, or cushion removed from a vehicle. It is also important to quickly identify or create a source of shade. Foliage is rarely available, so the shade structure must often be constructed from equipment on hand, such as a tarp with hiking poles or a vehicle parked either to create the shade or act as a base for the tarp. For longer-term survival in the desert, digging a trench will provide both protection from the surface heat and the sun. Three feet below the surface, the temperature may cool by as much as 30%.[2] A trench provides a cooler environment during the daytime desert heat and will also insulate and keep people warm in high-altitude deserts that can become very cool at night.

### Hydration

An ill or injured individual may no longer be in a state of mind to manage their own hydration. It is important that someone on the medical team monitor their intake as well as their urine output for adequate quantity and color. A patient who can orally hydrate should be encouraged to continue to do so, but intravenous hydration or resuscitation may be warranted if the patient is unable to tolerate oral intake. Fluids can be provided either as a bolus or continuously, depending on transport factors and patient acuity.

### Evacuation Considerations

The greatest challenge to patient evacuation in the desert environment is the continuous exposure to the heat and associated risk of heat illness and dehydration. A motorized vehicle is one of the best options. A car can protect from the heat, provide cooling, and remove the need for continued exertion while exposed to the heat. A UTV or motorbike may not offer all of those protections but it would be the next best as a way to transport someone without requiring any exertion. When a vehicle is not available, travel by pack animal is preferred to decrease physical exertion. However, limitations include continued exposure to the elements as well as the need for additional resources to manage the heat, nutritional, and hydration needs of the animal.[2]

If neither motorized vehicle nor animal travel is available and the rescuers, and possibly the patient, must travel by foot, then it is recommended to travel at night and rest during the day. The risks of traveling at night include injury from poor visibility and encounters with nocturnal animals. However, the advantages of traveling in significantly cooler temperatures without exposure to the sun outweigh these by significantly lowering the risk of heat illness, dehydration, and solar UV radiation.

Lastly, when choosing whereby to rest and travel, it is important to avoid what may look like a dry riverbed, narrow canyon, or ravine. These places may seem attractive because they often offer some natural shade sources, but they are at risk of flash flooding. Though it may take a few hours of heavy rainfall to generate a flash flood, the rainfall may be remote and not visible from your location, presenting no warning sign until it is too late to safely evacuate the area. While these may not be frequent events, the fatal consequences are too high to warrant the risk of spending prolonged periods of time resting or traveling in these areas.[2]

### Rescuer Preparation and Self-care

Rescuers are susceptible to the same harsh environment as the patients they are helping. It is important that they are well prepared for the desert environment to prevent rescuer injuries. These principles apply to both rescuers and one's general preparations before heading into the desert and will help prepare you to rescue yourself or another individual in need.

A rescuer should have appropriate clothing to protect them from the elements. This includes clothing that will provide solar protection, such as a hat with a brim and cloth extending to cover the neck, long sleeves, and long pants. These should be made of breathable materials that are light in color to reflect the sun and loose to allow for evaporative cooling directly from the skin. Gaiters can help keep sand and dust out of shoes to prevent blisters. A bandana can protect one's face from blowing sand and dust. Eye protection is important both to protect from the sun and blowing dust. Some may find the desert an environment not conducive to contact lens wear. It is important for a rescuer to know if they can comfortably and effectively use their contact lenses and to always keep prescription glasses with sun protection available as a backup.

A rescuer needs to carry adequate fluid supplies to stay hydrated throughout the rescue and should also be carrying additional water to help support others. Water and electrolyte needs for each individual can vary widely, and it is generally recommended to consume fluids at a rate that roughly matches water losses through sweating and urination. The rescuer should consider current weather conditions, the type of activity being performed, the duration of the activity, and the gear being worn or carried when identifying how much fluid they need to carry.[3] Though this is best learned through training in similar environments with similar equipment, the US Army has developed fluid replacement and work/rest guidelines for warm weather training conditions that offer a good generalizable place to start (**Table 1**).[4]

### Survival Kit

Each member of the group should have a kit of materials meant to improve survival in a broad spectrum of environments. Items should include those that are difficult to improvise or the tools needed to improvise materials for a variety of needs. When traveling in a desert environment, in addition to common survival kit contents, one may want to include additional sunscreen as well as a back-up source of eye protection, as these items can both be essential and very difficult to improvise (**Table 2**).

Water in the desert is a scarce resource. Though extra water should be carried, a survival kit should contain the tools needed to make a solar still to harvest water from the seemingly dry environment. To make the still, you will need to dig a hole and add a source of moisture (foliage, wet dirt, urine, or brackish water) as well as a collecting vessel. Cover the hole with plastic and place sand or dirt on the edges to

**Table 1**
Water requirements and soldier hydration[4]

| Wet Bulb Globe Temperature Index (°F) | Easy Work | | Moderate Work | | Hard Work | |
| | Walking on Hard Surface, 2.5 mph, <30 lb. load; Weapon Maintenance, Marksmanship Training. | | Patrolling, Walking in Sand, 2.5 mph, no load; Calisthenics. | | Walking in Sand, 2.5 mph, with load; Field Assaults. | |
| (WBGT) | Work/Rest Ratio (min) | Fluid Intake (qt/hr) | Work/Rest Ratio (min) | Fluid Intake (qt/hr) | Work/Rest Ratio (min) | Fluid Intake (qt/hr) |
|---|---|---|---|---|---|---|
| 78°–81.9° | No limit | 0.5 | No limit | 0.75 | 40:20 | 0.75 |
| 82° – 84.9° | No limit | 0.5 | 50:10 | 0.75 | 30:30 | 1 |
| 85° – 87.9° | No limit | 0.75 | 40:20 | 0.75 | 30:30 | 1 |
| 88° – 89.9° | No limit | 0.75 | 30:30 | 0.75 | 20:40 | 1 |
| > 90° | No limit | 1 | 20:40 | 1 | 10:50 | 1 |

Wet Bulb Globe Temperature (WBGT) - Calculation of heat stress on human body in direct sunlight based on temperature in the sun, humidity, wind speed, sun angle and cloud cover. In contrast, the Heat Index accounts for temperature in the shade and humidity only. work, rest, and fluid Intake recommendations are adequate for at least 4 hrs of work in that environment.

Hourly fluid intake not to exceed 1.5qt/hr and daily not to exceed 12qt.

Fluid needs very based on individual physiologic difference ± 0.25qt/hr and whether in direct sunlight v shade ± 0.25qt/hr

Body armor or protective equipment that is less breathable will increase effective WBGT.

Adaptation from Montain SJ, Ely M. Water requirements and soldier hydration. *Borden Institute Monograph Series*. 2010.

**Table 2**
**Suggested items for a desert survival kit[2]**

| | |
|---|---|
| Multi-Tool | Sunscreen |
| Parachute cord | Insect repellent |
| Compass | Rescue blanket |
| Topographic map | Sunscreen |
| First-aid kit | Eye protection |
| Plastic sheet/tarp | scarf, bandana, or dust mask |
| Duct tape | Hat |
| Plastic bags | Synthetic insulating jacket |
| Matches/fire starting tool | Waterproof jacket |
| Whistle | |
| Flashlight | |
| Water container | |
| Non-perishable food items | |

Source: Otten EJ. Desert Travel and Survival. Auerbach's Wilderness Medicine. 7 ed. 1280 to 1389:chap 61.

seal off the space below. Place a rock or other weight in the center of the plastic, directly over the collecting vessel. The heat will cause water to evaporate from the vegetation or other wet products and collect on the plastic. The rock will direct the water to run down the plastic and into the collecting cup. **Fig. 1** shows the steps in the development of a solar still.

## DESERT ENVIRONMENT-SPECIFIC MEDICAL CONDITIONS
### Heat Emergencies

#### Background and physiology
Heat-related deaths are one of the deadliest weather-related health outcomes in the United States. The acute presentation of heat illness is a significant, ongoing, and

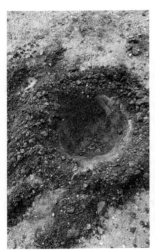
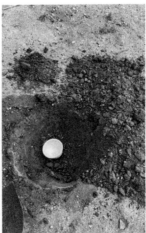
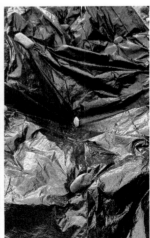

**Fig. 1.** Steps for solar still creation. (Author Geoff Comp's personal photo)

increasing cause of morbidity and mortality, especially in the desert regions. According to the CDC, from 2004 to 2018, there were 67,512 ED visits, 9235 hospitalizations, and 702 deaths due to heat-related illness on average per year.[5]

As body temperature increases, sweat production increases, and peripheral vasodilation in the skin occurs to augment and hasten heat transfer.[3] Continued repetitive exposure to heat stress results in heat acclimation and heat tolerance, which increase an individual's ability to withstand elevated temperatures and improve thermoregulation. These adaptations include improved sweating, improved vasodilation, lowered body temperatures, reduced cardiovascular strain, improved fluid balance, altered metabolism, and enhanced cellular protection.[6] These adaptations are especially important for those living or working in desert environments, as they provide some degree of protection against the elevated temperatures associated with these locations.

### Specific conditions and management

Heat emergencies represent a variety of disorders ranging from minor to severe when the environmental and metabolic heat burden outpaces an individual's thermoregulatory mechanisms for heat transfer, ultimately leading to increases in core temperature.[7] **Table 3** describes the range of heat related conditions, with a focus on symptoms and specific treatment considerations.

### Prevention

Those who spend time in desert locations should also take environmental considerations into account when preparing for work or recreation in these hot environments to prevent heat injuries. Many regional health departments and governmental organizations provide guidelines and strategies for preventing heat injuries, but it is up to the individual to take proactive measures to stop the onset of these conditions. General recommendations include wearing lightweight, loose-fitting clothing, attempting to stay in air-conditioned spaces, using fans or taking cool showers, and increasing social contact to prevent isolation.[10] Additionally, providing heat stress education to workers or athletes, such as staying well hydrated, replacing electrolytes lost in sweat and urine, taking frequent rest breaks, engaging in activities in the early morning hours, and limiting exertion in the hottest times of the day, are important preventative measures.[11,12]

### Dehydration/Volume Status

#### Background

Hydration refers to the total body water content. Total body water (TBW) is generally 45% to 75% of total body mass in a person of ideal body weight. Hydration is gained through oral intake of food and beverages as well as cellular metabolic processes. Water is lost through our respiratory effort, the gastrointestinal tract, sweat, and renal system. Maintaining a normal TBW is an important part of homeostasis in our cardiovascular system, thermoregulation, and a myriad of intracellular processes.[13] In the desert, all of these processes contribute to our ability to thermoregulate, making hydration an important factor in preventing hyperthermia and promoting cellular function.

Dehydration is often defined clinically as a hypertonic hypovolemia, meaning a greater loss of free water than electrolytes. One can also have isotonic or hypotonic hypovolemia, whereby equal solute and free water are lost or proportionally less solute than free water is lost, respectively.[14] In the desert, the greatest source of dehydration is sweating, which provides evaporative cooling. Normal sweat is hypotonic compared with plasma, partly because sweat glands have channels for the reabsorption of sodium and chloride. As sweating increases, eventually the level of reabsorption can no longer be increased. In situations of prolonged sweating in extreme heat,

**Table 3**
**Heat illness condition description[7-9]**

| Heat Illness Type | Description | Specific Notes on Treatment |
|---|---|---|
| Heat Edema | • Dependent edema and extremity swelling resulting from peripheral vasodilation. | • Extremity elevation and compression. Diuretics not indicated |
| Heat Cramps | • Painful involuntary muscle spasms experienced during exertional activity in hot environments are usually due to electrolyte depletion and muscular overuse | • Oral electrolytes as tolerated, stretching, and fluid replacement |
| Heat Rash (miliaria rubra) | • Cutaneous inflammatory response to heat exposure<br>• Papules or pustules primarily on the neck, upper extremities, and trunk | • Avoid hot environments and wear loose clothing.<br>• Glucocorticoids and antibacterial creams may be used if there is severe presentation or concern for infection<br>• Topical emollients not indicated |
| Heat Syncope | • Lightheadedness, diaphoresis, dizziness, or transient syncope immediately following the cessation of activity or with prolonged exertion caused by vasodilation and decreased vasomotor tone | • Rest in a supine position with leg elevation and rehydration.<br>• Prolonged recovery or a medical history or physical examination arousing concern about an alternative cause of syncope should prompt further evaluation |
| Heat Exhaustion | • Tachycardia, thirst, fatigue, nausea or vomiting, and diaphoresis<br>• The patient may have a normal or elevated core body temperature.<br>• No altered mental status | • Remove from heat source<br>• Evaporative, convective, and cooling<br>• Oral or intravenous isotonic or hypertonic fluid hydration.<br>• A delayed response to treatment may result in the development of heat stroke. |
| Heat Stroke | • Elevated core temperature (>40°C) and central nervous system abnormalities including altered mental status, ataxia, confusion, or stupor.<br>• Anhidrosis is not a diagnostic criterion<br>• High mortality if left untreated<br>• Severe thermoregulatory dysfunction: endotoxin leakage, systemic inflammatory response syndrome, cellular apoptosis, and multiorgan dysfunction or failure | • Evaluation and intervention of airway, breathing, and circulation<br>• Early active cooling: cold-water immersion, evaporative and convective cooling, cooled intravenous hydration |

Source: Refs.[7-9]

drinking too much water without supplemental electrolytes can lead to hypotonic hypovolemia, in particular hyponatremia.[15]

Excessive GI losses due to diarrhea or vomiting are the other significant factors that cause severe dehydration in the desert environment. GI losses have higher levels of electrolyte loss than sweat and lead to isotonic hypovolemia. If this is in addition to the sweat losses needed to maintain thermoregulation and the person is unable to tolerate oral liquids, they are at high risk of suffering from severe dehydration.

### Symptoms and effects

Common symptoms of dehydration include dizziness, headache, fatigue, and "brain fog." Signs of dehydration include tachycardia, delayed capillary refill, poor skin turgor, and sunken eyes. TBW loss of <2% does not generally have a significant effect on physiologic function. With every 1% increase in TBW loss, there is a 0.1 to 0.2°C increase in core body temperature, putting individuals at increased risk of hyperthermia.[15]

Exercise performance is also diminished in extreme heat or at altitude. After 90 minutes of exercise, the effect of dehydration increases disproportionately. This makes dehydration in a desert environment particularly concerning, as prolonged activity time results in increased dehydration and heat exposure, exponentially increasing one's risk of hyperthermia. In what is suspected to be a similar manner, studies have also shown dehydration to lead to decreased work productivity among firefighters and forest workers.[15] Protective clothing that blocks one's ability to perform evaporative cooling, as well as facial protective equipment that makes oral hydration more cumbersome, increase the overall risk of dehydration among laborers in these settings.

Cognitive performance in dehydration has been studied without clear results indicating whether there is dysfunction. However, in most situations, it is hard to separate the effects of hyperthermia from the effects of dehydration. Some studies show increased blood supply to the frontoparietal lobe during executive function. From this, it is hypothesized that, though cognitive function may not actually decline, it takes greater resources and energy, leading to increased total body stress, to achieve the same level of functioning.[15]

### Methods for monitoring hydration status

Symptoms of dehydration are very nonspecific, are usually late markers of dehydration, and thus may not allow for time to intervene prior to severe illness. The assessment of weight change, urine concentration, and color, along with thirst as surrogate markers, has been studied in athletes. In combination, weight, urine output, and thirst can be used as a reliable low-fidelity tool to allow early intervention in dehydration.[15,16] A deficit in 2 out of 3 markers makes dehydration likely, whereas a deficit in all 3 is highly suggestive of dehydration.[15,17]

### Prevention and treatment

Guidelines provide hydration recommendations, depending on the clinical or field setting. As hydration needs vary significantly with activity level, environmental conditions (temperature and humidity), and individual factors such as acclimation, sweat production, and sweat electrolyte content, it is difficult to present a simple plan that works for all. Later in discussion are principles to consider when developing an individualized plan.

- *How much to drink*: In most situations, drinking to thirst will provide adequate water intake. For activities that you expect to exceed 3 hours, a hydration plan should be developed.[15]
- *What to Drink*: In most situations whereby people are consuming normal meals and snacks, no supplemental electrolytes are needed.[13] For prolonged exercise,

supplementing with sodium (20–30mEq/L), potassium (2-5mEq/L) and carbohydrate (5%–10%) is necessary to replenish electrolytes lost through sweat.[15] While carbohydrate containing liquids help with sodium absorption, too much can slow gastric emptying, limiting water and electrolyte intake and absorption. When considering oral rehydration during illness, the WHO recommends an oral rehydration solution (ORS) with reduced osmolality. Their recommendation is for 75 mmol/L each of sodium and glucose, and 20 mmol/L potassium, with a total osmolality of 245 mmol/L (other components being chloride and citrate).[18] There are many commonly encountered commercial products including sports drinks, and electrolyte replacement solutions available that, when mixed per the directions, are within the WHO optimized osmolality range.[19] As volume and electrolyte loss may be worsened in the desert environment. It is critically important to maintain appropriate hydration and electrolyte intake.

- *Oral versus intravenous (IV) hydration*: If an individual can tolerate oral hydration, it has been shown to be just as effective as IV hydration.[8,15] IV hydration should be considered when a patient is unable to tolerate PO either due to vomiting, their mental state, or other injuries that would prevent oral intake. IV hydration or resuscitation can also be considered for excessively high fluid losses to augment oral rehydration if a patient is unable to keep up with the rate of fluid loss, as can occur in severe gastrointestinal illnesses.

### Solar Radiation Exposure

Acute sunburn, which results from prolonged exposure to the sun's harmful ultraviolet (UVA and UVB) rays, is one of the most prevalent ailments in desert medicine. Exposure to solar radiation puts patients at risk for short term injury as well as long term increases in skin cancer risk. Even though UVB rays are typically what cause sunburn, both UVB and UVA rays increase the risk of developing skin cancer.

In sunburn, endothelial cells are damaged, and prostaglandins are released that mediate an inflammatory response. Painful erythema of the skin is the hallmark sign and presents with warmth, blistering edema, or skin sloughing. Even a superficial sunburn can cause sweat pore clogging and decreased cooling ability. Severe cases can include nausea, vomiting, headaches, or general malaise. Cold water compresses, NSAIDs, and topical anesthetics can provide immediate relief from acute sunburn.[20]

Prevention includes avoiding prolonged exposure to direct sunlight by seeking shade, using protective clothing, and, when direct sunlight is unavoidable, using sunscreen. The two main types of sunscreens are organic compounds that absorb UV radiation and inorganic or physical filters that absorb, reflect, and scatter UV radiation.[21] The "Sun Protection Factor" (SPF) assesses a sunscreen's capacity to shield the skin from sunburn. This is defined as the ratio of UV radiation required to produce erythema in sunscreen protected skin versus unprotected skin. The time skin would be protected from burning with sunscreen can be determined by multiplying the time required to burn unprotected skin by the sunscreen's SPF factor. While sunscreen is effective at preventing sunburn and UV photodamage, its efficacy is dependent on the correct use of sunscreen. Underapplication, uneven application, and delayed application are common pitfalls that result in injury or unintended UV exposure.[21]

### Desert Animal Encounters

#### Background

Animals have evolved and adapted to the dry, arid desert climate and have become medically relevant as the human population has begun to urbanize the environment and live alongside them. The desert landscape is home to a tremendous variety of animal species, ranging from the harmless desert spiny lizard to the infamously venomous rattlesnake. Mammals such as the coyote and javelina occasionally collide with humans, while creatures such as the Bark Scorpion and the Gila Monster pose a smaller but more impactful threat. Prevention of injury from animal encounters is the best and first line of defense, but it is important for medical professionals to be well equipped with the knowledge to treat these injuries both in and out of the hospital setting.

### Reptiles

Venomous snakes inhabiting arid and desert environments globally exhibit unique adaptations to survive harsh conditions. In North American deserts, rattlesnakes including the western diamondback and Mojave species, showcase specialize behaviors and venom compositions. International examples include the horned viper, cobra variations, and saw scaled viper commonly found in African and Middle Eastern deserts, Brown snakes, and Taipans are found in Australia's arid regions, and multiple species in the *Bothrop* genus of crotalids and coral snakes can be encountered in Central and South American deserts.[22] These diverse species underscore the need for region-specific considerations in managing and treating venomous snake bites in desert environments.

According to the Centers for Disease Control, venomous snake bites occur in the United States on average between 7000 and 8000 times per year. Approximately 5 of those envenomations will be fatal, and 10% to 44% of them will have long-lasting morbidity.[23] The rattlesnake is responsible for the majority of this morbidity and mortality. Rattlesnakes belong to the family Crotalidae (Pit Viper), which is distinguishable by a depression or "pit" in the maxillary bone, vertical elliptical pupils, a triangular head, and a rattle in the tail.[24] Video 1 is a demonstration of the classic rattling of the tail. Common symptoms after a bite can include pain and swelling at the site, nausea, vomiting, and dizziness. More severe systemic effects include ecchymosis, hemorrhagic blebs, and bullae at the site of the bite. These can systematically progress into disseminated intravascular coagulopathy. It is imperative to quickly identify and treat a rattlesnake bite, both in the wilderness and at the hospital. Prehospital management is focused on minimizing tissue destruction and preventing these dangerous sequelae. If possible, splint the extremity and keep it at the level of the heart to prevent the venom from overwhelming a small, localized area of tissue. Remove any jewelry, such as rings or watches. Measure the circumference of the affected extremity every 15 minutes to track the spread of edema.[25]

In the hospital setting, the initial stabilization should include a rapid assessment of "airway, breathing, and circulation," especially if the bite involves the head or neck. Ultimately, the pillar of snakebite treatment is antivenom. The 2 types of antivenom used in the United States include Crotalidae Immune Equine (F9(ab')2, Fab2AV, "Anavip") and Polyvalent Crotalinae Ovine Immune Fab (FabAV, "CroFab"). Indications to use antivenom for a bite include progressing edema beyond the local bite, any edema around bites of the face, head, or neck, hemotoxicity (thrombocytopenia, hypofibrinogenemia, or prolonged prothrombin time), or systemic effects such as shock or severe bleeding. The determination of antivenom use should be done in conjunction with a toxicology consultation. After administration, the patient should be monitored closely for possible allergic or adverse medication reactions as well as the progression of symptoms indicating a need for the administration of additional antivenom (**Fig. 2**).[25,26]

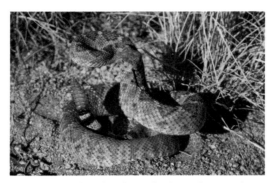

**Fig. 2.** Western diamondback rattlesnake. (Patrick Alexande, Crotalus atrox - Flickr - aspido-scelis. (2024, April 26). Wikimedia Commons. Retrieved from https://commons.wikimedia.org/w/index.php?title=File:Crotalus_atrox_-_Flickr_-_aspidoscelis_(13).jpg&oldid=871436117.)

A reptile that humans rarely encounter, the Gila Monster (*Heloderma suspectum),* is a colorful, nocturnal, slow-moving lizard that carries a strong, threatening bite. Gila monsters are non-predatory toward humans. They are slow-moving and will usually offer multiple warnings through hissing before they attack. When they do attack, they can turn their whole bodies and bite in an incredibly quick manner. Almost all re-ported incidents of Gila Monster's biting humans are the result of humans attempting to handle or harass a Gila Monster, which is illegal in all states in which they reside.[27]

Gila Monsters have large venom glands and deliver their venom with deeply grooved teeth. The lizards will tend to lock their jaws and relentlessly maintain their bite, so sometimes mechanical means are required to break free. The venom consists of enzymes that promote local tissue damage and edema. There are no neurotoxins or enzymes that interfere with coagulopathy.[27] Common symptoms include intense pain radiating up the extremity, edema surrounding the wound, and local blue discolor-ation. Severe edema, airway compromise, hypotension, and loss of consciousness are less frequent reactions. Although infrequent, these encounters can carry signifi-cant morbidity. One study reports 105 calls were made to the Arizona Poison Center regarding Gila Monster human encounters between the years 2000 and 2011. Of these cases, 16% were admitted to the hospital, 5 patients were admitted to the ICU, and 3 patients required airway management due to edema. There were no deaths reported from Gila monster bites.[28] Since most of these bites result in local inflammation and tissue damage, it is again imperative to know first aid management for wounds. The wound should be thoroughly irrigated and inspected for any embedded Gila monster teeth. More severe reactions should be managed symptomatically; there is no anti-venom for Gila Monster envenomation (**Fig. 3**).[27]

### *Arthropods*
Another clinically relevant category of desert species is the arachnids, which include desert spiders and scorpions. The bark scorpion, *Centruroides sculpturatus,* is a slightly translucent yellow/tan scorpion that contains a strong neurotoxin in its stinging tail. Fluorescent compounds in the exoskeleton of scorpions make the creatures glow when viewed under ultraviolet light. They are primarily found in the Southwestern United States and are the only scorpion in the U.S. that can cause a potentially life threatening reaction, especially in children. The signs and symptoms of scorpion sting envenomation are used to grade the severity and dictate treatment. Grade I is pain or paraesthesia at the site of the sting. Grade II is characterized by pain and paraesthesia

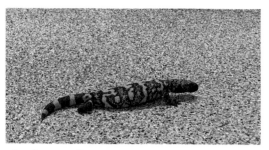

**Fig. 3.** Gila monster. (Author Geoff Comp's personal photo)

remote from the sting site, in addition to localized pain. Grade III is *either* cranial nerve dysfunction (opsoclonus, tongue fasciculation, slurred speech, and so forth) *or* somatic skeletal dysfunction (jerking motions of the extremities, arching of the back, and so forth). The most severe, Grade IV, is characterized by a combination of *both* cranial nerve dysfunction *and* somatic skeletal dysfunction.[29,30] In mild to moderate cases (usually grades I-II), localized inflammation can be treated with ice and NSAIDs. In severe cases (severe grade III or IV), a commercially available antivenom is available.[29] This can be used in conjunction with the judicious use of benzodiazepines or opioids for extreme agitation and pain (**Figs. 4** and **5**).

Tarantulas are a desert arachnid in the family Theraphosidae that can inflict injury through bites as well as with the urticarial hairs. While the venom from a tarantula bite contains compounds that can cause neurologic as well as local cytotoxic effects, most tarantula bites result in mild localized symptoms, including pain, swelling, and numbness. Tarantulas do, however, produce hairs that can be "flicked" by the animal toward an aggressor. These can be inflicted on humans as the tarantula is handled. They are particularly harmful if they contact mucosal membranes, resulting in soft tissue inflammation and local pruritis, or the eyes, causing keratoconjunctivitis. Treatment includes pain control, removal of all hairs, irrigation, ophthalmic antibiotic ointment, and prompt ophthalmology follow up as warranted (**Fig. 6**).[31]

### Other animal encounters
It is much rarer to encounter the mammals that roam the desert. These include the coyote, javelina, mule-deer, kit fox, Sonoran Pronghorn, and ground squirrel, who

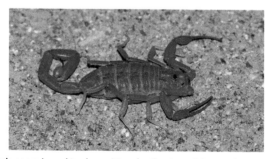

**Fig. 4.** Arizona bark scorpion. (Andrew Meeds, Centruroides sculpturatus. (2024, February 18). Wikimedia Commons. Retrieved from https://commons.wikimedia.org/w/index.php?title=File:Centruroides_sculpturatus_191624836.jpg&oldid=853168546.)

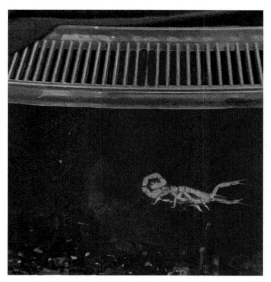

**Fig. 5.** Bark Scorpion under UV light. (Author Geoff Comp's personal photo)

all might cause occasional harm to humans. Many injuries from these mammals involve bites, but large animals may also inflict blunt trauma in attacks or trampling. They can be treated similarly to other canine or feline bites familiar to most medical providers. All injuries require careful inspection for fractures and foreign bodies, copious irrigation, and local wound care.[32] Up-to-date tetanus prophylaxis is indicated for all mammal bites that penetrate the skin. Antibiotic prophylaxis must be considered in wounds requiring primary closure or surgical repair, wounds near a bone or joint, those in an immunocompromised patient, or other risk factors that would make a patient more susceptible to infection.[33]

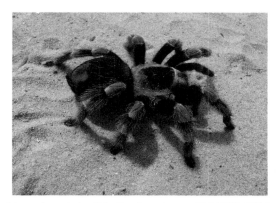

**Fig. 6.** Mexican red-knee tarantula. (File:Brachypelma smithi 2009 G09.jpg. (2024, April 12). Wikimedia Commons. Retrieved from https://commons.wikimedia.org/w/index.php?title=File:Brachypelma_smithi_2009_G09.jpg&oldid=867631603.)

## SUMMARY

The realm of desert medicine encapsulates a dynamic synergy between the environment and human health. The challenges presented by this extreme environment necessitate an understanding of the epidemiology of desert-related conditions, the impact of extreme temperatures, and how to manage the unique challenges posed by the arid landscape. The goal of this article is to equip medical practitioners with the essential knowledge and tools to adeptly navigate the complexities of desert medicine amidst these demanding terrains.

## CLINICS CARE POINTS

- Variations in temperature, humidity, and topography in desert climates predispose patients to medical conditions that practitioners in both rural and urban deserts must recognize and manage.

- When caring for patients in extreme heat and arid conditions, one must always take additional measures to prevent hyperthermia and dehydration during assessment and prolonged evacuation in both the patient and rescuer.

- Heat emergencies represent a variety of disorders ranging from minor to severe when the environmental and metabolic heat burden outpaces an individual's thermoregulatory mechanisms for heat transfer.

- Acclimation to heat occurs over a 10 to 14 day period and leads to increased sweat glands, sweating at lower body temperatures, and a decreased concentration of electrolytes in our sweat, allowing individuals to cool their core temperature more efficiently.

- Dehydration can be monitored through the 3 low fidelity tools of weight, urine concentration and color, and thirst.

- A normal diet and oral hydration with water are adequate to prevent dehydration in most situations. With prolonged exertion, oral hydration with electrolyte replacement in addition to water is advised.

- Severe complications of Pit Viper envenomation include coagulopathy and tissue destruction, which require prompt evaluation and treatment with antivenom.

- Scorpion envenomation can have severe sequelae, especially in at-risk populations such as children and elderly patients. Consider antivenom in serious envenomation.

- Sun exposure to UVA and UVB rays can have a wide range of effects, ranging from erythema to severe full thickness burns, and increase cancer risk over time. "Broad spectrum" sunscreen that protects from both UVA and UVB rays should be used liberally and reapplied often during times of sun exposure.

## DISCLOSURE

This author group has no conflicts of interest to disclose.

## SUPPLEMENTARY DATA

Supplementary data to this article can be found online at https://doi.org/10.1016/j.emc.2024.02.016.

## REFERENCES

1. Kowal-Vern A, Matthews MR, Richey KN, et al. "Streets of Fire" revisited: contact burns. Burns Trauma 2019;7:32.

2. Otten EJ. Chapter 61: Desert Travel and Survival, In: Auerbach's Wilderness Medicine, 7th edition, 1280–1389.
3. Wendt D, van Loon LJ, Lichtenbelt WD. Thermoregulation during exercise in the heat: strategies for maintaining health and performance. Sports Med 2007;37(8): 669–82.
4. Montain SJ and Ely M. Water requirements and soldier hydration, 2010, Borden Institute Monograph Series. Available at: www.govinfo.gov/content/pkg/GOVPUB-D104-PURL-gpo13944/pdf/GOVPUB-D104-PURL-gpo13944.pdf.
5. Vaidyanathan A, Malilay J, Schramm P, et al. Heat-Related Deaths - United States, 2004-2018. MMWR Morb Mortal Wkly Rep 2020;69(24):729–34.
6. Périard JD, Racinais S, Sawka MN. Adaptations and mechanisms of human heat acclimation: Applications for competitive athletes and sports. Scand J Med Sci Sports 2015;25(Suppl 1):20–38.
7. Lipman GS, Eifling KP, Ellis MA, et al, Wilderness Medical Society. Wilderness Medical Society practice guidelines for the prevention and treatment of heat-related illness: 2014 update. Wilderness Environ Med 2014;25(4 Suppl):S55–65.
8. Gauer R, Meyers BK. Heat-related illnesses. Am Fam Physician 2019;99(8): 482–9.
9. Sorensen C, Hess J. Treatment and prevention of heat-related illness. N Engl J Med 2022;387(15):1404–13.
10. Epstein Y, Yanovich R. Heatstroke. N Engl J Med 2019;380(25):2449–59.
11. Tustin A, Sayeed Y, Berenji M, et al. Prevention of Occupational Heat-Related Illnesses. J Occup Environ Med 2021;63(10):e737–44.
12. Casa DJ, DeMartini JK, Bergeron MF, et al. National Athletic Trainers' Association Position Statement: Exertional Heat Illnesses. J Athl Train 2015;50(9):986–1000.
13. Sawka MN, Burke LM, Eichner ER, et al. American College of Sports Medicine position stand. Exercise and fluid replacement. Med Sci Sports Exerc 2007; 39(2):377–90.
14. Lacey J, Corbett J, Forni L, et al. A multidisciplinary consensus on dehydration: definitions, diagnostic methods and clinical implications. Ann Med 2019;51(3–4): 232–51.
15. Kenefick RWC, Leon Samuel N, Lisa R, et al. Dehydration and Rehydration. Auerbach's Wilderness Medicine 2017;7:89.
16. Cheuvront SS, Michael. Hydration assessment of athletes. Sports Science Exchange 2005;18(2).
17. Sekiguchi Y, Benjamin CL, Butler CR, et al. Relationships Between WUT (Body Weight, Urine Color, and Thirst Level) Criteria and Urine Indices of Hydration Status. Sports Health Jul-Aug 2022;14(4):566–74.
18. World Health O. Oral rehydration salts : production of the new ORS. https://iris.who.int/bitstream/handle/10665/69227/WHO_FCH_CAH_06.1.pdf?sequence=1
19. Sollanek KJ, Kenefick RW, Cheuvront SN. Osmolality of Commercially Available Oral Rehydration Solutions: Impact of Brand, Storage Time, and Temperature. Nutrients 2019;11(7). https://doi.org/10.3390/nu11071485.
20. Miller DM, Brodell RT, Herr R. Wilderness dermatology: prevention, diagnosis, and treatment of skin disease related to the great outdoors. Wilderness Environ Med 1996;7(2):146–69 [0146:wdpdat]2.3.co;2.
21. Krakowski ACG. Chapter 16: Exposure to radiation from the sun, Auerbach's Wilderness Medicine, 7th edition, 335–353.
22. Warrell D. Bites by Venomous and Nonvenomous Reptiles Worldwide. Auerbach's Wilderness Medicine 2017;7.

23. Venomous Snakes. The National Institute for Occupational Safety and Health (NIOSH). Available at: https://www.cdc.gov/niosh/topics/snakes/default.html#:~:text=Venomous%20snakes%20found%20in%20the,die%20from%20a%20venomous%20bite.

24. Cardwell MD. Recognizing dangerous snakes in the United States and Canada: a novel 3-step identification method. Wilderness Environ Med 2011;22(4):304–8.

25. Gold BS, Dart RC, Barish RA. Bites of venomous snakes. N Engl J Med 2002; 347(5):347–56.

26. Lavonas EJ, Ruha AM, Banner W, et al. Unified treatment algorithm for the management of crotaline snakebite in the United States: results of an evidence-informed consensus workshop. BMC Emerg Med 2011;11:2.

27. Norris RLB, Sean P, Michael D. Bites by Venomous Reptiles in Canada, the United States, and Mexico. Auerbach's Wilderness Medicine 2017;7:35.

28. French R, Brooks D, Ruha AM, et al. Gila monster (Heloderma suspectum) envenomation: Descriptive analysis of calls to United States Poison Centers with focus on Arizona cases. Clin Toxicol (Phila) 2015;53(1):60–70.

29. Isbister GK, Bawaskar HS. Scorpion envenomation. N Engl J Med 2014;371(5): 457–63.

30. Klotz SA, Yates S, Smith SL, et al. Scorpion Stings and Antivenom Use in Arizona. Am J Med 2021;134(8):1034–8.

31. Boyer LVB, Greta J, Janice A. Spider Bites. Auerbach's Wilderness Medicine 2017;7:43.

32. Madadin M, Al-Abdulrahman R, Alahmed S, et al. Desert Related Death. Int J Environ Res Public Health 2021;18(21). https://doi.org/10.3390/ijerph182111272.

33. Stevens DL, Bisno AL, Chambers HF, et al. Practice guidelines for the diagnosis and management of skin and soft tissue infections: 2014 update by the infectious diseases society of America. Clin Infect Dis 2014;59(2):147–59.

# Endurance Sporting Events

Matt Golubjatnikov, MD, Anne Walker, MD, FAWM, DiMM*

## KEYWORDS

- Ultraendurance • Endurance medicine • Ultramarathon • Stage race
- Endurance sport

## KEY POINTS

- Endurance training results in long-term cardiovascular and neurologic benefits but can have acute injury risks.
- In athletes with sudden cardiac death, immediate CPR should be performed, and prioritization of automated external defibrillator use is the most lifesaving intervention.
- Suspect heat stroke if an athlete develops altered mental status, seizure or coma, and has a temperature over 40 C, treat with rapid ice water immersion.
- Severe hyponatremia should be treated with 100 mL of 3% normal saline over 3 minutes, repeated after 10 minutes up to 2 times until mental status improves or seizing stops.
- Most musculoskeletal injuries during competition only result in the athlete self-removing from competition usually due to severity of symptoms or inability to make time cutoffs.
- Athletes with tendon ruptures should not be allowed to continue in competition and should be splinted in tendon shortened position and told to remain nonweight-bearing until specialty follow-up.

## INTRODUCTION

There is variation among definitions of what constitutes an endurance athletic event and there is not one that is universally accepted. For the purposes of this article, we consider endurance events to be those between 30 minutes and 6 hours in duration and requiring continuous high-intensity exercise and anything over 6 hours are considered as an ultraendurance event. Endurance and ultraendurance sports encompass events such as marathons, ultramarathons, triathlons, long-distance cycling, swimming, skiing, and adventure races of all types. These sports have witnessed a surge in popularity over the last several decades. By challenging the limits of human physical achievement, they also call for a corresponding expanse of emergency medicine toward addressing the physiologic demands, associated injuries, and medical emergencies associated with its pursuit. This article reviews the history of emergency medicine in endurance races, reviews the most common causes of injury and illness related to

St Joseph's Medical Center, 1800 N California Street, Stockton, CA 95204, USA
* Corresponding author.
E-mail address: anne.m.walker88@gmail.com

Emerg Med Clin N Am 42 (2024) 581–596
https://doi.org/10.1016/j.emc.2024.02.017
0733-8627/24/© 2024 Elsevier Inc. All rights reserved.
emed.theclinics.com

endurance sport, and discusses considerations for medical directors/personnel associated with such events.

## HISTORY/BACKGROUND

As the human body has evolved, some of its adaptations have been proposed to select for more endurance-adapted bodies. Up to 2 million years ago, the genus *Homo* was observed to have characteristics thought to have evolved for long-distance running[1] which could have assisted in pursuing prey by persistence hunting.[2] As history continued, *Homo sapiens*, of all primates were identified, as most unique in the ability for endurance effort[3] evidenced by the evolution of longer legs with specialized tendons such as the Achilles tendon and the formation of the plantar arch (which act as springs) as well as mouth breathing, sweat glands, decreased body hair (allowing for greater temperature control), larger gluteus maximus musculature, slow-twitch muscle cell development, and hip/shoulder structure.[3]

According to legend, in 490 BC, Pheidippides, a Greek herald, ran from the battle of Marathon back to Athens to announce a key victory; however, immediately after delivering the news, he collapsed and died. This distance was thought to be close to the modern marathon distance, 26.2 miles. Whether Pheidippides was the original marathon runner and whether his death was due to cardiovascular cause, heat illness, electrolyte disturbance, or another cause is unconfirmed, but this legend showcases that health risks exist with pushing the body to the extreme in endurance pursuits. The first recorded marathon competition was not until the Olympic Games in Athens in 1896. Since then, long-distance endurance competitions have become quite popular among the public. For example, recreational trail running alone has seen a growth of approximately 23% over the last 10 years, with female participation increasing from 13% to 46% between 1997 and 2022.[4] Participation in extreme ultramarathons has also seen a rise, with participation in the Badwater ultramarathon seeing over a 50% increase in the 12 year period between 2000 and 2012.[5]

Endurance athletics, as they have become more popular, have simultaneously been more frequently studied by exercise physiologists and health care professionals. Although we primarily discuss the injurious health effects in this article, the research also points to several advantageous health benefits among those who participate in regular endurance training, most prominent among them being cardiac and neurologic advantages.

Endurance athletics, due to their more aerobic nature, involve stress on the heart which can cause adaptive physiologic changes over time. A recent study indicated that the human heart could evolve to different exercise stimuli, for those who primarily do resistance training, the heart adapts to better handle a pressure challenge, whereas for those who do endurance training, the heart adapts to better handle a volume stimulus.[6] Endurance training over 30 minutes per day of at least moderate effort, during 34 years of cohort follow-up demonstrated 7 to 8 year gains in life expectancy.[7]

The connection of brain health to endurance sports has also been researched in recent years with focus on several neurotrophic factors such as brain-derived neurotrophic factor (BDNF). This factor is stimulated by endurance exercise resulting in dendrite growth and strengthened connections between brain synapses creating positive effects on memory and overall cognitive function.[3]

Although there are many positive health effects of endurance exercise, there is also potential for both acute and long-term maladaptations and injuries. There are variations in injury prevalence across the variety of endurance sports and on different terrain. Ski injuries are more likely to involve sprains/strains followed by fractures and concussions.[8] Cross-country mountain bikers are most likely to get skin injuries such as abrasions and lacerations, followed by concussions,[9] and long-distance multiday running event competitors are most likely to get skin injuries primarily blisters, followed by musculoskeletal injuries and medical illnesses.[10] There is an expansive list of possible illnesses and accidents that may need emergency care during an event; here, we focus on the most serious and the most common: cardiac events, heat illness, dysnatremia, musculoskeletal injuries, and blisters.

## CARDIAC EVENTS

As mentioned previously the heart can evolve to different repetitive stimuli, this occurs in athletic training over time and is genetically variable among different individuals. This process is known as cardiac remodeling and it can be both structural and physiologic. Cardiac remodeling is seen not just in humans but across mammalian species; animals needing or choosing to run for prolonged periods are found to have increased heart size and mass[11] compared to those that are more sedentary which can be measured in echocardiograms. A large increase in cardiac output is needed in endurance aerobic activities to supply blood volume and thus oxygen to the muscles. The increase in cardiac output over time leads to cardiac remodeling. It is thought that these changes can be reversible in the absence of further training/stimuli. Vagal nerve stimulation also increases with endurance exercise which is why bradycardia is often seen in these athletes. Electrocardiogram (EKG) and Holter monitor studies have revealed a variety of bradyarrhythmias including sinus bradycardia, junctional bradycardia, first-degree atrioventricular block, and ectopy including premature atrial complexes and premature ventricular complexes.[12] Primarily, these are thought to be benign; however, there is crossover between the physiologic changes that happen with cardiac remodeling and pathologic changes.

Cardiac events overall are some of the most widely publicized and feared medical events in endurance sports. In terms of life-threatening conditions during competition, myocardial infarction (MI) and sudden cardiac death (SCD) are of primary concern for medical care providers.

### Myocardial Infarction

MI is caused by a partial or complete occlusion of blood flow to the coronary arteries resulting in significantly impaired cardiac function. Those who have existing coronary artery disease (CAD), hypertension, hyperlipidemia, diabetes, or are smokers have a greater risk. During endurance events, many of the tell-tale signs and symptoms of an impending myocardial event may be clouded by the physical manifestations from extreme physical exertion. Symptoms such as tachycardia, tachypnea, diaphoresis, and fatigue cannot be relied on in isolation to rule in or rule out cardiac risk; however, when coupled with findings such as chest pain, shortness of breath, nausea, and vomiting, a clearer picture of the underlying pathology can emerge.[13] In order, the most useful features for in-field clinical identification of MI are chest pain with radiation to both arms (Liklihood Ratio [LR] 7.1), presence of a third heart sound (LR 3.2), and hypotension (LR 3.1). Conversely, the most reliable features that decrease the probability of MI are pleuritic chest pain (LR 0.2), chest pain reproduced by palpation (LR range 0.2–0.4), sharp or stabbing chest pain (LR 0.3), and positional chest pain (LR 0.3).[14]

Research shows the greatest benefit in patients with MI when they are reperfused in the first 2 to 3 hours from the onset of symptoms.[15] For this reason, in the prehospital setting, an athlete with reported symptoms highly concerning for MI should be immediately removed from competition and transported for hospital evaluation. If an EKG or cardiac rhythm strip is available, these can be performed while awaiting transport and if there are no contraindications, aspirin can be administered.

### Sudden Cardiac Death

SCD is a general term for the abrupt and unexpected halt of cardiac function from various causes. Fortunately, the overall incidence of SCD is relatively low. In young athletes, the incidence is estimated to be 1 in 50,000[16]; however, the risk precipitously increases in older adults with an incidence of 1:7000.[17] As in MI, men tend to be at greater risk than women, with a relative risk (RR) approximately 9:1.[18] Caffeine use, stimulant medications, illegal drugs, and prolonged exercise are other factors that can increase the arrhythmic potential and thus risk of SCD during competition.[19]

The cause of SCD varies based on the athlete's age. In those less than or equal to 35 years old, the etiology of arrest in order of prevalence was primary electrical disease without cause, idiopathic left ventricular hypertrophy, anomalous origin of the coronary artery, heritable cardiomyopathy, myocarditis, and electrical cause, such as congenital or acquired prolonged QTc (the interval from the start of the Q wave on an EKG to the end of the T wave, corrected for heart rate). In those aged greater than 35 years, cause in order of prevalence was CAD, idiopathic left ventricular hypertrophy, heritable cardiomyopathy (hypertrophic or dilated), primary electrical causes, and myocarditis.[20] People with existing cardiac disease have a higher overall risk of SCD than those without but engaging in endurance activity is still very beneficial for this cohort. Although they have a greater instantaneous risk of a cardiac event during competition, the lifetime risk is decreased in these patients who regularly exercise at a moderate level.[12]

Owing to the inherently abrupt nature of SCD, the first symptom is typically outright collapse, most often toward the end of an event or shortly after it. Regardless of the plethora of potential cardiac etiologies, resuscitation revolves around effective implementation of advanced cardiopulmonary life support algorithms. The most significant interventions in the prehospital setting are (1) minimally interrupted chest compressions without delay, (2) prompt utilization of defibrillation or automated external defibrillator (AED), and (3) expedited delivery to a care facility.[21] Quality chest compressions have been shown to provide one of the greatest improvements in mortality in the prehospital setting. According to the American Heart Association (AHA), effective cardiopulmonary resuscitation (CPR) can double or triple survival rates.[14] It is widely recommended to have AEDs available in sporting events now. One study showed 89% survival rate after SCD in high school athletes if AED was available.[22] Another study showed 100% survival rate of 28 athletes with SCD treated with AED in Japanese marathons.[23] Expedited transport to a hospital preferably with an interventional cardiologist is a priority, especially in those aged greater than 35 years with SCD whose most common etiology, CAD, accounts for approximately 85% of deaths in this age cohort.[11]

## HEAT ILLNESS

Heat illnesses in athletes range from mild to severe. Mild heat illness such as heat cramps, head edema, and heat syncope/collapse will not be discussed here. Heat exhaustion is a moderate heat illness and is important to manage during endurance events to prevent progression. Exertional heat stroke is the most feared heat-related illness in endurance races and must be addressed immediately to prevent severe morbidity and mortality. Here, we discuss thermoregulation mechanics as well as assessment and management of heat exhaustion and heat stroke.

To understand the causes, prevention strategies and the treatments, it is important to discuss thermoregulation mechanics of the body. The muscles work by utilizing energy released by hydrolyzing adenosine triphosphate (ATP) on a cellular level; however, they only use about 20% to 25% of this energy and the rest must be dissipated to prevent hyperthermia in the body.[24] The body uses 4 main mechanisms to regulate temperature: conduction, convection, radiation, and evaporation. When doing normal daily activities or mild exertion in cooler temperatures, the body is generally using conduction, convection, and radiation as its primary thermal regulatory mechanisms. However, as either the ambient temperature increases or as a person's exertion level increases, evaporation becomes the primary mechanism. These mechanisms can fail in the setting of individual factors such as diseases affecting ability to tolerate heat, as well as in the case of acute illness, poor physical fitness, or lack of heat acclimatization. They can even occur in an optimized athlete in the case that evaporation is not possible such as an environment with both high humidity and ambient temperature.

### Heat Exhaustion

Heat exhaustion is defined as a heat-related injury characterized by hyperthermia associated with mild dysfunction in the central nervous system. Clinical manifestations of heat exhaustion typically include nausea, vomiting, headache, dizziness, and mild confusion. Physical examination often reveals pallor, excessive sweating, and dry mucous membranes. Vital signs commonly show an elevated body temperature (but still <40°C), tachycardia, and, in some cases, hypotension.[25] Diagnosis is primarily made based on clinical assessment. Treatment consists of supportive care, which includes discontinuing physical activity, moving the individual to a cooler environment, and removing excess clothing.[26] If an athlete improves with a short rest period, does not have persistent vital sign abnormalities and there is a conservative plan in place should symptoms recur, medical staff may consider allowing the athlete to continue the race after a discussion of potential risks. If the athlete is worsening despite passive methods, they may require active cooling such as ice/cool packs, cool water and fanning, and consideration of cool/cold water immersion.

### Heat Stroke

Heat stroke is considered the leading cause of death on athletic fields,[19] and it is the second most common overall cause of exertional sudden death, after cardiac causes.[17] Although less deadly than cardiac causes, heat stroke-related events were more common; one study revealed that for every single serious cardiac event in endurance athletics, there were 10 serious heat stroke events.[27] Heat stroke is characterized by hyperthermia (body temperature exceeding 40°C) associated with severe central nervous system dysfunction. The hallmark features of heat stroke distinguishing it from heat exhaustion are altered mental status (AMS), coma, or seizures associated with core body temperature greater than 40°C. Physical examination often reveals pallor, dry and hot skin, and dry mucous membranes; however, exertional heat stroke can also be present in a patient drenched with sweat. Vital signs exhibit hyperthermia (>40°C) which is frequently accompanied by tachycardia, rapid breathing, and low blood pressure. Heat stroke can cause heart strain ultimately leading to cardiac arrest. Beware of this when treating patients SCD and consider heat stroke as a potential etiology.[21] EKG changes may also be present in those with heat exhaustion and heat stroke; one study showed 15 of 56 subjects with heat illness had ST- or T-wave abnormalities on their initial EKG.[21] This highlights the importance of considering environmental factors in addition to cardiac etiology as a cause for collapse based on rhythm strip/EKG findings.

Treatment focuses on rapid cooling because in heat stroke, the time above core temperature of 40°C is correlated with a worse prognosis. Nothing should delay cooling, especially not transport or even obtaining a core temperature if a thermometer is not immediately available. Ice bath immersion is the preferred method for cooling given its decreased time to obtaining relative normothermia. Survival rate has been reported at near 100% when an ice bath is initiated within 10 minutes of symptom onset.[28] Total body cooling typically takes 20 minutes, but body temperature should be monitored and when temperature is at 38°C to 39°C, the subject should be removed from the ice bath to prevent overcorrection and hypothermia. In the absence of ice bath availability, tepid water immersion, water misting with aggressive fanning, cold intravenous (IV) fluid therapy, and ice packs placed in glabrous areas can be beneficial. Antipyretic medications are not effective in reducing hyperthermia in this context and can potentially cause harm. If a competitor is removed from competition due to heat stroke, they should abstain from exercise for at least 7 days or until cleared by their personal doctor but should not be allowed to rejoin competition, even if mental status has improved.[18]

## DYSNATREMIA

Sodium balance regulation is an important yet challenging task for competitors to manage during endurance and ultraendurance events. Although some symptoms can develop from high sodium levels in the blood (hypernatremia), more acute life-threatening illnesses in endurance sports occur from low sodium levels in the blood (hyponatremia). The typical cause of hyponatremia is excessive hypotonic fluid consumption rather than low sodium supplementation. In fact, excessive sodium supplementation has not been found to prevent exercise-associated hyponatremia (EAH).[29,30] EAH is more common in longer events, hotter events, and slower athletes within a given event.[21,31] A higher frequency of severe hyponatremia has been reported in female athletes.[32] Reports of hyponatremia are more common in running, swimming, and combination events such as triathlons rather than cycling only events.[25]

Clinical features of EAH range from mild to severe. Mild cases are usually asymptomatic and only found if sodium levels are checked for other reasons and found to be less than 135 mEq/L. Early symptoms include nausea, vomiting, headache, and dizziness. Severe cases cause confusion, stupor, ataxia, and seizures and are generally found with sodium levels less than 120 mEq/L. Death can occur with sodium levels less than 110 to 115 mEq/L.[25]

The most concerning presentation of hyponatremia is a collapsed competitor who is altered or seizing. The endurance athlete-specific differential diagnosis for the collapsed competitor includes heat stroke, hyponatremia, hypoglycemia, and cardiac collapse in addition to general emergency medicine differentials for syncope, collapse, and AMS. AMS in EAH is thought to be caused by hyponatremic encephalopathy due to cerebral edema,[33] and athletes may also have associated noncardiogenic pulmonary edema.

Although diagnosis in the emergency department primarily relies on blood tests, in many endurance/ultraendurance events, this may not be available and clinical suspicion must be relied upon. In select events, checking sodium levels can be achieved with portable blood analysis machines, but this may be challenging as they often only function within certain temperature ranges. Thus, caring for the collapsed competitor may mean simultaneously treating many potential causes with priority to the most clinically suspected. In a subject who is conscious, and when a history can be obtained, ascertain their hydration status including how much free water they have had, their electrolyte consumption, and their urine production amount/frequency. It is helpful to also assess for weight changes which competitors often check daily when scales are available at multiday stage races and evaluate for edema on physical examination. When differentiating the dehydrated patient versus the overhydrated patient with symptomatic hyponatremia, another tool to use is vital sign abnormalities. Although never to be solely relied upon, in general, a patient with dehydration, while symptomatic, will have tachycardia and/or hypotension, whereas a patient with hyponatremia tends to have normal vital signs. Similarly, hyponatremic patients do not improve in the Trendelenburg position whereas symptoms of dehydration generally do improve.[34]

Treatment of mild EAH involves fluid restriction and consideration of additional electrolyte consumption. Consider oral hypertonic saline solution which can be as effective as IV hypertonic saline in reversing mild EAH[35] or other solutions with high sodium concentration such as sports drinks, bouillon, or simply a saltwater mixture. Severe hyponatremia presenting with encephalopathy or seizure should be treated with IV 3% normal saline. Give 100 mL over 3 minutes and repeat up to 2 additional times at 10 minute intervals if symptoms persist.[27] The first reported treatment with this was in 2000 in a case series of 7, the 6 who were treated as above survived.[36] Although overly rapid correction of chronic hyponatremia carries a risk of osmotic demyelination, in EAH, which is by nature acute, this is not the case.

## MUSCULOSKELETAL INJURIES

Endurance athletes regularly push their bodies to the limit and, as a result, place considerable stress on muscles and tendons. Muscle sprains involve the overstretching or tearing of ligament fibers which are tissues connecting bone to bone. Muscle strains in contrast involve overstretching or tearing of muscle fibers or tendon fibers and tissues that connect muscle to bone. Typically, these injuries happen due to a combination of strenuous overuse coupled with poor warm-up and recovery or pushing in an activity at a level the tissues are unprepared for. Clinical features range from localized pain, tenderness, swelling, stiffness, and limited range of motion to severe pain, extensive swelling, and development of muscle weakness. It is important to remember that endurance events are not uniform, they vary significantly in terms of their overall distance, activity, organization (single continuous event vs stage race) and the surface on which they are conducted. With these considerations in mind, injury patterns certainly differ between events even within the same sport. A review article of musculoskeletal injuries noted this difference when comparing a 1005 km running road race which showed 31% of injuries involving the knee, 28% ankle, and 14% the lower leg with the overall most common diagnosis being patellofemoral pain syndrome (PFPS), while in a 65 km trail race 28.6% of patients had plantar fasciitis, with other most common injuries involving ankle sprains and knee injuries.[37] Tendonitis of foot dorsiflexors was most common in timed events.[31] In Olympic runners followed during several seasons of training, hamstring muscle strain was the muscular injury most likely to cause time loss of training followed by Achilles tendinopathy and soleus muscle strains.[38] A high percentage of athletes with a musculoskeletal injury will have previously had an injury to the same area, especially when involving the ankle/knee.[39] Diagnosis is primarily clinical, relying heavily on targeted history-taking and physical examination. Prevention strategies generally highlight proper warm-up, stretching, and conditioning techniques. Treatment involves RICE therapy (rest, ice, compression, and elevation) acutely, consideration of physical therapy, and, in cases of complete muscle tears or extensive tendon damage, surgery may ultimately be necessary. We discuss PFPS, iliotibial band syndrome (ITBS), and Achilles tendon injuries in the following.

### Patellofemoral Pain Syndrome

PFPS is a complex musculoskeletal strain pattern commonly associated with endurance sports such as running and cycling. PFPS in the general population is quite common with one study placing the incidence at 6%, and it disproportionately affects women.[40] The underlying pathophysiology is multifactorial but generally involves a misalignment of the patella compared to the femur as it slides during activity. The hallmark presentation of PFPS is pain around the anterior knee that worsens when the knee is flexed such as during weight-bearing activities. It is often described as a dull aching pain which starts gradually and is sometimes accompanied by popping or cracking when bending/straightening such as when climbing stairs.[41] History of pain in the anterior knee or deep to the patella that is worse with activity or when knees are kept in flexed position (movie theater sign)[35] should cause you to suspect this diagnosis. Athletes will sometimes also describe pain initially on activity which disappears after some time and then returns after finishing exercise. This can be tested on physical examination by having the patient squat, if this causes consistent reproducibility of pain, then a clinical diagnosis is made. An examiner should also check patellar alignment during standing and with knees bent, knee stability, range of motion, and assessment for cracking/popping during movements. RICE therapy is the mainstay of early intervention. Anti-inflammatory medication may be cautiously used during competition, giving consideration that nonsteroidal antiinflammatory drugs (NSAIDs) are not recommended during vigorous activity. It is not strictly necessary to remove an athlete with PFPS from competition, however a discussion with the athlete about the possibility of extended recovery time if they persist in the current event with continued pain may be prudent.[42] Physical therapy can be beneficial in the long term as weak quadriceps and tight hamstrings, and calves may be contributing factors.[35]

### Iliotibial Band Syndrome

Like PFPS, ITBS causes pain primarily during activity that improves after activity completion; however, pain with ITBS is located on the lateral portion of the knee rather than anterior. The mechanism behind ITBS is not fully understood, but several theories have been proposed such as friction against the lateral femoral epicondyle, compression of the fat and connective tissue deep to the iliotibial band, and chronic inflammation of the iliotibial band bursa.[43] Most commonly, ITBS is found in long-distance runners but also in cyclists, triathletes, and skiers. It is more likely to occur in athletes who have a high weekly mileage, spend time training on tracks, and do more interval training.[44] History is more important than physical findings in obtaining the diagnosis, but some tests may also be of aid. Physical examination is typically revealing for painful palpation of the distal iliotibial (IT) band 2 cm above the lateral joint line. The Noble's test is a physical examination maneuver that may lead to diagnosis of ITBS which involves extending the knee from 90° to 0° while palpating the lateral femoral epicondyle. A positive test is eliciting pain at 30°. Another proposed, although not universally agreed upon, provocative test is Ober's test which involves passive adduction of the hip of the affected leg in slight extension with the patient lying on the unaffected side with the unaffected knee flexed slightly. A positive test occurs when the affected leg is unable to be then moved to the table or if pain in the lateral knee occurs during manipulation.[45] A lateral meniscus injury is an important differential diagnosis. Examination findings such as swelling of the knee and pain with walking as well as running favor lateral meniscal injury.[37] Both ITBS and lateral meniscus injury can present with clicking/popping, however in ITBS these can be palpated over the iliotibial band superior to the knee. When this diagnosis is encountered during training, best treatment is cessation followed by slow increased progression of activity over days to weeks. Continuing to perform activity at decreased load is also possible. Like PFPS, a competitor does not need to be removed from competition if they are diagnosed with ITBS during an event unless they decide to remove themselves due to severity of pain.

Treatment options include pain relief with acetaminophen during activity or NSAIDs if the athlete has completed activity for the day and does not have contraindication, ice/cold therapy, and manual massage. Reduction of overpronation has been proposed as a way of decreasing pain with ITBS, this can be done with foot orthotics.[46] Trigger point release with 5 minutes of pressure applied with the thumb on distal ITB resulted in greater pain relief in one study and application of specialized tape in a way that provides support to the knee showed increased knee flexion and pain reduction in another study.[47] Most studies of treatments involve hip abduction strengthening and stretching of all upper leg muscles in addition to the abovementioned therapies.

### Achilles Tendon Injuries

The Achilles tendon is a unique tendon in the body in that it undergoes a high loading force. In in vitro measurements, the Achilles tendon was found to have a breaking stress of 100 mega pascal (mPA). Most tendons are found to undergo a peak stress of less than 30 mPA during activity; however, the Achilles has been measured at greater than 70 mPA during extreme plantar flexion illustrating why this tendon may be commonly injured.[48] Achilles tendon injuries range from Achilles tendinopathy to partial and complete ruptures. The threat of Achilles tendinopathy looms ominously in the world of sports in general, posing significant challenges to athletes and clinicians alike. Current data suggest that the incidence of Achilles tendinopathy may be as high as 24% in competitive athletes.[49] The pathophysiology of Achilles tendinopathy generally involves excessive tendon loading which causes repetitive microtraumas but may also involve chronic inflammation.[50] There may be high reinjury rates with 35% of marathon runners reporting a previous Achilles tendon injury within a year.[51] Achilles tendinopathy is primarily a clinical diagnosis. The most accurate diagnostic tests are pain on palpation of the Achilles tendon (84% sensitive, 73% specific) and subjective pain at the site of the Achilles tendon with activity (78% sensitive, 77% specific).[52] Differential diagnosis for Achilles tendinopathy should include bursitis, bone anomalies, partial or complete rupture, and tarsal tunnel syndrome.[46] The mainstay of treatment of Achilles tendinopathy is activity modification and exercise rehabilitation focused on decreasing excessive load on the Achilles tendon. Rest, ice, and heel inserts can be helpful in the short term. If these symptoms are encountered during an event, the degree of symptoms and loss of function can be used for decision on whether an athlete can continue in competition and this is primarily self-directed.

As opposed to tendinopathy which is a more subacute process characterized by gradual onset of heel pain and stiffness, Achilles ruptures, whether partial or complete, are acute events characterized by sharp onset of pain and inability to fully load the tendon following injury. Injured subjects will often report an accompanying audible pop. Partial Achilles tendon rupture may be difficult to distinguish from tendinopathy based on physical examination so history of onset should be a guiding factor.[53] Ultrasound if available can help distinguish these two entities. Partial tears can be treated with 2 cm heel lift, rest from running, and these patients should be referred to sports medicine/orthopedic follow-up with instructions to avoid stretching of the

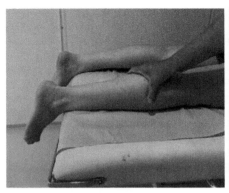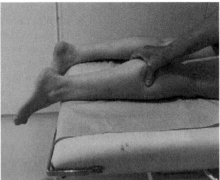

**Fig. 1.** Thompson test. (Larsson, E., Brorsson, A., Carmont, M. R., Fahlström, M., Zeisig, E., & Nilsson Helander, K. (2022). A narrative review of Achillestendon ruptures in racket sports. International Journal of Racket Sports Science, 4(1), x-x.)

tendon until then.[49] A complete Achilles rupture will have a similar historical story to a partial rupture with sudden pain, possible audible "pop" or snap. Examination may reveal swelling or bruising over the tendon; however, this is not always present. Feel for tenderness or a palpable gap along the tendon and assess active and passive range of motion. It is possible that some active plantar flexion will still be possible even in the case of complete tear due to the other tendons which traverse from the lower leg into the foot.[54] The best test to diagnose a complete rupture is the Thompson test (**Fig. 1**). To perform this test, the subject should be positioned either in a kneeling position or in a prone position with the feet and ankles hanging off the structure they are positioned on. The evaluator squeezes the calf muscle which should cause the foot to plantarflex. This should be trialed in the noninjured extremity for comparison. A positive test results in no plantarflexion with calf squeeze due to the muscles of gastrocnemius/soleus being disconnected from the foot.[50] Ultrasound in axial view over the Achilles tendon will reveal a loss in the continuity of the tendon fibers with a hypoechoic area between two edges.[55] If uncertain, ultrasound can be compared between the two extremities and can be tested through range of motion. Patients with partial or complete tendon rupture should not continue competition. Treatment includes splinting in position of Achilles tendon shortening such as with toes in slight plantar flexion, and they should be nonweight-bearing on that extremity until follow-up with orthopedics.

## BLISTERS

Although not generally life-threatening or significant from a long-term health perspective, blisters can be extremely painful and affect race performance. Blisters are more common in running events, especially those of longer distance and varying terrain compared to cycling events and swimming events. A friction foot blister incidence was reported at greater than 76% in an ultramarathon event[56] versus only 3% in marathons.[57] Most of the minimal research available on this subject thus focuses on marathons and ultramarathon competitors, and blister incidence is not commonly reported in other endurance research. A range of 6% to 16% of competitors who start but do not finish an ultramarathon cite blisters as the primary reason.[58] Blisters injuries occur due to friction which is primarily between footwear or socks and the skin. This friction or shearing stress occurs and propagates between the layers of the epidermis, eventually resulting in a cavity that becomes filled with a transudative fluid that we call a blister.[59] The use of athletic socks that separate toes, as well as the use of paper tape to pretape toes or blister prone areas of feet before competitions is some preventative strategies. Painful blisters are a common reason for visits to the medical tent at race events, in one study, blisters represented 20% of medical tent visits at marathons and 70% at ultramarathons.[58] If the blister is not painful it is generally advised to leave it alone or apply paper tape to it, unless it is very large or in a place where it is more likely to tear with continued competition. Drainage can be achieved with a clean needle, or safety pin, after cleansing skin with an alcohol swab or with soap and water, making 1 to 2 small holes and then expressing the drainage. Ideally, the area would be allowed to dry and then carefully covered with paper tape if on toes, or another athletic tape of choice such as Elastikon or KT tape if on other areas of the foot for the duration of the race, these materials can be cut to fit well on the foot and not cause wrinkles which could lead to other blisters. If the roof of a blister is completely torn off, options for care include applying second skin prior to taping or Compeed, although this should be used only when a competitor has positive experience with it in the past since if it needs to be removed it often causes some damage to the remaining skin around the blister. A special case is hemorrhagic blisters, which in general are not recommended to be drained due to theoretic concern for greater risk of infection. However, like in other blisters, if it is likely to burst on its own with continued competition or it is very large, it can be drained like nonhemorrhagic blisters after a risk benefit discussion with the competitor. The main blister complication to look for is cellulitis. Providing some daily soap/water for foot cleaning in multiday off-road events can be helpful to prevent this complication, and competitors can be instructed to self-evaluate blisters for signs of redness or discharge.

## CONSIDERATIONS FOR ENDURANCE EVENT MEDICAL DIRECTORS AND STAFF

As an endurance sport medical provider, preparedness is key to reducing anxiety and chaos surrounding events and providing high-quality care. As is often the case in medicine, the best treatment is prevention. One important method of preventing devastating events in organized endurance sports is proper screening for participants. To reduce the risk of SCD, the AHA and the American College of Cardiology recommend a set of guidelines for cardiac screening for participants that focuses on personal medical history, family medical history, and a focused physical examination.[60] Many ultraendurance events require clearance by a primary physician or specialist at the time of race enrollment. In all events but especially in more austere events, a health questionnaire should be completed by competitors and reviewed with the medical director including discussion of potential risks prior to the start of the event. Note any medications competitors are on chronically and assess if they will be continuing them during the race. Angiotensin-converting enzyme (ACE) inhibitors can impair thirst perception and contribute to dehydration and electrolyte imbalances. Opioids, selective serotonin reuptake inhibitors (SSRIs), carbamazepine, anticholinergics, and tricyclic antidepressants (TCAs) can impair central thermoregulation.[20] Antipsychotics, TCAs, and anticholinergics can also impair the normal sweating mechanisms leading to less heat dissipation during exercise.

A medical briefing is standard for austere and ultraendurance events especially if there are clear health risks such as high heat and humidity or other environmental hazards such as wind, lighting, chance of storm fronts, or animal encounters. Competitors and staff should be specifically educated on the early signs of heat illness and heat exhaustion and hyponatremia so they can appropriately care for themselves and prevent serious progression. On the days leading up to an event, wet-bulb globe temperature should be monitored to assess the risk level for exertional heat illness. Adjusting start times, cutoff times, or even event dates may be necessary to avoid widespread environmental caused morbidity/mortality.

A medical director should preplan to ensure that appropriate medical gear is available for daily issues such as foot care, skin issues such as chafing/sunburns, and musculoskeletal injuries as well as the more rare but life-threatening possibilities such as those previously described. An adequate number of AEDs can be determined based on course geography and race risks. Ideally, AEDs should be placed so that a provider can access one within 3 minutes[11]; however, this is often not logistically possible, so at minimum an AED should be available at the finish line and a halfway point or a location after which a greater amount of exertion is predicted to be required. The appropriate needed supplies for heat stroke should be on hand such as ice, material for a makeshift "tub" which can include materials such as troughs, tarps, and nonpenetrable bags such as conventional "body bags" and can include environmental resources such as known access to local cool streams. Supplies for intravenous access, cool fluids, and ability to create shade are also important. Hyponatremia supplies should include oral hypertonic solution and 3% saline IV solution. An Istat machine to evaluate blood for electrolyte levels including sodium should be brought if feasible. Musculoskeletal injury supplies can include a preferred kinesiotape brand, prehospital commercial splint which should be a product that becomes stiff when bent to supply support to the injured body part, splint padding such as a gauze wrap. ACE wraps and chemical cold packs can also be helpful.

It is important that all medical personnel are adequately trained on all the equipment available.

A plan of evacuation should be considered. In austere locations, nontraditional methods should be thought about such as off-road vehicles, all terrain vehicles (ATVs), use of animals, or a plan for use of Med Sled or air evacuation. Coordination should be implemented with local health centers and the most proximal trauma center and cardiac center to the event site.

## SUMMARY

Emergency medicine and its further specialization of training in wilderness and sports medicine neatly fill a unique niche called for by the specific needs of endurance athletes. Initially focusing on acute but simple injuries, emergency medicine has since expanded the scope of care for endurance athletes by focusing on such medical complications such as cardiac events, heat illness, electrolyte disturbances, and musculoskeletal injuries. The inherent competitive drive of endurance athletes to push the human body to its limit coupled with the sport's surging popularity has made it common practice to staff emergency medical personnel on standby at such events. With a proactive approach to injury prevention and athlete safety, the partnership between emergency medicine and endurance sports continues to evolve, and emergency physicians can guide and buttress the evolution of medical care in endurance sport.

## CLINICS CARE POINTS

- Endurance training results in long-term cardiovascular and neurologic benefits but can have acute injury risks.

- In athletes with sudden cardiac death, immediate CPR should be performed, and prioritization of automated external defibrillator use is the most lifesaving intervention.
- Suspect heat stroke if an athlete develops altered mental status, seizure or coma, and has a temperature over 40 C, treat with rapid ice water immersion.
- Severe hyponatremia can present with neurologic symptoms similar to heat stroke; these two entities can be differentiated by temperature, vital signs, and history of athlete's water intake and weight.
- Severe hyponatremia should be treated with 100 mL of 3% normal saline over 3 minutes, repeated after 10 minutes up to 2 times until mental status improves or seizing stops.
- Most musculoskeletal injuries during competition only result in the athlete self-removing from competition usually due to severity of symptoms or inability to make time cutoffs.
- Athletes with tendon ruptures should not be allowed to continue in competition and should be splinted in tendon shortened position and told to remain nonweight-bearing until specialty follow-up.

## DISCLOSURE

The authors have no commercial or financial conflicts of interest to declare.

## REFERENCES

1. Hunter P. The evolution of human endurance: Research on the biology of extreme endurance gives insights into its evolution in humans and animals. EMBO Rep 2019;20(11):e49396.
2. Liebenberg. The relevance of persistence hunting to human evolution. J Hum Evol 2008;55(6):1156–9.
3. Mattson MP. Evolutionary aspects of human exercise–born to run purposefully. Ageing Res Rev 2012;11(3):347–52.
4. Anderson J. The state of trail running 2022. Available at: 2022 https://runrepeat. com/the-state-of-trail-running-2022.
5. da Fonseca-Engelhardt K, Knechtle B, Rüst CA, et al. Participation and performance trends in ultra-endurance running races under extreme conditions - 'Spartathlon' versus 'Badwater'. Extrem Physiol Med 2013;2:15.
6. Shave RE, Lieberman DE, Drane AL, et al. Selection of endurance capabilities and the trade-off between pressure and volume in the evolution of the human heart. Proc Natl Acad Sci USA 2019;116:19905–10.
7. Li Y, Pan A, Wang DD, et al. Impact of healthy lifestyle factors on life expectancies in the US population. Circulation 2018;138:345–55.
8. Laver L, Pengas IP, Mei-Dan O. Injuries in extreme sports. J Orthop Surg Res 2017;12(1):59.
9. Buchholtz K, Lambert M, Corten L, et al. Incidence of injuries, illness and related risk factors in cross-country marathon mountain biking events: a systematic search and review. Sports Med Open 2021;7(1):68.
10. Krabak BJ, Waite B, Schiff MA. Study of injury and illness rates in multiday ultra-marathon runners. Med Sci Sports Exerc 2011;43(12):2314–20.
11. Shave R, Howatson G, Dickson D, et al. Exercise-Induced Cardiac Remodeling: Lessons from Humans, Horses, and Dogs. Vet Sci 2017;4(1):9.
12. Maron BJ, Pelliccia A. The heart of trained athletes: cardiac remodeling and the risks of sports, including sudden death. Circulation 2006;114(15):1633–44.

13. Lu L, Liu M, Sun R, et al. Myocardial Infarction: Symptoms and Treatments. Cell Biochem Biophys 2015 Jul;72(3):865–7.
14. Panju AA, Hemmelgarn BR, Guyatt GH, et al. The rational clinical examination. Is this patient having a myocardial infarction? JAMA 1998;280(14):1256–63.
15. Gersh BJ, Stone GW, White HD, et al. Pharmacological facilitation of primary percutaneous coronary intervention for acute myocardial infarction: is the slope of the curve the shape of the future? JAMA 2005;293:979–86.
16. Maron BJ, Gohman TE, Aeppli D. Prevalence of sudden cardiac death during competitive sports activities in Minnesota high school athletes. J Am Coll Cardiol 1998;32:1881–4.
17. Franklin BA, Thompson PD, Al-Zaiti SS, et al, American Heart Association Physical Activity Committee of the Council on Lifestyle and Cardiometabolic Health; Council on Cardiovascular and Stroke Nursing; Council on Clinical Cardiology; and Stroke Council. American Heart Association Physical Activity Committee of the Council on Lifestyle and Cardiometabolic Health; Council on Cardiovascular and Stroke Nursing; Council on Clinical Cardiology; and Stroke Council. Exercise-Related Acute Cardiovascular Events and Potential Deleterious Adaptations Following Long-Term Exercise Training: Placing the Risks Into Perspective-An Update: A Scientific Statement From the American Heart Association. Circulation 2020;141(13):e705–36.
18. Mannakkara NN, Sharma S. Sudden cardiac death in athletes. Cardiovascular problems 2020. https://doi.org/10.1002/tre.758.
19. Seely KD, Crockett KB, Nigh A. Sudden cardiac death in a young male endurance athlete. J Osteopath Med 2023;123(10):461–5.
20. Fanous Y, Dorian P. The prevention and management of sudden cardiac arrest in athletes. CMAJ (Can Med Assoc J) 2019;191(28):E787–91.
21. Brown AJ, Ha FJ, Michail M, et al. In: Watson TJ, Ong PJL, Tcheng JE, editors. Prehospital diagnosis and management of acute myocardial infarction. 2018.
22. Drezner JA, Peterson DF, Siebert DM, et al. Survival after exercise-related sudden cardiac arrest in young athletes: can we do better? Sports Health 2019;11:8.
23. Kinoshi T, Tanaka S, Sagisaka R, et al. Mobile automated external defibrillator response system during road races. N Engl J Med 2018;379:488–9.
24. Bouscaren N, Millet GY, Racinais S. Heat stress challenges in marathon vs. ultra-endurance running. Front Sports Act Living 2019;1:59.
25. Nichols AW. Heat-related illness in sports and exercise. Curr Rev Musculoskelet Med 2014;7(4):355–65.
26. Leyk D, Hoitz J, Becker C, et al. Health risks and interventions in exertional heat stress. Dtsch Arztebl Int 2019;116(31–32):537–44.
27. Yankelson L, Sadeh B, Gershovitz L, et al. Life-threatening events during endurance sports: is heat stroke more prevalent than arrhythmic death? J Am Coll Cardiol 2014;64(5):463–9.
28. Casa DJ, McDermott BP, Lee EC, et al. Cold water immersion: the gold standard for exertional heatstroke treatment. Exerc Sport Sci Rev 2007;35(3):141–9.
29. Lipman GS, Burns P, Phillips C, et al. Effect of Sodium Supplements and Climate on Dysnatremia During Ultramarathon Running. Clin J Sport Med 2021;31(6):e327–34.
30. Hoffman MD, Myers TM. Case Study: Symptomatic Exercise-Associated Hyponatremia in an Endurance Runner Despite Sodium Supplementation. Int J Sport Nutr Exerc Metabol 2015;25(6):603–6.
31. Nikolaidis PT, Veniamakis E, Rosemann T, et al. Nutrition in Ultra-Endurance: State of the Art. Nutrients 2018;10(12):1995.

32. Knechtle B, Chlíbková D, Papadopoulou S, et al. Exercise-Associated Hyponatremia in Endurance and Ultra-Endurance Performance-Aspects of Sex, Race Location, Ambient Temperature, Sports Discipline, and Length of Performance: A Narrative Review. Medicina (Kaunas) 2019;55(9):537.

33. Lau M, Choi Y. Exercise-Associated Hyponatremia: A Local Case Report. Hong Kong J Emerg Med 2009;16(2):88–92.

34. Vazquez-Galliano J, Mehech D, Vallejos CC, et al. Hydration Issues in the Athlete and Exercise Associated Hyponatremia. Essentials of Rehabilitation Practice and Science. 4/29/21.

35. Urso C, Brucculeri S, Caimi G. Physiopathological, Epidemiological, Clinical and Therapeutic Aspects of Exercise-Associated Hyponatremia. J Clin Med 2014; 3(4):1258–75.

36. Ayus JC, Moritz ML. Misconceptions and Barriers to the Use of Hypertonic Saline to Treat Hyponatremic Encephalopathy. Front Med 2019;6:47.

37. Scheer V, Krabak B, Villiger E, et al. Endurance and Ultra-Endurance Sports in Extreme Conditions: Physiological and Pathophysiological Issues. Front Physiol 2021;12.

38. Kelly S, Pollock N, Polglass G, et al. Injury and illness in elite athletics: a prospective cohort study over three seasons. Int J Sports Phys Ther 2022;17(3):420–33.

39. Prieto-González P, Martínez-Castillo JL, Fernández-Galván LM, et al. Epidemiology of sports-related injuries and associated risk factors in adolescent athletes: an injury surveillance. Int J Environ Res Publ Health 2021;18(9):4857.

40. Glaviano NR, Kew M, Hart JM, et al. Demographic and epidemiological trends in patellofemoral pain. Int J Sports Phys Ther 2015;10(3):281–90.

41. Cosca DD, Navazio F. Common problems in endurance athletes. Am Fam Physician 2007;76(2):237–44.

42. Collins NJ, Crossley KM, Darnell R, et al. Predictors of short and long term outcome in patellofemoral pain syndrome: a prospective longitudinal study. BMC Muscoskel Disord 2010;11:11.

43. Strauss EJ, Kim S, Calcei JG, et al. Iliotibial band syndrome: evaluation and management. J Am Acad Orthop Surg 2011;19(12):728–36.

44. Beals C, Flanigan D. A Review of treatments for iliotibial band syndrome in the athletic population. J Sports Med 2013;2013:367169. Hindawi Publ Corp.

45. Willett GM, Keim SA, Shostrom VK, et al. An Anatomic Investigation of the Ober Test. Am J Sports Med 2016;44(3):696–701.

46. Dodelin D, Tourny C, Menez C, et al. Reduction of foot overpronation to improve iliotibial band syndrome in runners: a case series. Clin Res Foot Ankle 2018; 6:272.

47. Trevlaki E, Dimitriadou S, Trevlakis E. Physical therapy approaches for the treatment of iliotibial band syndrome: a systematic review. International Journal of Advanced Health Science and Technology 2022;2(5).

48. Kongsgaard M, Aagaard P, Kjaer M, et al. Structural Achilles tendon properties in athletes subjected to different exercise modes and in Achilles tendon rupture patients. J Appl Physiol 2005;99(5):1965–71.

49. Kujala UM, Sarna S, Kaprio J. Cumulative incidence of Achilles tendon rupture and tendinopathy in male former elite athletes. Clin J Sport Med 2005;15(3): 133–5.

50. Dakin SG, Newton J, Martinez FO, et al. Chronic inflammation is a feature of Achilles tendinopathy and rupture. Br J Sports Med 2018;52:359–67.

51. Starbuck C, Bramah C, Herrington L, et al. The effect of speed on Achilles tendon forces and patellofemoral joint stresses in high-performing endurance runners. Scand J Med Sci Sports 2021.

52. Hutchison AM, Evans R, Bodger O, et al. What is the best clinical test for Achilles tendinopathy? Foot Ankle Surg 2013;19(2):112–7.

53. Gatz M, Spang C, Alfredson H. Partial achilles tendon rupture—a neglected entity: a narrative literature review on diagnostics and treatment options. J Clin Med 2020;9(10):3380.

54. Boyd R, Dimock R, Solan MC, et al. Achilles tendon rupture: how to avoid missing the diagnosis. Br J Gen Pract 2015;65(641):668–9.

55. Aminlari A, Stone J, McKee R, et al. Diagnosing achilles tendon rupture with ultrasound in patients treated surgically: a systematic review and meta-analysis. J Emerg Med 2021;61(5):558–67.

56. Scheer BV, Reljic D, Murray A, et al. The enemy of the feet: blisters in ultraendurance runners. J Am Podiatr Med Assoc 2014;104(5):473–8.

57. Yang HR, Jeong J, Kim I, et al. Medical support during an Ironman 70.3 triathlon race. F1000Res 2017;6:1516.

58. Lipman GS, Sharp LJ, Christensen M, et al. Paper tape prevents foot blisters: a randomized prevention trial assessing paper tape in endurance distances II (Pre-TAPED II). Clin J Sport Med 2016;26(5):362–8.

59. Knapik JJ, Reynolds KL, Duplantis KL, et al. Friction blisters. Pathophysiology, prevention and treatment. Sports Med 1995;20(3):136–47.

60. Hainline B, Drezner J, Baggish A, et al. Interassociation consensus statement on cardiovascular care of college student-athletes. J Am Coll Cardiol 2016;67(25):2981–95.

# Tick-Borne Illnesses in Emergency and Wilderness Medicine

Michael D. Sullivan, MD[a], Kyle Glose, MD[a], Douglas Sward, MD[b],*

## KEYWORDS

- Tick-borne • Lyme • Ticks • Anaplasmosis • Ehrlichiosis • Babesiosis • RMSF

## KEY POINTS

- Tick-borne illnesses are responsible for the majority of vector-borne disease in the United States, and the geographic distribution of these diseases is expanding.
- Many tick-borne illnesses have overlapping, nonspecific symptoms and rely on serology testing for laboratory diagnosis, making diagnosis in the emergency or wilderness setting challenging.
- Tick-borne illnesses can be associated with mortality if treatment is delayed, and antibiotics should be administered if there is high clinical suspicion, even before laboratory confirmation of diagnosis.

## INTRODUCTION

Ticks are responsible for over 95% of vector-borne disease cases in the United States.[1] As tick-borne illnesses are being reported in increasingly large geographic areas, it is essential that emergency medicine clinicians are familiar with the presentation, diagnosis, and treatment of the most common tick-borne infections.[2,3] It is hypothesized that climate changes are altering the geographic distribution of these ticks, which may change the spatial relationship of tick-borne illnesses in years to come. Case incidence data show that tick-borne illnesses can occur in areas that are not associated with known tick vector habitats.[4] This text serves as a guide for emergency medicine providers to review the pathogenesis, clinical features, diagnosis, and treatment of the most common tick-borne illnesses.

[a] Department of Emergency Medicine, University of Maryland Medical Center, 6th Floor, Suite 200, 110 South Paca Street, Baltimore, MD 21201, USA; [b] Department of Emergency Medicine, University of Maryland School of Medicine, 6th Floor, Suite 200, 110 South Paca Street, Baltimore, MD 21201, USA
* Corresponding author.
*E-mail address:* DSward@som.umaryland.edu

Emerg Med Clin N Am 42 (2024) 597–611
https://doi.org/10.1016/j.emc.2024.02.018
0733-8627/24/© 2024 Elsevier Inc. All rights reserved.

## LYME DISEASE
### Introduction

Lyme disease is the most common vector-borne disease in the United States, with approximately 30,000 cases reported to the Centers for Disease Control and Prevention (CDC) every year, though the true number of infections is estimated to be 10-fold higher. The disease was first described in 1977 when a group of Yale researchers noticed an increase in incidence of juvenile rheumatoid arthritis around Lyme, Connecticut.[5,6]

### Causative Organisms

Lyme disease is caused by spirochete bacteria known as *Borrelia burgdorferi*, with a majority of cases occurring in the Northeastern United States. The bacteria are most frequently transmitted to human hosts through bites from *Ixodes* species ticks, specifically the *I scapularis* tick in the Northeast and Midwest United States, while the *I pacificus* is more prevalent in transmission that occurs along the West Coast (**Fig. 1**).[5,6] While *B burgdorferi* has been found in a large number of tick species, only *Ixodes* ticks are known to be capable of transmitting the infection to new hosts.[7]

Humans are non-obligate hosts of the *B burgdorferi* life cycle, thus acting as a "dead end" for the bacteria. Transovarial (vertical) transmission of *B burgdorferi* is thought to be non-existent, and thus ticks are born without infection. The first chance that ticks have to become infected with *B burgdorferi* occurs during their first blood meal when the ticks latch onto an infected host, most commonly the white-footed mouse.[8] While nymph and adult ticks can both transmit the bacteria, it is thought that nymphs transmit a majority of *B burgdorferi* to humans, given that they are smaller and more difficult to detect.[6]

### Clinical Features/Presentation

Lyme disease has 3 clinical stages: early localized, early disseminated, and late disseminated. The early localized disease is characterized by the hallmark erythema migrans (EM) rash, resembling a "bull's eye." This rash is not typically tender or pruritic. The EM rash will most often appear in the first weeks after infection (**Fig. 2**).[9,10]

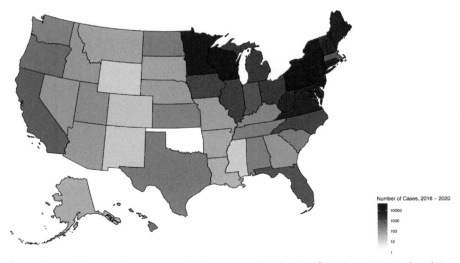

Number of Cases, 2016 – 2020

10000
1000
100
10
1

**Fig. 1.** Cases of Lyme disease reported by states to the Centers for Disease Control and Prevention (CDC) between 2016 and 2020. (CDC NNDSS.)

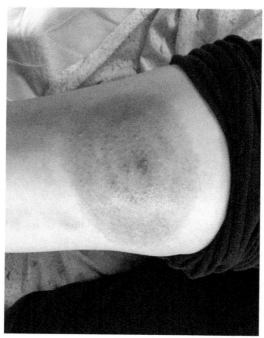

**Fig. 2.** Erythema migrans rash.

The second and third stages of Lyme disease encompass a wider range of disease manifestations, including multiple EM lesions, Lyme neuroborreliosis, Lyme carditis, and Lyme arthritis.[7,11] The second phase, early disseminated Lyme, can involve multiple EM lesions or an objective finding such as Lyme carditis, while late disseminated Lyme tends to involve Lyme arthritis. However, the second and third phases of Lyme disease can have overlapping syndromes, and the distinction is not always consistent with clinical findings.[7] Lyme neuroborreliosis is a constellation of symptoms including headache, nuchal rigidity, and facial nerve palsy. The facial nerve palsy can be unilateral or bilateral, and is frequently mistaken for Bell's palsy.[11] Patients can also go on to develop Lyme carditis, characterized by heterogeneous cardiac involvement that can cause shortness of breath, palpitations, chest pain, lightheadedness, or even arrhythmogenic syncope. One of the principal features of Lyme carditis is an atrioventricular block that can have fluctuations and rapid progression. Lyme carditis can also manifest as atrial fibrillation or sick sinus syndrome.[9,12] While Lyme carditis appears to be extremely rare, several cases of sudden cardiac death have been attributed to cardiac involvement of Lyme disease.[13]

Lyme arthritis, the most common sequalae of disseminated spirochetal infection, presents as a monoarticular or oligoarticular joint involvement with swelling, large effusions, and mild pain.[14] The knee is the most common joint to be affected, but large or small joints can be affected. It is rare for only small joints to be involved.[15] Symptoms tend to resolve with antibiotic therapy, though some patients are noted to have persistent synovitis which is termed "post-infectious, antibiotic-refractory Lyme arthritis." This causes continued symptoms through an unclear mechanism. Antibiotic-refractory Lyme arthritis typically resolves within approximately 1 year.[14]

Of note, the term "chronic Lyme" is now used in the United States to refer to persistent fatigue, pain, or other neurocognitive complaints without evidence of previous Lyme borreliosis.[7,12] Individuals who diagnose patients with chronic Lyme disease argue that accepted laboratory tests are unreliable, and patients may be prescribed prolonged and unusual treatment courses in an effort to provide relief. It has been well documented that these treatments are potentially dangerous, leading to morbidity and even mortality.[16,17] Separate from "chronic Lyme" disease, some patients with true Lyme disease will have persistent, nonspecific symptoms even after a complete course of antibiotics. The term "post-treatment-Lyme-disease-syndrome" (PTLDS) refers to patients with greater than 6 months of fatigue, articular pain, and cognitive difficulties after a documented, confirmed case of early or late Lyme disease. The important distinction to be made is that patients with PTLDS have a prior, documented history of Lyme disease.[12]

### Diagnosis

The only clinical finding that is diagnostic of Lyme disease is an EM rash, but patients may present with arthritic, neurologic, or cardiac symptoms without having a clear history of tick exposure or EM rash. *B burgdorferi* has difficult culture requirements and it will not grow on routine blood cultures. Serologic testing is the key to diagnosis; however, these tests involve immunoassays that will generally not result in time to assist the emergency medicine provider.[9,15] Diagnostic testing previously consisted of an enzyme-linked immunosorbent assay followed by a Western blot confirmation test; however, Lyme diagnostic testing guidelines were updated in 2019 given the development of new serologic assays, which now allow for a second sensitive enzyme immunoassay to be used in the testing for Lyme disease rather than a Western blot.[18] While this testing method results in sufficient sensitivity and specificity, immunoassays still have shortcomings such as difficulty in identifying active versus previous infection, as well as detection of early disease when relying on antibody response.[15]

### Treatment

Treatment of Lyme disease is meant to shorten duration of symptoms—early manifestations of Lyme disease will resolve spontaneously without antibiotics.[15] The 2020 Infectious Disease Society of America (IDSA) treatment recommendations for Lyme disease are stratified by the type of presenting symptoms. For patients presenting with EM rash, the IDSA recommends oral antibiotic therapy with doxycycline, amoxicillin, or cefuroxime, for a 10-day to 14-day course. If a patient is unable to take any of these agents, azithromycin can be used, but it is not recommended as a first-line agent.[15,19]

For patients who have Lyme neuroborreliosis, the recommendation is to treat with intravenous (IV) ceftriaxone, cefotaxime, penicillin G, or oral doxycycline for a 14-day to 21-day course. When a patient develops Lyme arthritis, the overall course is increased to 28 days, and these patients can take oral antibiotics rather than intravenously. Symptoms can be initially managed with nonsteroidal anti-inflammatory drugs, though the IDSA also recommends referral to a rheumatologist for persistent joint swelling to rule out other causes of arthritis.[9]

## ROCKY MOUNTAIN SPOTTED FEVER
### Introduction

The first tick-borne illness to be recognized in the United States, *Rickettsia rickettsii* was identified as the causative agent for a syndrome of malaise and fever, which was coined Rocky Mountain spotted fever (RMSF), in the early 1900s.[20,21] While the disease was originally discovered in the Rocky Mountains, the disease name is somewhat of a misnomer—the highest incidence of the disease is in the Southeast and mid-Atlantic United States (**Fig. 3**). Cases have also been reported in Canada, as well as

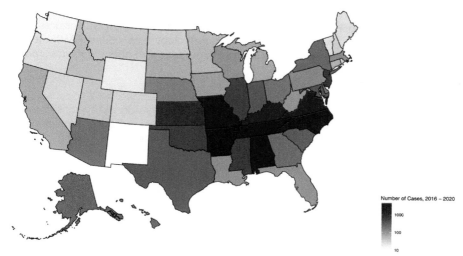

**Fig. 3.** Cases of Rocky Mountain spotted fever reported by states to the CDC between 2016 and 2020. (CDC NNDSS.)

Central and South America.[22,23] The primary vector for Rocky Mountain spotted fever is the *Dermacentor variabilis*, or the American dog tick.[23]

### Causative Organisms

The causative agent of RMSF is *R rickettsii,* gram-negative, obligate intracellular bacteria which can be maintained in ticks through transovarial transmission.[24] Of note, the *Rickettsia* genus also contains the causative agent for typhus (*R typhi*). There are several other *Rickettsial* bacteria that cause diseases known as spotted fever group rickettsioses (SFGR), of which RMSF is the most severe. In untreated Rocky Mountain spotted fever by *R rickettsii,* mortality may approach 20%.[21,24] Infections from SFGR tend to produce overlapping clinical features with RMSF, and differentiating the causative bacteria for these diseases is difficult, given nonspecific syndromes as well as serologic cross-reactivity when using R rickettsii assays.[25] RMSF is not typically associated with eschar formation at the site of inoculation, while many other SFGR have this symptom.

### Clinical Features/Presentation

The clinical syndrome for RMSF is non-specific—a recent study of 340 patients with the diagnosis of RMSF revealed that 86% of the patients with available data had fever and 80% had rash, which was primarily maculopapular or petechial in appearance. Although RMSF rash classically includes the palms and soles, it should be noted that only 58% of the patients were noted to have this rash on their palms or soles.[21] Patients will also often have nonspecific viral symptoms such as headaches, fever, weakness, fatigue, nausea, vomiting, and photophobia. Patients presenting with these symptoms should be asked about potential tick exposures in their history, but the reported history of a tick bite is only present in 50% to 60% of patients with RMSF.[22]

More severe findings of RMSF can include cardiopulmonary disease such as myocarditis, congestive heart failure, dysrhythmia, and pneumonia. These sequalae are not likely to occur until after the fifth day after symptom onset, and are less common in patients who are treated early.[22] Patients can also develop acute renal failure, cutaneous necrosis, acute respiratory distress syndrome (ARDS), seizures, and meningoencephalitis. The wide spectrum of pathology can cause RMSF to be mistaken for other disease syndromes such as thrombotic thrombocytopenic purpura, vasculitis, or viral meningitis.[26,27]

### Diagnosis

The diagnosis of RMSF relies on serologic testing. Patients do not typically have a positive antibody response until 7 to 10 days after disease onset, but serum immunofluorescence antibody tests should be obtained. Negative serology does not rule out RMSF, and positive tests are only able to confirm that the patient has been exposed to the disease in the past, not to confirm an active infection.[22,28] It is possible to take immunohistochemical stains of biopsied specimens, but these are only able to be processed in specific laboratories and unlikely to provide diagnostic information in the acute, emergency, or wilderness setting.[25,28]

### Treatment

Doxycycline is used to treat all patients with RMSF, or any tick-borne rickettsial disease. For adults, the recommended dose is 100 mg twice daily, orally or intravenously, for a 5-day to 7-day course. This course can be extended for more critically ill patients, until the patient has been afebrile for 3 days. Prompt initiation of treatment is essential because delays in treatment can lead to long-term sequalae or death.[22,26,29] Doxycycline is the only recommended agent for RMSF. Chloramphenicol is the only additional agent that has been used, but data suggest that patients have higher mortality when treated with chloramphenicol over doxycycline.[26] If a patient is allergic to doxycycline, the allergy reaction should be assessed. If the patient's reaction is life-threatening, consultation with an allergy and immunology specialist for rapid desensitization should be pursued. Patients with non-life-threatening reactions should be strongly considered to receive doxycycline in an observed setting, but determinations must be made based on each individual patient's clinical status.

The recommendation for doxycycline also applies to pediatric patients, including those under 8 years of age. Research suggests that the short course used to treat RMSF does not result in significant discoloration of the teeth, and the CDC recommends initiation of treatment with doxycycline for patients of all ages.[26,30] An expert review of doxycycline in pregnancy based on observational studies suggested that there is likely low teratogenic risk, but there is not enough evidence to conclude there is no risk. Counseling of risks versus benefits for doxycycline treatment is strongly advised in the setting of a potentially fatal case of RMSF in a pregnant patient.[26]

## EHRLICHIOSIS AND ANAPLASMOSIS
### Introduction

Anaplasmosis and ehrlichiosis share similar clinical presentations, and prior to the advent of polymerase chain reaction (PCR), shared a common diagnostic criterion—the visualization of morulae within infected immune cells on a peripheral blood smear. Even immune-competent hosts can develop severe illness requiring hospitalization, which is thought to occur in approximately 1% to 3% of cases of anaplasmosis and in up to 42% of cases of ehrlichiosis.[31–33]

### Causative Organisms

Ehrlichiosis is primarily caused by the bacteria *Ehrlichia chaffeensis* and *E ewingii,* though *E muris eauclairensis* has recently been identified as a clinically relevant subspecies.[34] Anaplasmosis is caused by *Anaplasma phagocytophilum* (formerly *E phagocytophilum*).[35] The lone-star tick, *Amblyomma americanum*, is responsible for transmission of ehrlichiosis caused by *E chaffeensis* and *E ewingii*; however, the newly emerging subspecies of *E muris euaclairensis* is transmitted by the deer tick, *I scapularis*. *A phagocytophilum* is transmitted exclusively by the *I scapularis* tick. The distribution of infections correlates roughly, though not entirely, with tick populations since multiple vector species are responsible for the spread of these diseases (**Fig. 4**).[36]

### Clinical Features/Presentation

Ehrlichiosis and anaplasmosis share overlapping clinical syndromes, although the prevalence of severe disease is significantly greater in ehrlichiosis. Patients with mild disease are often misdiagnosed with viral illness, as they present with fever, headaches, myalgias, and arthralgias. Rash is common in ehrlichiosis, though more so in children, and spares the palms, soles, and face. Rash is uncommon in anaplasmosis, occurring in fewer than 10% of cases. Laboratory abnormalities include leukopenia/thrombocytopenia, elevated aspartate trasaminase/alanine transaminase, and mild hyponatremia.[26,37,38]

Severe manifestations of these diseases can be life-threatening, even in immune-competent hosts, highlighting the importance of early recognition and treatment of these diseases. Case-fatality in ehrlichiosis approaches 3%, while it is less than 1% for anaplasmosis.[26,33,39,40] Severe manifestations include ARDS, meningitis/meningoencephalitis, acute renal failure, myocarditis, and hepatic failure.[37,41,42] There are reports of Anaplasma-induced hemophagocytic lymphohistiocytosis.[43]

### Diagnosis

Although confirmatory testing is available, the treatment of anaplasmosis/ehrlichiosis should not be delayed if clinical suspicion is high. Delays in definitive treatment are associated with increased incidence of severe disease and higher mortality. Laboratory testing includes serologic assays, PCR, and morulae detection in peripheral blood smears. Morulae, intracellular clusters of organisms, can be observed in peripheral

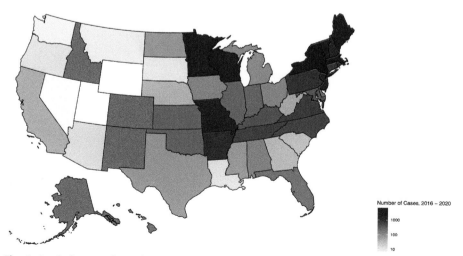

Number of Cases, 2016 – 2020

1000

100

10

**Fig. 4.** Pooled cases of anaplasmosis and ehrlichiosis reported by states to the CDC between 2016 and 2020. (CDC NNDSS.)

blood monocytes, neutrophils, and rarely eosinophils, though morulae formation is only seen in approximately 20% of cases. Serologic testing is available, though immunoglobulin (Ig)G and IgM titers may be falsely undetectable in early disease. Whole-blood PCR is effective at diagnosing active disease, though often it is not readily available.

### Treatment

Doxycycline is the first-line treatment for both ehrlichiosis and anaplasmosis. Prompt initiation of treatment can significantly reduce the severity of symptoms and prevent complications. Current guidelines recommend a 10-day course of therapy.[44] Rifampin has been suggested as an alternative for pregnant patients and patients with a history of drug allergy to doxycycline. As discussed, short courses of doxycycline in pediatric patients do not appear to cause tooth discoloration and should be considered for pediatric patients.

## BABESIOSIS
### Introduction

Babesiosis, caused by protozoa of the *Babesia* genus, is an important emerging tick-borne disease. The prevalence has been increasing worldwide, especially in the United States and Europe, and the disease is becoming a more common cause of hospitalization due to tick exposure. It is transmitted to humans by the bites of infected ticks.

### Causative Organisms

In the United States, the vast majority of infections are due to *B microti*, which is spread by the *I scapularis* tick.[45] Due to the common vector, coinfections with *B burgdorferi*, the causative agent of Lyme disease, may occur.[46] Rarely, infections with *B duncani* have been reported in the Pacific Northwest United States—though the vector is unknown, it is thought to most likely be *I pacificus* (**Fig. 5**).[47]

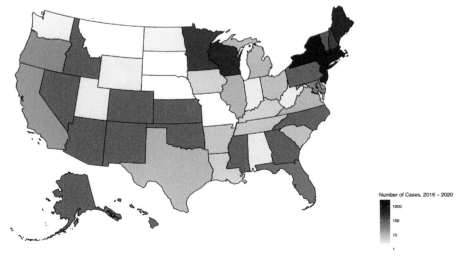

**Fig. 5.** Cases of babesiosis reported by states to the CDC between 2016 and 2020. (Centers for Disease Control and Prevention. National Notifiable Diseases Surveillance System (NNDSS) AnnualSummary Data for years 2016 to 2019, United States. Accessed August 16, 2023. http://wonder.cdc.gov/nndss-annual-summary.html.)

## Clinical Features/Presentation

Babesiosis often presents with nonspecific symptoms like other tick-borne illness, making diagnosis challenging. Typical clinical manifestations include high fever, chills, and myalgias. Most patients will begin to experience symptoms after an incubation period of 1 to 4 weeks following their exposure to an infected tick.[47] Patients who are asplenic or otherwise immunosuppressed may present with features of severe infection, typically characterized by a high parasitic burden on peripheral blood smear and mild to severe hemolytic anemia (caused by the parasite erupting from within erythrocytes during its replication cycle), requiring hospitalization. Hospitalized patients are at risk for development of ARDS, disseminated intravascular coagulation, multi-system organ failure, and atraumatic splenic rupture.[45,47,48] Furthermore, in patients treated with doxycycline for anaplasmosis or Lyme disease whose symptoms fail to resolve, consideration should be given to babesiosis as all 3 diseases share a common vector.[44]

## Diagnosis

The diagnosis of babesiosis is confirmed by the identification of intraerythrocytic parasites, often in ring forms, on peripheral blood smear. The classic finding on peripheral blood smear is that of a "maltese cross" (a tetrad merozoite form of the organism), although this is rare.[47] Other testing options include real-time PCR, indirect immunofluorescence, and serologic testing.[49,50]

## Treatment

The treatment of babesiosis varies with the severity of the infection. For uncomplicated cases, the first-line treatment is a combination of azithromycin and atovaquone. The combination of clindamycin and quinine is considered second-line.[51,52] In patients with severe disease, defined as those with high-grade parasitemia (>10%), severe hemolytic anemia, or pulmonary/hepatic/renal disease, exchange transfusion should be considered both to reduce the parasitic burden and to limit the severity of intravascular hemolysis.[52]

# OTHER TICK-BORNE DISEASES
## Tularemia

Tularemia, also known as Q fever, is a rare disease which can present as one of many different clinical syndromes depending on the route of exposure. Tick bite is not the only method of transmission. Caused by the gram-negative coccobacillus *Francisella tularensis*, tularemia infection can range from mild disease easily managed with antibiotics to life-threatening illness. It is rare in the United States, with roughly 250 naturally-occurring infections reported annually.[53] If contracted via tick bite, tularemia typically presents with localized lymphadenopathy and may also manifest with a cutaneous ulcer at the site of exposure. In addition, it presents with nonspecific symptoms including fever, malaise, headache, myalgias, anorexia, abdominal pain, and sore throat. Definitive diagnosis is microbiological, though *F tularensis* is a slow-growing organism and the diagnosis may be supported by immunohistochemical testing or PCR.[54] Doxycycline is the only Food and Drug Administration (FDA)-approved therapy for the disease; however, gentamicin and ciprofloxacin have also been used successfully in cases where doxycycline was contraindicated.[55] Notably, for severe infection (ie, hospitalized patients), the World Health Organization guidelines recommend treatment with gentamicin as first-line.[56]

### Tick-Borne Encephalitis and Powassan Virus

Powassan virus (POWV) and tick-borne encephalitis virus (TBEV) are 2 closely related flaviviruses that belong to the tick-borne encephalitis complex. These viruses are primarily transmitted through the bite of infected ticks and are a rare cause of encephalitis in humans, with a notable potential for severe neurologic disease.

POWV is a member of the Powassan virus lineage within the tick-borne encephalitis virus complex. It is primarily transmitted by *I scapularis* and *I cookei* ticks in North America. TBEV is the prototype virus of the complex and is prevalent in Europe and Asia.[57]

Both viruses can cause febrile illnesses. TBEV generally causes a more severe clinical course, including meningoencephalitis. Powassan virus can lead to severe neurologic complications, such as encephalitis and meningitis, with a fatality rate of up to 15% in reported cases.[58] Symptoms are typical of encephalitis, beginning after an incubation period of approximately 2 to 4 weeks. Early symptoms include fatigue before progressing to severe neuroinvasive disease, with hallmark symptoms of headache, confusion, and focal neurologic deficits. Rarely, chorioretinitis, ophthalmoplegia, and flaccid paralysis have been reported. Diagnosis is secured with PCR-based detection in cerebrospinal fluid.[59]

Vaccines are available for TBEV in endemic regions, contributing significantly to disease prevention, although no specific antiviral treatments exist for either virus, emphasizing the importance of tick avoidance and early diagnosis. Care is supportive, and the role for steroids or intravenous immunoglobulin (IVIG) has been proposed but not borne out in data.[60] In patients who survive severe disease, roughly one-third develop permanent neurologic deficits.

### Alpha-Gal Syndrome

First described in 2009,[61] alpha-gal syndrome, an IgE-mediated allergic reaction to the carbohydrate galactose-α-1,3-galactose (α-Gal), has emerged as a condition substantially associated with exposure to tick bites.[62] Colloquially, it may be known as "meat allergy" due to the presence of α-Gal in most mammalian meats. An estimated 110,000 cases were identified in the United States based on the detection of anti-α-Gal IgE antibodies in serum specimens submitted to the CDC.[63] Its incidence overlaps heavily with the habitat of the lone star tick, though conclusive evidence linking this specific tick to the disease is lacking.[62] Despite its growing recognition as a disease entity, a recent survey of US primary health care providers demonstrated a low level of knowledge about the disease. On average, patients experienced a delay of 7.1 years from symptom onset to diagnosis.[64] Symptoms of alpha-gal syndrome may vary from purely gastrointestinal symptoms (abdominal pain/cramping, diarrhea, and nausea) to pruritis, hives, angioedema, or anaphylaxis. The diagnosis can be made based on a history of delayed allergic reactions after the consumption of pork, lamb, or beef, as well as a positive serologic test for anti-α-Gal IgE.[64] Notably, skin-prick tests have been shown to be unreliable.[61] Treatment consists of allergen avoidance. Long-acting oral antihistamines such as fexofenadine or levocetirizine can be used, though the quality of evidence is low.[64]

## TICK-BITE PREVENTION AND REMOVAL

Addressing ways to prevent tick bites, and therefore reduce transmission of tick-borne illnesses, is an area for public health intervention, and emergency medicine clinicians can provide education to patients regarding tick bite prevention and prompt recognition of symptoms.[65] Ticks quest for meals by waiting in tall grass for a potential host to walk by, and will attach to any portion of clothing or skin that brushes close enough to make contact. They will often attach on the scalp, abdomen, axillae, groin, and along the belt or sock line.[66,67] Removing the tick as soon as possible is critical to reducing the risk of transmission. The CDC recommends a variety of actions to prevent tick bites, including the treatment of clothing with permethrin and skin with N, N-diethyl-meta-toluamide or similar Environmental Protection Agency-registered insect repellents, avoiding areas with high grass, and checking clothing and skin for ticks after returning home from the outdoors. These approaches are based on common sense and expert opinion, without strong underlying evidence.[68,69]

For a patient presenting with a tick attached to their person, removing the tick as soon as possible can help lower the chance of transmission of tick-borne pathogens. The CDC recommends removing any tick found attached to the skin as quickly as possible; using clean, fine tipped tweezers, the tick should be grasped as close to the skin as possible and removed with gentle, outward pressure. Efforts should be made to remove the whole tick without leaving parts of the mouth behind, but *Ixodes* species produce a substance to cement their mouths to the skin which can make entire removal difficult. If parts of the mouth are left behind, they can safely be left in the skin.[70] There are commercial devices available for assisting in tick removal, including low-energy radiofrequency devices or slightly heated forceps that can be used as available. It is not recommended to crush a tick with fingers, and the CDC recommends against home remedies such as painting the tick with nail polish or petroleum jelly.[70,71]

## SUMMARY

Tick-borne illnesses represent an emergent threat to human health in the United States, and it is important that wilderness and emergency medicine providers be aware of the common epidemiology, presentations, diagnoses, treatments, and prevention practices associated with these illnesses. While many of the clinical syndromes can appear overlapping, a discerning history and physical examination can provide clues about the etiology of each individual illness. Prompt treatment can oftentimes help prevent morbidity and mortality, and wilderness providers are in a unique position, given that there is a tendency to take care of individuals in areas where they might be exposed to ticks. As the geographic distribution of tick habitats changes over time, it will become even more important to be aware of these clinical syndromes to provide the highest quality care and wilderness medicine.

## CLINICS CARE POINTS

- Tick-borne illnesses can present without confirmed history of tick exposure. Keep these illnesses on the differential when evaluating patients with fever, rash, and nonspecific symptoms.

- Many tests for tick-borne illness are based on serology and will not be immediately available for emergency medicine and wilderness providers. Antibiotics should not be delayed if there is high clinical suspicion based on history and physical examination.

- Doxycycline is the first-line treatment for Lyme, RMSF, anaplasmosis, ehrlichiosis, and tularemia, and evidence suggests minimal side effects with short courses (even in pediatric patients).

- Removing ticks as soon as possible can reduce disease transmission.

## DISCLOSURE

The authors have no financial disclosures.

## REFERENCES

1. Rochlin I, Toledo A. Emerging tick-borne pathogens of public health importance: a mini-review. J Med Microbiol 2020;69(6):781–91.
2. Diaz JH. Emerging tickborne viral infections: what wilderness medicine providers need to know. Wilderness Environ Med 2020;31(4):489–97.
3. Eisen RJ, Kugeler KJ, Eisen L, et al. Tick-borne zoonoses in the united states: persistent and emerging threats to human health. ILAR J 2017;58(3):319–35.
4. Alkishe A, Raghavan RK, Peterson AT. Likely geographic distributional shifts among medically important tick species and tick-associated diseases under climate change in north america: a review. Insects 2021;12(3):225.
5. Bobe JR, Jutras BL, Horn EJ, et al. Recent progress in lyme disease and remaining challenges. Front Med 2021;8:666554.
6. Forrester JD, Vakkalanka JP, Holstege CP, et al. Lyme disease: what the wilderness provider needs to know. Wilderness Environ Med 2015;26(4):555–64.
7. Stanek G, Wormser GP, Gray J, et al. Lyme borreliosis. Lancet 2012;379(9814): 461–73.
8. Barbour AG. Infection resistance and tolerance in Peromyscus spp., natural reservoirs of microbes that are virulent for humans. Semin Cell Dev Biol 2017;61: 115–22.
9. Applegren ND, Kraus CK. Lyme disease: emergency department considerations. J Emerg Med 2017;52(6):815–24.
10. Schell E, Saks M. Erythema migrans in a healthy female. Vis J Emerg Med 2018; 13:125–6.
11. Cardenas-de la Garza JA, De la Cruz-Valadez E, Ocampo-Candiani J, et al. Clinical spectrum of lyme disease. Eur J Clin Microbiol Infect Dis 2019;38(2):201–8.
12. Radolf JD, Strle K, Lemieux JE, et al. Lyme disease in humans. Curr Issues Mol Biol 2021;42:333–84.
13. Marx GE, Leikauskas J, Lindstrom K, et al. Fatal lyme carditis in new england: two case reports. Ann Intern Med 2020;172(3):222–4.
14. Arvikar SL, Steere AC. 5. Diagnosis and treatment of lyme arthritis. Infect Dis Clin North Am 2015;29(2):269–80.
15. Stanek G, Strle F. Lyme borreliosis–from tick bite to diagnosis and treatment. FEMS Microbiol Rev 2018;42(3):233–58.
16. Lantos PM. Chronic lyme disease. Infect Dis Clin North Am 2015;29(2):325–40.
17. Holzbauer SM, Kemperman MM, Lynfield R. Death due to community-associated clostridium difficile in a woman receiving prolonged antibiotic therapy for suspected lyme disease. Clin Infect Dis 2010;51(3):369–70.
18. Mead P, Petersen J, Hinckley A. Updated CDC recommendation for serologic diagnosis of lyme disease. MMWR Morb Mortal Wkly Rep 2019;68. https://doi.org/10.15585/mmwr.mm6832a4.
19. Lantos PM, Rumbaugh J, Bockenstedt LK, et al. Clinical Practice Guidelines by the Infectious Diseases Society of America (IDSA), American Academy of Neurology (AAN), and American College of Rheumatology (ACR): 2020 Guidelines for the Prevention, Diagnosis and Treatment of Lyme Disease. Clin Infect Dis 2021;72(1):e1–48.
20. Spencer RR. Rocky mountain spotted fever. J Infect Dis 1929;44(4):257–76.

21. Jay R, Armstrong PA. Clinical characteristics of rocky mountain spotted fever in the united states: a literature review. J Vector Borne Dis 2020;57(2):114.

22. Gottlieb M, Long B, Koyfman A. The evaluation and management of rocky mountain spotted fever in the emergency department: a review of the literature. J Emerg Med 2018;55(1):42–50.

23. Lin L, Decker CF. Rocky mountain spotted fever. Dis Mon 2012;58(6):361–9.

24. Hardstone Yoshimizu M, Billeter SA. Suspected and confirmed vector-borne rickettsioses of north america associated with human diseases. Trop Med Infect Dis 2018;3(1):2.

25. Wood H, Artsob H. Spotted fever group rickettsiae: a brief review and a Canadian perspective. Zoonoses Public Health 2012;59(Suppl 2):65–79.

26. Biggs HM, Behravesh CB, Bradley KK, et al. Diagnosis and management of tick-borne rickettsial diseases: rocky mountain spotted fever and other spotted fever group rickettsioses, ehrlichioses, and Anaplasmosis — United States. MMWR Recomm Rep (Morb Mortal Wkly Rep) 2016;65. https://doi.org/10.15585/mmwr.rr6502a1.

27. Archibald LK, Sexton DJ. Long-Term Sequelae of Rocky Mountain Spotted Fever. Clin Infect Dis 1995;20(5):1122–5.

28. Dantas-Torres F. Rocky mountain spotted fever. Lancet Infect Dis 2007;7(11): 724–32.

29. Kirkland KB, Wilkinson WE, Sexton DJ. Therapeutic delay and mortality in cases of rocky mountain spotted fever. Clin Infect Dis 1995;20(5):1118–21.

30. Todd SR, Dahlgren FS, Traeger MS, et al. No visible dental staining in children treated with doxycycline for suspected rocky mountain spotted fever. J Pediatr 2015;166(5):1246–51.

31. Bakken JS, Dumler JS. Human granulocytic anaplasmosis. Infect Dis Clin North Am 2015;29(2):341–55.

32. Stone JH, Dierberg K, Aram G, et al. Human monocytic ehrlichiosis. JAMA 2004; 292(18):2263.

33. Dumler JS, Bakken JS. Ehrlichial diseases of humans: emerging tick-borne infections. Clin Infect Dis 1995;20(5):1102–10.

34. Pritt BS, Munderloh UG, McElroy KM, et al. Emergence of a new pathogenic ehrlichia species, Wisconsin and Minnesota, 2009. N Engl J Med 2011;365(5):422–9.

35. Dumler JS, Barbet AF, Bekker CP, et al. Reorganization of genera in the families Rickettsiaceae and Anaplasmataceae in the order Rickettsiales: unification of some species of Ehrlichia with Anaplasma, Cowdria with Ehrlichia and Ehrlichia with Neorickettsia, descriptions of six new species combinations and designation of Ehrlichia equi and "HGE agent" as subjective synonyms of Ehrlichia phagocytophila. Int J Syst Evol Microbiol 2001;51(6):2145–65.

36. Centers for Disease Control and Prevention. National Notifiable Diseases Surveillance System (NNDSS) AnnualSummary Data for years 2016-2019, United States. http://wonder.cdc.gov/nndss-annual-summary.html. [Accessed 16 August 2023].

37. Olano JP, Hogrefe W, Seaton B, et al. Clinical manifestations, epidemiology, and laboratory diagnosis of human monocytotropic ehrlichiosis in a commercial laboratory setting. Clin Diagn Lab Immunol 2003;10(5):891–6.

38. Ismail N, Bloch KC, McBride JW. Human ehrlichiosis and anaplasmosis. Clin Lab Med 2010;30(1):261–92.

39. Olano JP, Masters E, Hogrefe W, et al. Human monocytotropic ehrlichiosis, Missouri. Emerg Infect Dis 2003;9(12):1579–86.

40. Paddock CD, Childs JE. Ehrlichia chaffeensis: a prototypical emerging pathogen. Clin Microbiol Rev 2003;16(1):37–64.

41. Kobayashi KJ, Weil AA, Branda JA. Case 16-2018: a 45-year-old man with fever, thrombocytopenia, and elevated aminotransferase levels. In: Cabot RC, Rosenberg ES, Pierce VM, et al, editors. N Engl J Med 2018;378(21):2023–9.

42. Sykes DB, Zhang EW, Karp Leaf RS, et al. Case 10-2020: An 83-year-old man with pancytopenia and acute renal failure. N Engl J Med 2020;382(13):1258–66.

43. Scribner J, Wu B, Lamyaithong A, et al. Anaplasmosis-induced hemophagocytic lymphohistiocytosis: a case report and review of the literature. Open Forum Infect Dis 2023;10(5):ofad213.

44. Wormser GP, Dattwyler RJ, Shapiro ED, et al. The clinical assessment, treatment, and prevention of lyme disease, human granulocytic anaplasmosis, and babesiosis: clinical practice guidelines by the infectious diseases society of America. Clin Infect Dis 2006;43(9):1089–134.

45. Waked R, Krause PJ. Human babesiosis. Infect Dis Clin North Am 2022;36(3):655–70.

46. Diuk-Wasser MA, Vannier E, Krause PJ. Coinfection by ixodes tick-borne pathogens: ecological, epidemiological, and clinical consequences. Trends Parasitol 2016;32(1):30–42.

47. Kjemtrup AM, Conrad PA. Human babesiosis: an emerging tick-borne disease. Int J Parasitol 2000;30(12–13):1323–37.

48. Patel KM, Johnson JE, Reece R, et al. Babesiosis-associated Splenic Rupture: Case Series From a Hyperendemic Region. Clin Infect Dis 2019;69(7):1212–7.

49. Ryan R, Krause PJ, Radolf J, et al. Diagnosis of babesiosis using an immunoblot serologic test. Clin Diagn Lab Immunol 2001;8(6):1177–80.

50. Teal AE, Habura A, Ennis J, et al. A new real-time PCR assay for improved detection of the parasite Babesia microti. J Clin Microbiol 2012;50(3):903–8.

51. Krause PJ, Lepore T, Sikand VK, et al. Atovaquone and azithromycin for the treatment of babesiosis. N Engl J Med 2000;343(20):1454–8.

52. Krause PJ, Auwaerter PG, Bannuru RR, et al. Clinical practice guidelines by the infectious diseases society of america (IDSA): 2020 guideline on diagnosis and management of babesiosis. Clin Infect Dis 2021;72(2):e49–64.

53. CDC. Tularemia data and surveillance | CDC. centers for disease control and prevention. 2022. https://www.cdc.gov/tularemia/statistics/index.html. [Accessed 24 August 2023].

54. Maurin M. Francisella tularensis, tularemia and serological diagnosis. Front Cell Infect Microbiol 2020;10:512090.

55. Johansson A, Berglund L, Sjöstedt A, et al. Ciprofloxacin for treatment of tularemia. Clin Infect Dis 2001;33(2):267–8.

56. World Health Organization. WHO guidelines on tularaemia. 2007:115.

57. Gritsun TS, Lashkevich VA, Gould EA. Tick-borne encephalitis. Antiviral Res 2003;57(1–2):129–46.

58. Hermance ME, Thangamani S. Powassan virus: an emerging arbovirus of public health concern in North America. Vector Borne Zoonotic Dis Larchmt N 2017;17(7):453–62.

59. Piantadosi A, Solomon IH. Powassan virus encephalitis. Infect Dis Clin North Am 2022;36(3):671–88.

60. Raval M, Singhal M, Guerrero D, et al. Powassan virus infection: case series and literature review from a single institution. BMC Res Notes 2012;5:594.

61. Commins SP, Satinover SM, Hosen J, et al. Delayed anaphylaxis, angioedema, or urticaria after consumption of red meat in patients with IgE antibodies specific for galactose-α-1,3-galactose. J Allergy Clin Immunol 2009;123(2):426–33.e2.

62. Young I, Prematunge C, Pussegoda K, et al. Tick exposures and alpha-gal syndrome: a systematic review of the evidence. Ticks Tick-Borne Dis. 2021;12(3): 101674.
63. Thompson JM, Carpenter A, Kersh GJ, et al. Geographic distribution of suspected alpha-gal syndrome cases — United States, January 2017–December 2022. MMWR Morb Mortal Wkly Rep 2023;72(30):815–20.
64. Commins SP. Diagnosis & management of alpha-gal syndrome: lessons from 2,500 patients. Expert Rev Clin Immunol 2020;16(7):667–77.
65. Eisen L. Personal protection measures to prevent tick bites in the United States: Knowledge gaps, challenges, and opportunities. Ticks Tick-Borne Dis 2022; 13(4):101944.
66. Leal B, Zamora E, Fuentes A, et al. Questing by tick larvae (acari: ixodidae): a review of the influences that affect off-host survival. Ann Entomol Soc Am 2020; 113(6):425–38.
67. Felz MW, Durden LA. Attachment sites of four tick species (acari: ixodidae) parasitizing humans in georgia and south carolina. J Med Entomol 1999;36(3):361–4.
68. CDC. Preventing tick bites on people. CDC. Centers for Disease Control and Prevention; 2020. https://www.cdc.gov/ticks/avoid/on_people.html. [Accessed 23 August 2023].
69. Eisen L, Dolan MC. Evidence for Personal protective measures to reduce human contact with blacklegged ticks and for environmentally based control methods to suppress host-seeking blacklegged ticks and reduce infection with lyme disease spirochetes in tick vectors and rodent reservoirs. J Med Entomol 2016;tjw103. https://doi.org/10.1093/jme/tjw103.
70. Garber B, Glauser J. Tick-borne illness for emergency medicine providers. Curr Emerg Hosp Med Rep 2019;7(3):74–82.
71. Tick CDC. removal | CDC. centers for disease control and prevention. 2022. https://www.cdc.gov/ticks/removing_a_tick.html. [Accessed 24 August 2023].

# Plant Dermatitis

Veronica Diedrich, DO, Kara Zweerink, MD, Brandon Elder, MD*

## KEYWORDS

- Plant dermatitis • Poison ivy • Poison oak • Poison sumac • Contact dermatitis
- Phytophototoxic dermatitis • Phytophotoallergic dermatitis • Pseudophytodermatitis

## KEY POINTS

- The most common cause of plant dermatitis in North America comes from exposure to the chemical urushiol secreted from the *Toxicodendron* species (poison ivy family).
- Mortality of plant dermatitis is typically low, but the morbidity can be significant from a health care cost and economic impact.
- The categories of plant dermatitis are irritant, allergic contact, contact urticaria, phytophototoxic, and photoallergic. Pseudophytodermatitis can also cause cutaneous reactions and mimic true plant dermatitis.
- Prevention of exposure by barrier protection (clothing, appropriate protective gear, and gloves) is the best means of addressing this health condition for those who work and recreate in areas, where these plants thrive.
- The mainstays of treatment for plant dermatitis are supportive with corticosteroids and antihistamines. Soaps and Inactivating chemicals have shown mild efficacy if used close to the timing of chemical exposure.

## BACKGROUND, PREVALENCE, AND HEALTHCARE IMPACT

North America has a wide variety of poisonous plants. The Toxicodendron genus, which includes poison ivy, poison oak, and poison sumac, is the most common cause of diagnosed acute allergic contact dermatitis in North America, and it is estimated to affect approximately 10 to 50 million Americans per year.[1,2] It is estimated that 85% of the United States population is allergic and approximately 10% to 15% are extremely allergic to poison ivy and its relatives.[1] Studies have suggested that sensitization to the offending chemical found in the Toxicodendron genus species plants, urushiol, typically occurs in adolescence, between the ages of 8 and 14, and that infants are not as susceptible (**Figs 1** and **2**).[3]

While the mortality from plant dermatitis is usually low, the morbidity, as well as cost of care and loss of wages related to this condition can be significant. For example, a visit to an urgent care for a plant-related dermatitis or injury has been estimated to cost

Department of Emergency Medicine, 2301 Holmes Street, Kansas City, MO 64108, USA
* Corresponding author. Department of Emergency Medicine, 2301 Holmes Street, Kansas City, MO 64108.
*E-mail address:* brandon.elder.md@gmail.com

Emerg Med Clin N Am 42 (2024) 613–638
https://doi.org/10.1016/j.emc.2024.03.001
0733-8627/24/© 2024 Elsevier Inc. All rights reserved.

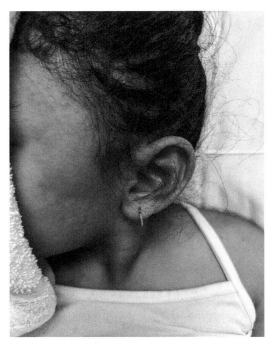

**Fig. 1.** Facial/Auricular plant dermatitis - 7 year old female with Poison Ivy "Toxicodendron radicans" exposure. (Photo credit: Brandon Elder, MD.)

just under $200, while an emergency department visit can incur costs of up to 3 times as much.[4] The Centers for Disease Control and Prevention (CDC) reported that the number of emergency department visits related to allergic contact dermatitis due to poison ivy was 929,290 in 2012, which is nearly doubled from 2002, which recorded 472,000 visits.[5] This is a concerning trend as our general population continues to explore the outdoors more and climate volatility has facilitated increasing atmospheric $CO_2$ levels, which has led to increased biomass of the plants and increased urushiol potency that cause plant dermatitis.[6] The United States Forest Services reported that dermatitis from Toxicodendron genus plants resulted in 10% loss of time due to injury related rash.[7] In areas of the country, where there are significant forest fire efforts, such as California, Oregon, and Washington, it has been estimated that one-third of firefighters are afflicted with dermatitis related to Toxicodendron species each fire season. According to the state of California, in 2014, the cost for worker's compensation related to plant dermatitis is approximately 1% of the 11.4 billion dollar budget, annually.[8]

This article will explore the known types of plant dermatitis, standard treatments, prevention, and novel advances in care of patients at risk for and afflicted by these conditions.

## CLASSIFICATIONS

Plant dermatitis can be classified into several different categories: Irritant, allergic contact, contact urticaria, phytophototoxic, and photoallergic. Pseudophytodermatitis can also cause cutaneous reactions and mimic true plant dermatitis (**Table 1**).

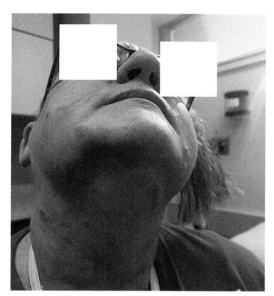

**Fig. 2.** A mild case of facial plant dermatitis (Poison Ivy "Toxicodendron radicans" exposure). (Photo Credit: Veronica Diedrich, DO.)

### Irritant Contact Dermatitis

Irritant contact dermatitis is the most common cause of contact dermatitis, causing approximately 80% of all reactions.[18] Irritant dermatitis can further be subclassified based on mechanism into mechanical and chemical. Mechanical dermatitis is due to traumatic injury of tissues. Trauma is usually caused by sharp structures that scratch, impale, or lacerate the skin and result in wounds and excoriations.[18] Trichomes (hairs), glochids (barbed hairs), spines, and thorns are common causes of mechanical dermatitis.[18,19] While mechanical dermatitis is due solely to trauma and does not, by nature, involve host immune response, it can play an important role in enhancing penetration and in chemical irritant and allergic effects.[18]

Chemical irritant dermatitis is due to an inflammatory response localized to cutaneous tissues.[18] Presentations vary greatly based on the characteristics of the irritant, volume and duration of exposure, and host-protective factors. Common chemical irritants and presentations are listed in **Table 2**. Irritant contact dermatitis does not cause an antigen specific immune response but does cause proinflammatory cytokine release leading to inflammation.[18]

Photoirritant, or phototoxic dermatitis, is another type of irritant dermatitis. In this reaction, cutaneous irritation happens from light activated irritants. Reactions include erythema, edema, and bullae. This is caused by necrosis of keratinocytes.[20] More mild reactions can also be seen resulting only in hyperpigmentation or lichenoid reactions.[20] In contrast to photoallergic dermatitis, reactions occur on first exposure to substances and symptoms take minutes to days to occur.[20]

### Allergic Contact Dermatitis

Allergic contact dermatitis is caused by an immune mediated response to molecular allergens in plants. This is a type IV delayed hypersensitivity reaction.[21] The causative haptens are usually water insoluble and found in plant resins, or oleoresins.[19] The

**Table 1**
**Types of plant dermatitis**

| Subtype of Plant Dermatitis | Example of Offending Agent | Example of Clinical Manifestation |
|---|---|---|
| Mechanical | Cactus bristles can cause a mechanical plant dermatitis[8] Photo credit: *Veronica Diedrich, DO* | Mechanical plant dermatitis, with linear and punctate lesions, from willow bushes Photo credit: Kara Zweerink, MD |

Irritant contact

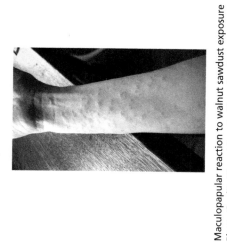

Maculopapular reaction to walnut sawdust exposure

Photo Credit: Kiera. I love it, I hate it. The Bennett House. December 20, 2012. Accessed September 6, 2023. http:// bennetthousediary.blogspot.com/2012/12/i-love-it-i-hate-it.html.

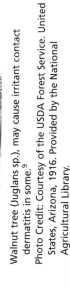

Walnut tree (Juglans sp.), may cause irritant contact dermatitis in some.[9]

Photo Credit: Courtesy of the USDA Forest Service. United States, Arizona, 1916. Provided by the National Agricultural Library.

(continued on next page)

**Table 1**
*(continued)*

| Subtype of Plant Dermatitis | Example of Offending Agent | Example of Clinical Manifestation |
|---|---|---|
| Allergic contact | <br>Poison ivy and poison oak (Toxicodendron spp) are the most common cause of plant dermatitis.[10–12]<br>Photo Credit: Robert H. Mohlenbrock. USDA SCS, 1991, Southern wetland flora: Field office guide to plant species. | <br>Mild Plant Derm - Poison Ivy "Toxicodendron radicans" exposure<br>Photo Credit: Brandon Elder, MD<br>6/13/23 |

Contact urticaria

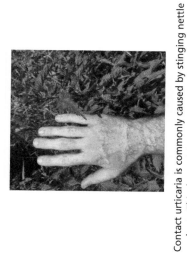

Stinging nettle (Urtica dioica), a common cause of contact urticaria.[10–12]

Photo Credit: Shari Hagwood, United States, Idaho, Bureau of Land Management Jarbridge Resource Area, June 25th 2003.

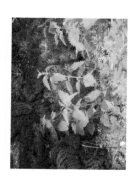

Contact urticaria is commonly caused by stinging nettle plants. This dermatitis presents as raised lesions with surrounding edema and erythema[10–12]

(continued on next page)

**Table 1**
*(continued)*

| Subtype of Plant Dermatitis | Example of Offending Agent | Example of Clinical Manifestation |
|---|---|---|
| Phytophototoxic contact | 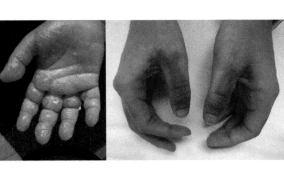 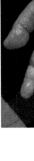 Lime tree (Tilia sp.), the juice of limes reacts upon sun exposure. [13]<br>Photo Credit: Smithsonian open access database, John G Jack 8/28/21 | 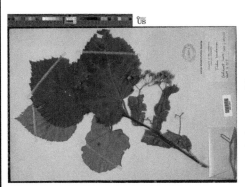 Limes are a common cause of phytophototoxic dermatitis, with the often dubbed "Margarita rash" presenting as significant erythema, possible bullae, and hyperpigmentation [13]<br>Photo Credit: *Phytophotodermatitis- Marjanovic D. Category:phytophotodermatitis. Wikimedia Commons. December 7, 2008. Accessed September 1, 2023.* https://commons.wikimedia.org/wiki/Category: Phytophotodermatitis. |

Phytophotoallergic contact

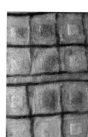

Musk ambrette (Abelmoschus moschatus), a common fragrance additive in perfumes, may cause photoallergic reactions.[14]

Photo Credit: Tracey Slotta. Provided by ARS Systematic Botany and Mycology Laboratory.

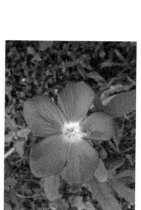

A photoallergic reaction may occur due to various perfume fragrances including musk ambrette. This can present as a variety of dermatoses including maculopapular, blistering, and hives. Patch testing can help identify these allergens.[14]

Photo Credit: Sviineviken (https://commons.wikimedia.org/wiki/File:2+_reaction.jpg), "2+ reaction", https://creativecommons.org/publicdomain/zero/1.0/legalcode

(continued on next page)

**Table 1**
*(continued)*

| Subtype of Plant Dermatitis | Example of Offending Agent | Example of Clinical Manifestation |
|---|---|---|
| Pseoudophytodermatitis | **ACARINA > PEDICULOIDIDAE** *Pyemotes ventricosus* (Newport) (female, dorsal aspect)<br><br>Straw itch mite (Acari and Pyemotes), the causative organism. An example of "Grain itch" rash, secondary to straw itch mites. Often mistaken for phytodermatitis due to recent plant exposure.[15–17]<br>Photo Credit: Straw itch mites. www.agric.wa.gov.au. Accessed August 19, 2023. https://www.agric.wa.gov.au/feeding-nutrition/straw-itch-mites | Erythematous vesiculopapular lesions caused by *Pyemotes ventricosus.*<br>Photo Credit: Parsons P. Details - public health image library(phil). Centers for Disease Control and Prevention. Accessed September 1, 2023. https://phil.cdc.gov/Details.aspx?pid=20199. |

*Data from refs.[9–17]*

**Table 2**
Irritant contact dermatitis

| Irritant | Mechanism of Action | Cutaneous Symptoms | Common Sources |
|---|---|---|---|
| Calcium oxalate | Mechanical irritation from sharp raphides (needlelike crystal bundles of salt), allow penetration of other plant chemical toxins and irritants, and induce histamine release from mast cells | Pruritus, erythema, vesicular, and bullous eruptions are most common on fingertips and hands | Dieffenbachia, flower bulbs |
| Protoanemonin | Ranunculin (a glycoside) hydrolyzes on maceration of plant tissue to protoanemonin. This combines with sulfhydryl groups in skin and disrupts disulfide bonds. | Transient contact-skin warmth, burning, and irritation<br>Sustained contact-erythema, edema, vesiculation, bullae, ulceration, and residual hyperpigmentation | Ranunculaceae (buttercup) family |
| Isothiocyanates | Myrosinase from plant injury hydrolyzes glucosides to isothiocyanates, which react with amino-groups of proteins | Transient burning, erythema, and urticaria | Brassicaceae mustard oils |
| Diterpene esters (phorbol, daphnane, diterpene) | Corrosive irritation, activate intracellular protein kinase C, and can cause tumorigenesis | Pain, erythema, edema, bullae, conjunctivitis, and blindness | Euphorbiaceae (spurges) |
| Bromelain | Contains proteases, phosphatases, and peroxidase that cause proteolysis. | Cutaneous irritation, fissures, and loss of fingerprints | Pineapple (ananas comosus) |
| Capsaicin/alkaloids | Alkaloid that binds with vanilloid receptors on neurons, resulting in sensation of heat and pain | Cutaneous burning and erythema, smooth muscle stimulation, glandular secretion, vasodilation, and does not blister as only nerves are affected. | Solanaceae family, Narcissus |
| Juglone | Aromatic naphthoquinone causing irritating and staining chemical injury | Irritant dermatitis and noninflammatory hyperpigmentation | Juglandaceae (walnut trees) |

*Data from* Refs.[18,19]

most common causes of allergic contact dermatitis are from plants in the *Toxicodendron* genus: poison ivy, poison oak, and poison sumac.[21] Urushiol is the major allergen found in the *Toxicodendron* species. This chemical can be found well distributed about the plant including the leaves, stems, and root systems. Exposure can be through direct contact with the plant or by indirect contact with contaminated items such as clothing, gloves, shoes, or pets.[22] Numerous substances from a variety of plant species can cause this reaction (**Table 3**).

### Contact Urticaria

Contact urticaria is a non-immunologic reaction thought to be due to irritation from chemical or mechanical trauma.[21] This is a type 1 hypersensitivity reaction.[19] The name of the reaction urticaria comes from the stinging nettle plant, which is from the family Urticaceae. The plant has stinging trichomes, which inject histamine, formic acid, and acetylcholine into the skin. This causes pruritus and erythema that can last up to 12 hours.[21] Ricin, a poisonous substance found in castor bean seeds, is also a common cause contact urticaria.[19]

### Phytophotodermatitis

Exposure to furanocoumarin from plants and ultraviolet A (UVA) light causes a phototoxic reaction known as phytophotodermatitis.[21] Psoralens are the active particles in furanocoumarins and are commonly found in plants in the Rutacea family (lemons and limes), parsley, celery, and carrots.[21,23] In phytophotodermatitis reactions, psoralen intercalates into double stranded DNA and causes intrastrand cross-linking when exposed to UVA light.[21] This leads to erythema, blistering, epidermal necrosis, and desquamation.[23] Symptoms usually occur about 24 hours after exposure and peak in 48 to 72 hours.[23] After the initial reaction, post-inflammatory hyperpigmentation can occur due to both melanin ingestion by melanophages and increase in the number of functional melanocytes and melanosomes.[23]

### Photoallergic Dermatitis

Photoallergic dermatitis is caused by a delayed hypersensitivity reaction to light activated antigens.[21] Chromophores in the plants absorb radiant energy, producing a photochemical change. This photoproduct then conjugates to a protein carrier, where it can be processed by antigen presenting cells and activate the immune response.[20] Clinically, photoallergic dermatitis presents as an eczematous response with pruritus and erythema.[20] Reactions do not occur on first exposure but require previous sensitization. On subsequent exposures, onset of symptoms is typically 24 to 48 hours.[20] Implicated causes are musk ambrette, sandalwood oil, diallyl disulfide, alantolactone, *Arnica montana*, sesquiterpene, lactone, pyrethrum, and *Tanacetum vulgare*.[23]

### Pseudophytodermatitis

Pseudophytodermatitis is not mediated by plants themselves, but secondarily applied substances or plant inhabitants. These commonly include waxes, dyes, insecticides, or arthropods.[21] Mites, which frequently infect grains or other foods, can cause dermatitis. For instance, the North American itch mite, *Pymotes ventricosus*, has a bite that causes a hemorrhagic and papular eruption. This rash is often mistakenly believed to have been caused by contact with straw.[24] Pseudophytophotodermatitis may also be seen. Celery is the most frequent plant implicated. A phytophotodermatitis-like reaction such as severe sunburns can be caused as a result of contact with Celery infected with pink rot. Furocoumarin made by the fungus, *Sclerotinia sclerotiorum* is the underlying etiology of both pink rot and this photosensitization reaction.[24]

**Table 3**
Allergic contact dermatitis

| Molecular Allergen | Clinical Symptoms | Common Sources |
|---|---|---|
| Urushiol | Pruritus, erythematous papules, plaques, and vesicles in linear distribution, black dot dermatitis | Anacardiaceae: Toxicodendron (poison ivy, poison oak, or poison sumac) |
| Sesquiterpene lactones | Erythema and scaling on face, neck, and upper chest, may progress to photosensitivity and chronic actinic dermatitis or erythroderma | Compositae/Asteraceae (ragweed, sneezeweed, orchrysanthemums) |
| Tulipalin A (α-methylene-ɣ-butyrolactones) | Dysesthesias, pulpitis with hyperkeratosis and fissuring of fingertips, and paronychia | Alstroemeriaceae, Liliaceae (tulip) |
| Unknown:Daffodil itch | Erythema, urticarial appearing papules, and eczematous dermatitis | Amaryllidaceae (daffodil) |
| Phenylacetaldehyde (hyacinthine) | Erythema and erythematous papular dermatitis | Thought to be hapten for hyacinth |
| Allicin and diallyl disulfide | Hyperkeratotic and fissured dermatitis of first 3 fingers on non-dominant hand | Alliaceae (garlic, chives, and onions) |
| Primin (2-methoxy-6-pentylbenzoquinone) | Edematous to papulovesicular lesions on fingertips, dorsal fingers, and hands, streaky or linear eruption | Primula obconica (primrose) |
| D nigra (R-4-methoxydalbergione) | Irritation and dermatitis | Dalbergia nigra (brazilian rosewood/Jacaranda) |
| Colophony (rosin) | Irritation, and dermatitis | Pinaceae (pine trees) |
| Sandalwood and ylang-ylang | Irritation dermatitis | Evergreen trees |

Data from refs.[19,21]

## PREVENTION

Individuals who engage in outdoor activities for recreation or occupation can take various precautions to protect themselves against plant dermatitis. Prevention is the best defense for plant dermatitis and relies on providing public health and patient specific education on ways to minimize exposure. One method for minimizing exposure is the use of clothing barriers. Clothing barriers may include gardening gloves, long pants and sleeves, and boots.[25,26] Some plants require a specific material of barrier. For instance, Toxicodendron irritants are soluble in rubber or latex, so vinyl or leather gloves may be recommended.[21,27–29] Alternatively, the allergen of the Peruvian lily penetrates most materials other than nitrile gloves.[30] Additionally, the allergic substance urushiol maintains its potency, even when dried or dead, and can be harbored in fingernails, clothing, and pet fur.[5,29,31] Specifically, warm or wet clothing may actually trap the toxin against the skin, causing an aggressive allergic reaction.[29,31,32]

Topical barrier creams have variable efficacy. Acting as a barrier of sorts, organoclay preparations may limit patient response when applied prior to exposure.[26] Various ingredients in barrier creams may limit movement of plant antigens and toxins prior to contact with skin.[21] For Toxicodendron species, application of Food and Drug Administration (FDA)-approved quaternium-18 bentonite lotion 5% has been shown to minimize or negate dermatitis.[2,21,27] Additional studies have shown statistically significant reduction in overall dermatitis for the following products: Stokogard (Stockhausen), Hollister Moisture Barrier (Hollister Inc.), and Hydropel (Genesis Pharmaceuticals).[2]

Phytophotodermatitis prevention relies on minimizing sun exposure and application of effective sunscreens that block both UVA and ultraviolet B (UVB) rays. For instance, UVA light activates psoralen-mediated dermatitis after only 30 minutes on skin.[21] Additionally, physicians may provide patient education on recognizing offending plants to further prevent exposure. This may include public health efforts to remove such plants from local parks or personal gardens.[26] After exposure occurs, washing with dish soap may help minimize absorption or reaction to the irritant. The sooner after exposure the better, at 10 minutes 50% of urushiol can be removed, while at 1 hour washing is no longer effective at removing the toxin.[32]

## TREATMENT

There is an enormous amount of lore surrounding plant dermatitis that goes beyond "Leaves of three, let them be". Myths recommend putting bleach or alcohol on rashes to help them dry up. As with any caustic material the application of these to the skin will only further irritate. Additional concerns arise due to the belief that the rash is contagious. If the oil has been washed off with soap and contaminated clothing removed, plant dermatitis rashes are merely an allergic manifestation with no contagious properties.[26]

After lore suggesting that Native Americans chewed poison ivy leaves to become desensitized, a small randomized controlled trial was conducted over 5 weeks showing that chewing leaves had no change in sensitization compared to placebo.[26] Rather, ingestion of the material often caused potent gastroenteritis.[33]

For all plant contact dermatitis patients, topical steroids can be given to reduce pruritus and improve overall symptoms (**Box 1**). Topical steroids are most effective early in disease course, applying clobetasol 0.05% BID may help symptoms. However, once vesicles develop, topical steroids are of little utility. Additionally, steroids are not recommended for sensitive areas such as face, genitals, or intertriginous regions.[30,34,35] In severe cases, systemic steroids may be considered. It is recommended to start oral therapy for severe cases such as: those involving 20% body surface area; involvement of face, hands, or genitals; and severe blistering or itching (**Table 4**).

---

**Box 1**
**Potency of topical Corticosteroids[37,38]**

   I. Ultra-high Potency
      Betamethasone dipropionate 0.05%
      Clobetasol propionate 0.05%
      Diflorasone diacetate 0.05%
      Fluocinonide 0.1%
      Halobetasol propionate 0.05%
      Amcinonide 0.1%

  II. High potency
      Desoximetasone (0.05%–0.25%)
      Fluocinonide 0.05%
      Halcinonide 0.1%

 III. Medium to high potency
      Fluticasone propionate 0.005%
      Triamcinolone acetonide 0.5%
      Betamethasone valerate 0.1%
      Fluocinolone acetonide 0.025%
      Hydrocortisone butyrate 0.1%

 IV. Medium potency
      Hydrocortisone valerate 0.2%
      Mometasone furoate 0.1%
      Triamcinalone acetonide (0.1%–0.025%)
      Alclometasone dipropionate

  V. Low to medium potency
      Flurandrenolide 0.05%
      Fluocinolone acetonide 0.025%

 VI. Low potency
      Desonide 0.05%
      Fluocinolone 0.01%

VII. Least potent
      Hydrocortisone (1%–2.5%)

Typically, ointment formulations have the highest potency, followed by creams, then gels or solutions.

(Note: classification may vary by source.)

*Data from* Refs.[39,40]

---

A 3 week course with taper is recommended to prevent rebound dermatitis.[26,36] An expert recommended regimen may include Prednisone at 1 mg/kg per day with slow tapering; however, there are few evidence based guidelines on this subject.[26,30,34,37] Discussing medication side effects with patients may help manage expectations. Specifically, these long courses of steroids can cause weight gain, mood instability, insomnia, and nausea.[38]

Additional supportive therapy includes cold compresses, oatmeal baths, and antihistamines for symptomatic relief.[21] However, antihistamines may be of questionable utility for some subtypes of plant dermatitis. For instance, the allergic response to urushiol may not be mediated by antihistamines, but rather the interleukin system and mast cells.[29,30,42]

Additional symptomatic therapy may include calamine lotion or diluted aluminum acetate solutions such as Burrow's solution. Use of topical antihistamines or anesthetics is not recommended due to risk for sensitization.[26,42]

**Table 4**
**Characteristics and potency of oral steroids[41]**

| Glucocorticoid | Relative Equivalent Dosage (mg) | Glucocorticoid: Mineralocorticoid Activity | Duration of Action (hrs) | Other Information |
|---|---|---|---|---|
| Hydrocortisone | 20 | 1:1 | 8–12 | Short acting and used more for adrenal insufficiency |
| Cortisone | 25 | 0.8:0.8 | 8–12 | Short acting |
| Prednisone | 5 | 4:0.8 | 12–36 | Intermediate acting and excellent anti-inflammatory agent |
| Prednisolone | 5 | 4: 0.8 | 12–36 | Intermediate acting and excellent anti-inflammatory agent |
| Methylprednisolone | 4 | 5:0 | 12–36 | Intermediate acting and excellent anti-inflammatory agent |
| Triamcinolone | 4 | 5:0 | 12–36 | Intermediate acting and excellent anti-inflammatory agent |
| Dexamethasone | 0.75 | 30:0 | 36–72 | Long acting, reserved for short-term use in extremely acute situations |
| Betamethasone | 0.6 | 30:0 | 36–72 | Long acting |

Recommendations for systemic therapy in plant dermatitis typically come from intermediate acting agents with high glucocorticoid:mineralocorticoid activity. *Data from* Refs.[41]

Occasionally, patients may present with anaphylactic reactions to various irritants from plants. In contrast to the typical presentation of rash 24 to 72 hours after exposure (a Type IV hypersensitivity reaction), an anaphylactic reaction would occur rapidly after exposure (a Type I hypersensitivity reaction). This would be managed as is typical - with intramuscular epinephrine, followed by steroids and Histamine-1/Histamine-2 blocking agents. Additional anaphylactoid reactions are possible, presenting like anaphylaxis with variable response to treatment (bradykinin-mediated).[30]

Any plant dermatitis consisting of open wounds should receive tetanus prophylaxis. Immunocompromised patients may be at risk for superinfection with bacterial or fungal components. These patients should take extra care in keeping rashes and wounds clean and dry. Additionally, the risks and benefits of further immunosuppression secondary to systemic steroids must be addressed depending on the etiology of immunosuppression. Patients on chronic steroids represent an interesting subgroup of the immunocompromised. Some individuals who are immunocompromised may have difficulty mounting a sufficient T-cell mediated response to truly have symptoms. Those with asthma have been noted to have decreased susceptibility. The true cause of this is unknown, but hypotheses include avoidance of outdoor activities due to asthma symptoms and decreased immune function at baseline.[6,21]

## COMPLICATIONS OF MECHANICAL PLANT INJURY

Mechanical plant injury leaves affected individuals at risk for secondary infections. This can be due to disruption of the protective barrier of the skin and subcutaneous tissue or through direct inoculation of infectious organisms from the spines, hairs, or thorns themselves.[18] Infectious complications can be classified into bacterial and fungal etiologies (**Table 5**). In addition to secondary infection, the body's immune system can cause complications from mechanical plant injury. For example, implanted cactus needles have been implicated as a cause of aseptic foreign body granulomas.[24] Thorns have also been found to cause periosteal reactions when embedded near bones and can mimic tumors.[24]

## PUBLIC HEALTH ADVANCES IN PLANT DERMATITIS MANAGEMENT

While plant dermatitis is often a broad public health concern, there is little in the way of research driving future dermatologic advances. Some recent research suggests that the itching component of plant dermatitis is often modulated independently of histamine receptors, and is rather interleukin mediated, specifically IL-33.[3,30] Topical tacrolimus and pimecrolimus have shown some promise in recent small scale studies, leading to reduced itchiness associated with contact dermatitis.[3] The use of topical JAK/STAT inhibitors has been suggested as a new potential modality to augment the cytokine pathway and inflammation induced plant dermatitis conditions. It is currently approved for psoriatic and rheumatoid arthritis, but it is currently being studied in its role for numerous other skin conditions - further, large scale studies are required before adopting this as a mainstay treatment.[3,30]

Additionally, there are further studies on barrier creams that may be effective, particularly in chemical warfare situations that could subsequently be applied to plant dermatitis conditions.[42,47,48] Specifically, a military Topical Skin Protectant substance has been tested on animals to protect against chemical warfare, but experiments in humans have used urushiol patch testing to emulate an exposure.[47,48] In post-exposure prophylaxis, over the counter urushiol inactivating chemicals and soaps, like Tecnu and Zanfel, have shown mild efficacy if used within a short duration from time of exposure, but some studies suggest a longer duration of papules and longer

**Table 5**
Common sources and symptoms for mechanical plant injury complications

| Organism | Type | Common Introducing Mechanism | Clinical Symptoms |
|---|---|---|---|
| Clostridium tetani | Bacterial | Spines and thorns | Generalized muscular rigidity, muscle contractions, and autonomic instability |
| Staphylococcus aureus | Bacterial | Black thorns | Cellulitis (erythema, warmth, or tenderness), abscesses |
| Mycobacteria (kansasii, marinum, ulcerans) | Bacterial | Kansasii-blackberry bushes Marinum-cactus spines Ulcerans-tropical vegetation | Lymphadenitis, marinum-localized erythema and granuloma formation of digits, hands, and forearms Ulcerans- Buruli ulcer (large areas of skin involvement, deep ulceration, marked disfiguration) Kansasii-large fibrocavities in apex of lung, cellulitis |
| Actinomyces | Bacterial | Vegetable fragments | Progressive, painless, indurated mass, possible bluish coloration of overlying skin, multiple abscesses with sinus tract formation, and yellow sulfur granule drainage |
| Sporothrix schenckii | Fungal | Rose thorns, sphagnum moss, grasses, and cornstalks | Nodular eruption at inoculation site and draining lymphatics |

Data from Refs.[18,43–46]

duration of signs and symptoms when topical soaps are used as primary treatment.[30,32] After further research was conducted on the biochemistry of urushiol, The University of Mississippi recently developed a prototype for the "Poison Ivy Vaccine" - a synthetic version of the active component of urushiol (PDC-APB).[49]

Similar to the North Americas, some countries are taking public health action and removing invasive causes of plant dermatitis from public areas.[6]

## CLIMATE CHANGE AND NEW CHALLENGES

Unfortunately, climate change has, and will continue to have, an effect on plant dermatitis. For example, elevated levels of carbon dioxide have induced the native *Toxicodendron* genus to produce a more allergenic form of urushiol, the oil-toxin responsible for the rash.[6,49,50] Additionally, during forest fires, urushiol can become aerosolized and cause airway inflammation and diffuse dermatitis.[50] Giant hogweed has also become more invasive secondary to rising temperatures and carbon dioxide-labels. The sap can cause photodermatitis with blistering; a condition with increasing prevalence amongst outdoor workers.[2,10,11,51]

---

**Table 6**
**Invasive dermatitis-causing plants and their distributions**

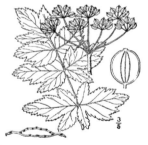

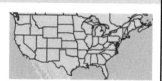

Distribution of invasive spread of wild Parsnip

Wild Parsnip (*Pastinaca sativa*). An invasive cause of phytophotodermatitis.
Photo Credit: Britton, N.L., and A. Brown, 1913, An illustrated flora of the northern United States, Canada and the British Possessions. 3 vols. Provided by Kentucky Native Plant Society, New York. Scanned By Omnitek Inc.

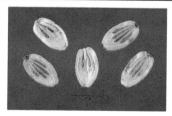

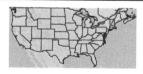

Distribution of invasive spread of Giant Hogweed

Seeds of Giant Hogweed (Heracleum mantegazzianum) an invasive cause of phytodermatitis
Photo Credit: Steve Hurst ARS Systematic Botany and Mycology Laboratory. Belgium, Gembloux

---

*Data from refs.[9,47]*

**Table 7**
**A selection of native dermatitis-causing plants and their distribution**

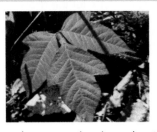

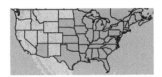

Native distribution of common poison ivy

*T. Radicans* (common poison ivy and eastern poison ivy)
Photo Credit: Common poison ivy - Anderson J. *Toxicodendron Radicans (L.) Kuntze Eastern Poison Ivy.*; 2001. Accessed August 31, 2023. https://plants.usda.gov/home/plantProfile?symbol=TORA2

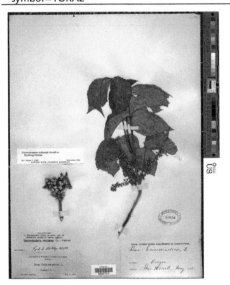

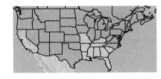

Native distribution of western poison ivy

*T. Rydbergii* (Western Poison Ivy).
Photo Credit: Western Poison Ivy- Howell T. *Toxicodendron Radicans Subsp. Rydbergii (Small & Rydb.).* (Löve A., Löve D., eds.).; 2019. Accessed August 31, 2023. Provided by Smithsonian Open Access, https://www.si.edu/object/toxicodendron-radicans-subsp-rydbergii-small-rydb-love-d-love:nmnhbotany_14861558

(*continued on next page*)

**Table 7**
*(continued)*

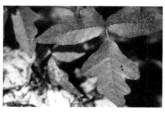

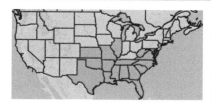

Native distribution of eastern poison oak

*T. toxicarium* and *T. pubescens* (eastern poison
oak and Atlantic poison oak)
Photo Credit: Eastern poison oak - Mohlenbrock
RH. *Toxicodendron Pubescens Mill. Atlantic
Poison Oak.*; 1991. Accessed August 31, 2023.
https://plants.usda.gov/home/plantProfile?
symbol=TOPU2

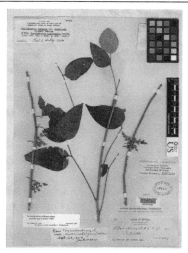

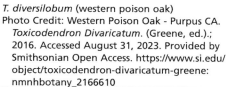

Native distribution of western poison oak

*T. diversilobum* (western poison oak)
Photo Credit: Western Poison Oak - Purpus CA.
*Toxicodendron Divaricatum.* (Greene, ed.).;
2016. Accessed August 31, 2023. Provided by
Smithsonian Open Access. https://www.si.edu/
object/toxicodendron-divaricatum-greene:
nmnhbotany_2166610

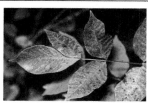

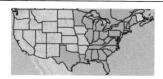

Native distribution of poison sumac

*T. Vernix* (poison sumac)

*(continued on next page)*

| Table 7 |
| --- |
| (*continued*) |
| Photo Credit: Robert H. Mohlenbrock. USDA SCS, 1991, Southern wetland flora: Field office guide to plant species. Provided by USDA NRCS Wetland Science Institute (WSI), Fort Worth.USDA, NRCS. 2023. PLANTS Database (https://plants.sc.egov.usda.gov/, 08/30/2023). National Plant Data Team, Greensboro, NC 27401–4901 USA.<br>D |

*Data from ref.*[9]

Many species that cause plant dermatitis are classified as invasive in the environments they thrive (**Table 6**). As these plants continue to grow and outcompete native flora, more episodes of dermatitis are expected. Multiple causes of phytophotodermatitis are non-native: The Giant Hogweed (H. mantegazzianum) is native to Asia, but aggressive in New York and surrounding areas; Wild Parsnip (Pastinaca sativa) is native to Asia and Europe, but is invasive in the United States.[2,50] To adequately address this issue, it is important to monitor the distribution of the most common, native, and dermatitis-inducing species (eg, *Toxicodendron*,) as they compare to the evolving distribution of invasive and dermatitis-inducing species (**Table 7**).[2,50,52–54]

If there are to be strides made against plant dermatitis, clinicians must realize that the continued volatility of the climate pushes imbalance to our ecosystems, and thus, complicates the care of our patients and perpetuates the medico-financial burden onto the North American populace.

## SUMMARY

Plant dermatitis is a common, usually low-mortality condition that can have significant morbidity and impact on healthcare burden and cost in North America. It is of the utmost importance for today's clinician to be familiar with the types of plant dermatitis and the common flora associated with this condition in their region.

The best way to address this condition is through prevention by reduction in exposure to common urushiol secreting plants, such as the *Toxicodendron* species, and dawning appropriate personal protective equipment and barrier clothing. The mainstays of treatment continue to be supportive care with corticosteroids and antihistamines, though pre- and post-exposure prophylaxis agents including soaps, inactivating chemicals, immunomodulators, and vaccines have shown some efficacy in condition improvement, but further studies are needed for validation.

The continued disruption of our ecosystem's homeostasis by climate change and increasing carbon dioxidelevels in the atmosphere is resulting in increased biomass of common plant-dermatitis-causing species and increases in chemical potency of urushiol. If any progress is to be seen against plant dermatitis, clinicians, and our society, must unite against the ever-looming threat of global warming.

## CLINICS CARE POINTS

- Plant dermatitis affects 10 to 50 million Americans per year with just under 1 million emergency department visits per year

- Plant dermatitis can be classified into several different categories: echanical, irritant, allergic contact, contact urticaria, phytophototoxic, and photoallergic. Pseudophytodermatitis can also cause cutaneous reactions and mimic true plant dermatitis.
- Plant dermatitis can be caused by a variety of processes, including traumatic injury of tissues, local inflammation, immune responses, and exogenous activation of benign structures
- Toxicodendron (poison ivy and its relatives), the most common genus of plant causing plant dermatitis in the United States, causes a type IV hypersensitivity reaction leading to an allergic contact dermatitis
- Prevention via clothing, barrier creams, and patient education is paramount to minimizing the effects of plant dermatitis. Treatment starts with thorough washing of skin and can be expanded to both topical and oral steroid regimens. Complications of secondary bacterial infections are not uncommon.
- Plant dermatitis can lead to break down of the body's innate immune system and predispose to secondary infections.
- New areas of research in Plant Dermatitis include immunomodulator treatments and an early phase "poison ivy vaccine"
- Climate change has been noted to cause increase in Urushiol potency (the oil-toxin responsible for rash) in the Toxicodendron genus.

## DISCLOSURE

The authors have no disclosures or conflicts of interest to report.

## REFERENCES

1. American Skin Association. Poison ivy, sumac and oak. 2020. Available at: https://www.americanskin.org/resource/poisonivy.php.
2. Gladman AC. Toxicodendron dermatitis: poison ivy, oak, and sumac. Wilderness Environ Med 2006;17:120–8.
3. Fisher A, Mitchell J. Toxicodendron plants and spices. In: *Fisher's contact dermatitis*. 4th edition. Baltimore (MD): Williams & Wilkins; 1995. p. 461–523.
4. Zomorodi N, Butt M, Maczuga S, et al. Cost and diagnostic characteristics of Toxicodendron dermatitis in the USA: a retrospective cross-sectional analysis. Br J Dermatol 2020;183:772–3.
5. Labib A, Yosipovitch G. Itchy Toxicodendron Plant Dermatitis. Allergies 2022; 2(1):16–22.
6. Mohan JE, Ziska LH, Schlesinger WH, et al. Biomass and toxicity responses of poison ivy (Toxicodendron radicans) to elevated atmospheric $CO_2$. Proc Natl Acad Sci USA 2006;103(24):9086–9.
7. Oltman J, Robert H. Poison oak/ivy and forestry workers. Clin Dermatol 1986;4: 213–6.
8. Epstein WL. Occupational poison ivy and oak dermatitis. Clin Dermatol 1994;12: 511–6.
9. Cactus Dermatitis. Available at: https://escholarship.org/content/qt87v8v850/cholla2.html. [Accessed 19 August 2023].
10. Foti C, Romita P, Angelini G, et al. Allergic contact dermatitis to walnut (Juglans Regia) husk. Indian J Dermatol 2015;60(6):622.
11. USDA, NRCS. PLANTS Database. Greensboro (NC): National Plant Data Team; 2023. Available at: https://plants.sc.egov.usda.gov/.
12. Sharma VK, Sethuraman G. Parthenium Dermatitis. Dermatitis 2007;18(4):183–90.

13. Kim Y, Flamm A, ElSohly MA, et al. Poison Ivy, Oak, and Sumac Dermatitis: What Is Known and What Is New? Dermatitis 2019;30(3):183–90.
14. Abugroun A. Lime-induced phytophotodermatitis. Oxford Medical Case Reports 2019;2019(11). Available at: https://academic.oup.com/omcr/article/2019/11/470/5670819. [Accessed 19 August 2023].
15. Photocontact Dermatitis — DermNet. dermnetnz.org, Available at: https://dermnetnz.org/topics/photocontact-dermatitis. Accessed September 11, 2023.
16. Straw itch mites. Available at: https://www.agric.wa.gov.au/feeding-nutrition/straw-itch-mites. [Accessed 19 August 2023].
17. Itch mites. Available at: https://www.missouribotanicalgarden.org/gardens-gardening/your-garden/help-for-the-home-gardener/advice-tips-resources/pests-and-problems/insects/mites/itch-mites. [Accessed 19 August 2023].
18. Modi GM, Doherty CB, Katta R, et al. Irritant contact dermatitis from plants. Dermatitis 2009;20(2):63–78. Available at: https://search-ebscohost-com.proxy.library.umkc.edu/login.aspx?direct=true&db=cmedm&AN=19426612&site=ehost-live&scope=site. [Accessed 31 July 2023].
19. Sheehan MP. Plant Associated Irritant & Allergic Contact Dermatitis (Phytodermatitis). Dermatol Clin 2020;38(3):389–98. https://doi.org/10.1016/j.det.2020.02.010.
20. DeLeo V. Photocontact Dermatitis. Immunol Allergy Clin 1997;17(3):451–69. https://doi.org/10.1016/S0889-8561(05)70321-0.
21. Watchmaker L, Reeder M, Atwater AR. Plant Dermatitis: More Than Just Poison Ivy. Cutis 2021;108(3):124–7. https://doi.org/10.12788/cutis.0340.
22. Lee NP, Arriola ER. Poison ivy, oak, and sumac dermatitis. West J Med 1999;171:354.
23. Baugh WP. Phytophotodermatitis. Medscape.. 2021. Available at: https://emedicine.medscape.com/article/1119566-overview#a4. [Accessed 1 August 2023].
24. Stoner JG, Rasmussen JE. Plant dermatitis. J Am Acad Dermatol 1983;9(1):1–15. https://doi.org/10.1016/s0190-9622(83)70104-0.
25. Plant dermatitis | DermNet NZ. dermnetnz.org, Available at: https://dermnetnz.org/topics/plant-dermatitis. Accessed September 11, 2023.
26. Sadovsky R. Poison Ivy, Oak and Sumac Contact Dermatitis. Am Fam Physician 2000;61(11):3408. Available at: https://www.aafp.org/pubs/afp/issues/2000/0601/p3408.html.
27. Marks JG, Fowler JF, Sherertz EF, et al. Prevention of poison ivy and poison oak allergic contact dermatitis by quaternium-18 bentonite. J Am Acad Dermatol 1995;33:212–6.
28. UpToDate, Beyond the Basics Patient Education, Available at: https://www.uptodate.com/contents/poison-ivy-beyond-the-basics/print. Accessed September 11, 2023.
29. Grevelink SA, Murrell DF, Olsen EA. Effectiveness of various barrier preparations in preventing and/or ameliorating experimentally produced Toxicodendron dermatitis. J Am Acad Dermatol 1992;27(2 Pt 1):182–8.
30. Vaught CK, Mold JW. Poison ivy: How effective are available treatments? J Fam Pract 2016;65(11):801–9. Available at: https://pubmed.ncbi.nlm.nih.gov/28087871/. [Accessed 17 August 2023].
31. Bolognia J, Jorizzo JL, Schaffer JV, McGovern TW. Dermatoses due to plants. *Dermatology*. 3rd ed. Philadelphia, PA: Elsevier Saunders; 2012. p. 273–89.
32. Stibich AS, Yagan M, Sharma V, et al. Cost-effective post-exposure prevention of poison ivy dermatitis. Int J Dermatol 2000;39(7):515–8.

33. Lofgran T. and Mahabal G., Toxicodendron Toxicity. PubMed, Available at: https:// www.ncbi.nlm.nih.gov/books/NBK557866/, 2020. Accessed September 11, 2023.
34. Vernon HJ, Olsen EA. A controlled trial of clobetasol propionate ointment 0.05% in the treatment of experimentally induced Rhus dermatitis. J Am Acad Dermatol 1990;23(5 Pt 1):829–32.
35. Goodall J. Oral corticosteroids for poison ivy dermatitis. CMAJ (Can Med Assoc J) 2002;166(3):300–1.
36. Wallis C. A Vaccine against Poison Ivy Misery Is in the Works as Scientists Also Explore New Treatment Paths. Sci Am. Available at: https://www.scientific american.com/article/a-vaccine-against-poison-ivy-misery-is-in-the-works-as-scientists-also-explore-new-treatment-paths/. [Accessed 17 August 2023].
37. Brodell RT, Williams L. Taking the itch out of poison ivy. PGM (Postgrad Med) 1999;106(1):69–70.
38. Neill BC, Neill JA, Brauker J, et al. Postexposure prevention of Toxicodendron dermatitis by early forceful unidirectional washing with liquid dishwashing soap. J Am Acad Dermatol 2019;81(2):e25.
39. Ference JD, Last AR. Choosing Topical Corticosteroids. Am Fam Physician 2009; 79(2):135–40. Available at: https://www.aafp.org/pubs/afp/issues/2009/0115/ p135.html#afp20090115p135-b24. [Accessed 19 August 2023].
40. Table: Relative Potency of Selected Topical Corticosteroids. Merck Manuals Professional Edition. Available at: https://www.merckmanuals.com/professional/ multimedia/table/relative-potency-of-selected-topical-corticosteroids. [Accessed 19 August 2023].
41. Liu D, Ahmet A, Ward L, et al. A practical guide to the monitoring and management of the complications of systemic corticosteroid therapy. Allergy Asthma Clin Immunol 2013;9(1):30.
42. Klein PA, Clark RAF. An Evidence-Based Review of the Efficacy of Antihistamines in Relieving Pruritus in Atopic Dermatitis. Arch Dermatol 1999;135(12). https://doi. org/10.1001/archderm.135.12.1522.
43. You AX, Carden DL, Moll J. Tetanus. In: Tintinalli JE, Ma O, Yealy DM, et al, editors. Tintinalli's Emergency Medicine: a Comprehensive Study Guide, 9e. New York, NY: McGraw Hill; 2020. p. 456–7. Accessed August 09, 2023.
44. Kelly E.W., Soft Tissue Infections, In: Tintinalli J.E., Ma O., Yealy D.M., et al., Tintinalli's Emergency Medicine: a Comprehensive Study Guide, 9e, 2020, McGraw Hill, New York, NY, 436- 441. Available at: https://accessmedicine-mhmedical-com.proxy.library.umkc.edu/content.aspx?bookid=2353&sectionid=220292152 (Accessed 9 August 2023).
45. Winburn B, Sharman T. Atypical Mycobacterial Disease. 2022. Available at: https://search-ebscohost-com.proxy.library.umkc.edu/login.aspx?direct=true& db=cmedm&AN=32310577&site=ehost-live&scope=site. [Accessed 9 August 2023].
46. Sharma S., Hashmi M.F. and Valentino I.I.I.D.J., Actinomycosis, In: Valentino D.J., III, Koirala J. and Tobin E.H., StatPearls, 2023, StatPearls Publishing; Treasure Island (FL), 1 - 7.
47. Liu D, Wannemacher RW, Snider TH, et al. Efficacy of the topical skin protectant in advanced development. 1999. Available at: https://doi.org/10.1002/(sici)1099-1263(199912)19:1+%3Cs40::aid-jat614%3E3.0.co;2-h.
48. Vidmar DA, Iwane MK. Assessment of the ability of the topical skin protectant (TSP) to protect against contact dermatitis to urushiol (Rhus) antigen. Am J Contact Dermatitis 1999;10(4):190–7.

49. Derriak J. Heracleum mantegazzianum and Toxicodendron succedaneum: plants of human health significance in New Zealand and the National Pest Plant Accord. N Z Med J 2007;120(1259). Available at: http://www.nzma.org.nz/journal/120-1259/2657/. [Accessed 17 August 2023].

50. Giant Hogweed – New York Invasive Species Information. Nyis.info., Available at: https://nyis.info/invasive_species/giant-hogweed/, 2022. Accessed September 15, 2023.

51. Giant Hogweed and Lookalikes: Giant Hogweed: Horticulture: APH: Maine ACF. Available at: https://www.maine.gov/dacf/php/horticulture/hogweedlookalikes.shtml. [Accessed 19 August 2023].

52. Daw S., Pacific Poison Oak. NPS.gov, Available at: https://www.nps.gov/articles/000/pacific-poison-oak.htm, 2020. Accessed September 15, 2023.

53. Fertig W. Plant of the Week: Western Poison-ivy (Toxicodendron rydbergii). U.S. Forest Service USDA. Available at: https://www.fs.usda.gov/wildflowers/plant-of-the-week/toxicodendron_rydbergii.shtml. [Accessed 17 August 2023].

54. Mazza G, Tricarico E, Genovesi P, et al. Biological invaders are threats to human health: an overview. Ethol Ecol Evol 2013;26(2–3):112–29.

# Animal Bites and Attacks

Sarah Schlein, MD[a,*], Andrew Park, DO[a], Sameer Sethi, MD[a]

## KEYWORDS

- Bites • Wounds • Rabies • Bats • Bears

## KEY POINTS

- Prevention of injury and illness from animal bites and attacks involves heightened awareness around animals and appropriate postexposure prophylaxis.
- Thorough irrigation, debridement, and cleansing with povidone-iodine is standard management for all animal bites and wounds.
- A bat found in a sleeping space upon waking requires rabies vaccine for all patients and rabies immunoglobulin for all non–previously immunized individuals.
- Rabies postexposure prophylaxis in non–previously immunized individuals includes human rabies immunoglobulin, 20 IU/kg, injected at the bite site, plus the 4-series rabies vaccine injected at a distant site.
- When threatened by a brown bear, the recommendation is to avoid eye contact and play dead if attacked. When threatened by a black bear, the recommendation is to be loud and aggressively fight back.

## INTRODUCTION

The human-animal interface is a source of complex health risks, including unique infectious disease vectors as well as blunt and penetrating trauma. Prevention, risk, and medical management of animal-human injuries are reviewed in later discussion. Detailed considerations for wild and domestic animal bites and wounds will give readers confidence in their management, both in wilderness settings and in the clinical environment. Particular care is taken to describe situations of rabies exposure risk, prophylaxis, and postexposure management. This review of risk and prevention provides appropriate responses to a selection of animal attacks, from both large and small animals. This text is divided into sections on animal bites, rabies, and animal attacks.

## ANIMAL BITES
### Background and Epidemiology

According to the 2017 to 2018 US Pet Ownership and Demographics Sourcebook, there are approximately 76.8 million dogs and 58.3 million cats owned in the United

[a] Larner College of Medicine, University of Vermont, 111 Colchester Avenue, Burlington, VT 05401, USA
* Corresponding author. 111 Colchester Avenue, Burlington, VT 05401.
E-mail addresses: sarah.schlein@uvmhealth.org; sarahmschlein@gmail.com

Emerg Med Clin N Am 42 (2024) 639–652
https://doi.org/10.1016/j.emc.2024.02.019
0733-8627/24/© 2024 Elsevier Inc. All rights reserved.

emed.theclinics.com

States.[1] Although some attacks are predatory in nature, the vast majority are caused by animals fearing humans.

Dog bites are most commonly seen among boys aged 5 to 9 years, whereas cat bites are generally seen in elderly women.[1] Veterinary and animal control workers are at a unique risk for injuries. Recommendations on the management of animal bites are largely based on data available from domestic dogs and cats. Animal bites can cause a variety of injuries, including puncture wounds and crush injuries. Because of oral flora, animal bites are typically polymicrobial and can lead to serious infection.

### General Wound Management

Early wound management for all animal bites is instrumental in reducing the risk of bacterial and viral infections. Irrigation should be completed with 1% to 5% povidone-iodine in normal saline, if available.[2] In out-of-hospital settings, potable water (preferably boiled and cooled) is a reasonable option, especially if wound care will otherwise be significantly delayed. Ideally, irrigation should be delivered with at least 7 psi of pressure via syringe.[2] Diluted, soapy water is another alternative, but should be followed by irrigation with nonsoapy water. Debridement of crushed and devitalized tissue is a key step in wound care, as it removes contaminants more effectively than irrigation alone. Irrigation of deep puncture wounds is less effective. Plain films can help evaluate for fractures and retained foreign bodies.[2]

### Antibiotic Prophylaxis

There is mixed evidence regarding the use of antibiotic prophylaxis to reduce the risk of infection. The use of prophylactic antibiotics has the strongest evidence in distal extremity wounds, especially of the hands. High-risk wounds, as well as patients at high risk for infection, should be considered for prophylactic antibiotics (**Table 1**). High-risk wounds include puncture wounds, wounds associated with crush injury, and wounds on the hands or feet, or over a joint. Asplenia, diabetes, immunocompromised state, and chronic heavy alcohol use are associated with high risk of infection.[2] Antibiotic

**Table 1**
**Infection risk associated with patient and wound factors**

| Factor | High Risk | Low Risk |
|---|---|---|
| Species | Cat<br>Monkey<br>Human | Dog (excluding hands and feet)<br>Rodent |
| Wound location | Hand<br>Foot | Face<br>Scalp |
| Wound type | Puncture<br>Crush<br>Devitalized tissue<br>Delayed presentation >6 h<br>Closed primarily | Laceration<br>Superficial |
| Patient factors | Age >50 y<br>Diabetes<br>Renal failure<br>Liver disease<br>Alcohol use disorder<br>Immunocompromise | |

*Adapted from* Walls R, Hockberger R, Gausche-Hill M, Erickson TB, Wilcox SR. Rosen's Emergency Medicine - Concepts and Clinical Practice E-Book: 2-Volume Set. 10th ed. Elsevier; 2022.

recommendations are summarized in **Table 2**. For wounds that are at higher risk of infection in the backcountry when definitive care is delayed and antibiotics are not available, honey can be applied to the wound for its antibiotic properties.[3,4] Routine wound cultures at the time of injury have not been shown to be predictive of a causative organism in an infection.[2]

## Wound Closure

The decision to complete primary closure of wounds from animal bites must be made after consideration of the risk of infection and the importance of the cosmetic outcome. Facial wounds heal well, with a lower risk of infection, but with an increased concern for good cosmetic outcome.[5] Primary closure after appropriate wound care is recommended in most facial wounds. A single-layer closure is optimal to reduce the risk of infection.[2] Glue is not advised. Conversely, hand or foot bites have a much higher risk of infection.[6] Most evidence suggests that primary closure of hand wounds is associated with an increased risk of infection and thus not advised.[7] Wounds with high-risk features and wounds in high-risk patients (see **Table 1**) can be left open for healing by secondary intention.[2]

## Tetanus

Tetanus immunization should be administered according to the patient's prior immunization status, most recent booster, and degree of wound contamination to prevent infection from *Clostridium tetani*. In clean wounds, no additional immunization is needed if the patient received a previous full course of tetanus immunization and a booster in the last 10 years. In a deep or contaminated wound, a patient should have received a full course of tetanus immunization and a booster in the last 5 years.[7] If the patient is unsure about their immunization status or has not received a childhood series, they should receive 0.5 mL of the diphtheria-tetanus or Tdap booster as well as 250 to 500 IU of tetanus human immune globulin.[2]

## Species Considerations

### Dogs

Dogs account for the vast majority of animal bites—upwards of 90% in some studies.[8] Dogs less than 1 year of age are most often involved. Young children are particularly

---

**Table 2**
**Empiric antibiotic options for bite wound prophylaxis and treatment**

| Antibiotic | Adult Dosing[a] | Pediatric Dosing (per dose)[a] |
|---|---|---|
| A. Amoxicillin-clavulanate (1st line) | 875/125 mg bid | 45 mg/kg bid |
| B. Metronidazole (2nd line with D, E, F, G, or H) | 500 mg tid | 10 mg/kg tid |
| C. Clindamycin (2nd line with D, E, F, G, or H) | 450 mg tid | 10 mg/kg tid |
| D. Doxycycline | 100 mg bid | Not preferred if < 8 y old |
| E. Trimethoprim-sulfamethoxazole | 160/800 mg bid | 4–5 mg/kg bid |
| F. Penicillin VK | 500 mg qid | 12.5 mg/kg qid |
| G. Cefuroxime | 500 mg bid | 10 mg/kg bid |
| H. Moxifloxacin | 400 mg qd | Not preferred in children |

[a] Duration of therapy for prophylaxis is 3 to 5 d, whereas treatment is 7 to 10 d.
*Adapted from Auerbach PS, Cushing TA, Harris NS. Auerbach's Wilderness Medicine, 2-Volume Set. 7th ed. Elsevier - Health Sciences Division; 2021.*[7]

susceptible owing to their small size and unintentional provoking of pets. *Pasteurella* spp are the most common pathogens implicated in dog bites, but *Staphylococcal* spp and *Streptococcal* spp are commonly seen as well.[9] Although relatively rare, *Capnocytophaga* spp are gram-negative rods and opportunistic pathogens implicated in invasive sepsis, putting immunocompromised patients at particular risk.[9]

### Cats

Although they have a weaker biting force than dogs, domestic cats account for about 5% to 15% of treated bites.[8] They also possess sharper teeth that lead to deeper puncture wounds and thereby pose an increased risk of infection. Cat bites inoculate many of the same organisms as dog bites, and therefore, antibiotic coverage is similar. However, cat bites are also associated with other diseases, in both immunocompetent and immunocompromised individuals.

*Bartonella henselae* is the causative agent in cat-scratch disease (or cat-scratch fever). Generally, cat-scratch disease is caused by scratches from cats, and there is an incubation period of 3 to 10 days. The diagnosis of cat-scratch disease relies on the presence of 3 out of 4 of the following features[7]:

1. Single or regional lymphadenopathy (usually in the affected extremity) leading to lymphadenitis
2. History of contact with a cat
3. An inoculation site
4. A positive skin test for cat-scratch

The skin test has largely fallen out of favor, so this is generally a clinical diagnosis. In most cases, symptoms resolve in 6 to 12 weeks.[7] Treatment is indicated in immunocompromised patients and those with severe or prolonged symptoms; however, some also recommend treatment in immunocompetent patients with a 5- to 10-day course of azithromycin.[7]

### Rodents

The risk of infection from rodent bites is cited as low as 2% and as high as 10%.[10] Rat-bite fever (or rat-bite disease) is a rare illness resulting from *Streptobacillus moniliformis* infection, a part of the normal oral flora in rodents. Symptoms include flulike symptoms, local lymphadenitis, and occasionally, septic arthritis. This is followed by a morbilliform or petechial rash often involving the palms of the hands and soles of the feet, and finally, a migratory polyarthritis. The disease process can be complicated by pericarditis, endocarditis, pneumonitis, and sepsis. The treatment of choice is penicillin.[7]

### Monkeys

Monkey bites have a high rate of infection despite prophylactic antibiotics. Herpes B virus infections must be considered in monkey bites, especially when macaque monkeys are involved. Bites, scratches, and exposure to blood or tissue (especially the brain) are primary modes of transmission. In the United States, occupational exposure is the primary risk factor. The incubation period is from 2 days to 5 weeks, after which a vesicular lesion at the site of exposure erupts with flulike symptoms. This is followed by symptoms of central nervous system (CNS) dysfunction, including paresthesias, muscle weakness, and ataxia. Prevention includes thorough wound decontamination immediately after exposure and prophylaxis with valacyclovir. Postexposure prophylaxis (PEP) should be offered for up to 5 days after exposure. Treatment of an active infection includes intravenous acyclovir or ganciclovir.[11]

## Summary

Although animal bites have the potential to lead to significant morbidity and mortality, most of them are avoidable with the appropriate precautions. Patient factors, location of the wounds, and particular species involved will determine the risk of infection. These factors will help determine whether a wound is closed by primary or secondary intention, and whether prophylactic antibiotics are indicated. The most important intervention is timely and thorough cleansing and debridement of the wound in order to reduce the risk of infection.

## CLINICS CARE POINTS—ANIMAL BITES

- Irrigation and debridement of an animal bite is a key and time-sensitive step in wound care, regardless of the location, patient factors, use of antibiotics, closure strategy, or setting.
- Wounds to the distal extremities are at highest risk of infection and should generally be left open and treated with prophylactic antibiotics.
- Wounds sustained from cat bites or scratches have a higher risk of infection and are associated with additional disease processes, such as cat-scratch disease.
- Although uncommon, monkey bites are at high risk of bacterial infection as well as infection with Herpes B virus, which carries a high morbidity and mortality.

## RABIES
### Background

Rabies is caused by the neurotropic RNA rabies virus, part of the Lyssavirus genus, Rhabdoviridae virus family. It causes at least 59,000 human deaths annually and is almost always fatal once symptoms appear. Rabies remains a large public health issue globally in places where domestic dogs are not widely vaccinated. In North America, most transmission comes from bats, raccoons, foxes, and skunks. Any mammal could carry rabies. Appropriate knowledge of when and how to treat possible bites and exposures can prevent more than 99% of deaths.[12] Once a person develops symptoms, the mean time to death is 17 days.[13]

Transmission can occur from a bite, mucus membrane contact, or, rarely, by high-quantity aerosolized inhalation.[14] Contact with urine, blood, or feces does not transmit the rabies virus; however, there has been one possible case of transmission from a mother to a breastfed infant.[14] Transplacental infection has been reported in skunks, cows, dogs, and bats and in some human case reports, whereas other case reports describe healthy human neonates despite active rabies infections in the mother.[14–18] The virus spreads from the exposure site to the CNS via retrograde axonal transport.[14] Antemortem diagnosis requires testing from multiple sources, including cerebral spinal fluid, nuchal skin biopsy, saliva, and serum. The post-mortem diagnosis gold standard is a brain biopsy.[19] Successful prevention requires vigilance to treat possible exposures before the virus penetrates the CNS.[14]

### Epidemiology

In 2019, 4690 of the 94,770 animals submitted for rabies testing in the United States tested positive. Of the total positive animals, 91.8% were wild, and the majority were bats, raccoons, foxes, and skunks. Of the few infected domestic animals, greater than 80% were dogs and cats. Other domesticated cases included cattle, horses, goats, sheep, ferrets, and a llama.[13] From 2000 to 2020, a total of 52 human rabies cases were confirmed in the United States. The mean age was 40, and 77% of human cases were in male patients. Foreign exposures, later diagnosed upon return to the United States, accounted for 14 of the 52 cases. Of the cases acquired in the United States, 82% were from bats, and 4 cases were from raccoons.[13] Only 35 of the 52 cases reported a known animal bite or contact. A total of 5 of the 52 cases were recipients of organ and tissue donation from 2 separate infected donors (through kidney, liver, and corneal transplants), leaving 12 of the 52 cases with unknown rabies exposure.[13,14] In India, dogs account for 95% of all reported cases. The most common reservoirs in South Africa are dogs and mongooses, whereas in Europe, foxes and raccoons are of greatest concern.[14]

### Signs/Symptoms

Rabies can present either with an encephalitis marked by hyperexcitability, hallucinations, bizarre behavior, disorientation, autonomic dysfunction, and hypersalivation or in a paralytic form that is characterized by weakness in the bitten extremity, with a risk of progression to paralysis.[14] Hydrophobia, a perceived appearance that the patient is unable to drink water, is present in 50% of patients. This is due to spasms of the larynx, pharynx, and diaphragm.[20] Death ultimately results from complications of respiratory failure, cardiac dysfunction, or autonomic dysfunction.[21]

### Preexposure Prophylaxis

Human rabies vaccines are all inactivated virus vaccines. The Centers for Disease Control and Prevention recommends either the human diploid cell culture vaccine (HDCV) or the produced chick embryo cell culture vaccine (PCECV).[22] There is no contraindication for vaccine administration, and it can be given safely in pregnancy and to very young children. Preexposure vaccination is important for high-risk professions such as veterinarians, laboratory workers, children in high-risk areas who play with unvaccinated dogs, and wildlife workers working directly with mammals. A 2-dose preexposure prophylaxis (PrEP) schedule has replaced the 3-dose PrEP schedule to protect for up to 3 years.[21]

### Postexposure Prophylaxis

Any possible exposure to the saliva of a wild animal or unvaccinated domestic mammal is an indication for PEP. In cases where a wild animal is vaccinated, such as in a wildlife rehabilitation program, PEP is still indicated, as the vaccine is only proven to be effective in domestic dogs and cats. Even if there are no bite wounds, any person found to have a bat in the room upon waking should receive PEP.[21]

Cleaning and irrigation of wounds with soap and water, and ideally a virucidal agent such as povidone-iodine, should be used for all wounds. For nonimmunized individuals, PEP includes both the rabies vaccine and the rabies immunoglobulin. The rabies vaccine is given in four 1-mL doses of HDCV or PCECV and should be administered intramuscularly (IM) to previously unvaccinated persons on days 0, 3, 7, and 14. The vaccine is administered in the deltoid for adults and the anterolateral thigh in children. The gluteal area results in lower neutralizing antibody titers so should not be used. PEP is not contraindicated in pregnant patients and unimmunized babies in the first few weeks of life. Immunosuppressive agents should not be administered during postexposure therapy unless essential for the treatment of other conditions. When PEP is administered to an immunosuppressed person, they should receive the current 4-dose vaccines schedule with an additional dose of vaccine on day 28 (1 mL IM in deltoid on days 0, 3, 7, 14, and 28).

All nonimmunized patients, of all ages, should also receive human rabies immunoglobulin (HRIG), 20 IU/kg, infiltrated in the area around and into the wounds with any remaining volume injected IM at a site distant from vaccine administration. For unvaccinated persons, HRIG and vaccine should be initiated regardless of the time interval between exposure and initiation of PEP. If PEP has been initiated and appropriate laboratory diagnostic testing indicates that the animal that caused the exposure was not rabid, PEP can be discontinued. Corticosteroids, immunosuppressive agents, and antimalarials can interfere with the development of active immunity after vaccination and should be avoided if possible. If HRIG was not administered when vaccination was begun, it can be administered up to 7 days after the administration of the first dose of the vaccine. In immunized patients, wounds still need to be thoroughly irrigated and cleaned with povidone-iodine—although no HRIG is indicated, they still require a 2 series (days 0 and 3) of the vaccine. A summary of PEP is provided in **Table 3**.

## Treatment

Patients with clinical rabies can be offered either supportive therapy or an aggressive treatment plan. There is no single effective treatment for rabies once clinical signs are evident. Although rabies has a mortality of nearly 100%, there are 20 cases of survivors reported globally.[21] The Milwaukee Protocol, which involves withholding vaccine/immunoglobulin, deep sedation, antiviral use, maintaining electrolyte balance, and management of vasoconstriction, has reported 10 survivors, all of whom were ages 4 to 17 years.[23]

## Summary

Rabies is an RNA virus that is almost uniformly fatal once symptoms appear. Any mammal can transmit rabies via a bite or mucus membrane contact. The virus spreads from the exposure site to the CNS via retrograde axonal transport. Signs and symptoms include encephalitis marked by hyperexcitability, hallucinations, bizarre behavior, disorientation, autonomic dysfunction, and hypersalivation; a paralytic form is characterized by weakness in the bitten extremity, with a risk of progression to paralysis. Management depends on the vaccination status of the patient. All wounds should be thoroughly irrigated and cleaned with povidone-iodine, and tetanus should be updated as indicated. Immunized patients should receive a 2 series (days 0 and 3) of the vaccine, without HRIG. Nonimmunized patients should receive a 4-series vaccine administration (days 0, 3, 7, 14), as well as 20 IU/kg of HRIG infiltrated in the area around and into the wounds, with any remaining volume injected IM at a site distant from vaccine administration.

**Table 3**
**Rabies postexposure prophylaxis based on vaccination status**

| Vaccination Status | Previously Vaccinated | NOT Previously Vaccinated |
|---|---|---|
| Wound cleansing | Immediately clean all wounds, irrigate with povidone-iodine | |
| Human rabies immunoglobulin (HRIG) | NO HRIG indicated | If possible, infiltrate full HRIG dose (20 IU/kg) into wound[b] |
| Vaccine | 2 SERIES (1 mL deltoid[a] day 0 and 3) | 4 SERIES (1 mL deltoid[a] day 0, 3, 7, 14) |

[a] Administer on the opposite side of the bite/exposure; for children, use the anterolateral thigh.
[b] Any remaining volume can be injected IM at a site distant from vaccine administration.
 *Adapted from CDC, Reference to specific commercial products, manufacturers, companies, or trademarks does not constitute its endorsement or recommendation by the U.S. Government, Department of Health and Human Services, or Centers for Disease Control and Prevention.*[21]

## CLINICS CARE POINTS—RABIES

- Any mammal can transmit rabies via a bite or mucus membrane contact. Appropriate knowledge of when and how to treat possible bites and exposures can prevent more than 99% of deaths if administered soon after the exposure.
- All wounds need to be thoroughly irrigated and cleaned with povidone-iodine, and tetanus vaccination needs to be updated as indicated.
- Immunized patients: human rabies immunoglobulin is not indicated; administer a 2 series (days 0 and 3) of the vaccine.
- Nonimmunized patients: a 4-series vaccine administration (days 0, 3, 7, 14), 20 IU/kg of human rabies immunoglobulin, infiltrated in the area around and into the wounds with any remaining volume is injected intramuscularly at a site distant from vaccine administration.

## ANIMAL ATTACKS
### Moose

Moose are tall animals with large body masses. Most attacks occur when people use poor judgment and/or are in unexpected proximity, especially when there are moose calves nearby. Dogs also provoke moose to attack, even if the dog is not approaching the moose. If an individual senses that a moose attack is imminent, they should hide behind some large object. If an individual has been knocked to the ground, they should assume the fetal position and protect their head.

### Yak

Yaks are encountered by many people when trekking in the Himalayas. They are beautiful animals but can weigh more than 900 kg. Yaks are like other animals when it comes to protecting their young and will act more aggressively if encountered with their young. Along the trails where people are most likely to have the greatest frequency of encounters with yaks, the best place to position oneself is on the uphill side of the trail. This is so that the individual is in a safer position than along the cliffside in the case of a yak collision.

### Bears

Bears can be found in most parts of the world, apart from Antarctica and Australia. Bear attacks typically occur when people encounter bears unexpectedly. The natural response of the bear is to remove the threat to themselves or their territory, such as people stopping to see bears near a roadway.[24] This kind of attack is typically more brief and less severe. A female bear with cubs typically responds to threats more aggressively. This kind of attack is also more common, accounting for 80% of all bear attacks.[25] Bears will also attack when provoked. Hunters who have wounded a bear are in an especially dangerous situation as they approach an injured bear; bears will attack with more aggression and for a prolonged time when in survival mode. Photographers also tend to get in dangerous proximity to bears, and this is often seen as an act of aggression by the bear.

### General concepts
**Prevention.** There are several steps one can take to help prevent unwanted interactions with bears in the wild. Making noise while out and walking around lets the bear know that people are in the area. Still, certain environmental factors may prevent

bears from sensing human presence. Individuals may need to make louder noises when traveling near a stream and in places where visibility is limited, such as in thick brush (where the bear will not be able to see humans approaching). Pay attention to clues that bears have been close by, such as watching for tracks, scat, or evidence of a fresh carcass.[26]

**Confrontations.** If confronted by a bear, one should avoid direct eye contact but let the bear know they are there by talking calmly, out loud. Remain visible and do not run.[27] These methods help the bear know that an individual is present, but that they are not aggressive and are willing to stand their ground.

**Management.** A victim of a bear attack should undergo a trauma evaluation for blunt injuries, in addition to other penetrating wounds. After wound debridement and irrigation, broad-spectrum antibiotics should cover for *Staphylococcus aureus* and gram-negative rods, in addition to anaerobes.

### Brown bears
Brown bear, including grizzly bear, attacks occur more frequently in recreational areas in national parks during peak tourist seasons and hunting seasons. There have been stable trends in most places over the last few decades, with some areas like Wyoming and Alaska experiencing increasing rates of bear encounters correlating with their increasing bear populations.[24]

**Confrontations.** If attacked by a brown bear, one should not run, fight back, or climb a tree. Bear spray should be the initial response to a close encounter with an aggressive bear. In one study of Alaskan bear attacks, bear spray was found to be 98% effective in deterring aggressive behavior and preventing injury from an attack.[28] If the bear continues an attack, one should lay prone or in a fetal position and cover their head with their hands over their ears. Do not look at the bear, partly because of the intimidation factor, but also to not expose the face. One should wait until they feel the bear has left the area to look around and go in the opposite direction.[29] If the bear has not left the area, attempting to flee can precipitate a second and even worse attack.

### Black bears
Black bears are the most widespread species of bears. They can be found in 30 of the lower 48 states. There is a trend of increasing bear sightings in different states, likely because of the adaptability of black bears. Black bear attacks typically result in less severe injuries when compared with other bears. With aggressive restriction of human food availability for bears, the number of bear encounters has declined significantly.[30]

**Confrontations.** If one is attacked by a black bear, aggressive actions are warranted. The individual should use bear spray, make loud noises, and make themselves appear larger than they are. They should fight back, yell, and throw rocks or other objects. Do not lie down and wait for the black bear to go away.

### Polar bears
Polar bears exist and hunt in the ice-covered seas of the arctic circle. Their diet consists primarily of seals. There are less reported attacks by polar bears primarily because there are less opportunities to interact with humans in these remote environments. Polar bear attacks are divided into 2 categories. Younger groups of polar bears typically display predatory behavior, whereas attacks from a mother bear protecting her cubs tend to be of the typical protective behavior.[31]

**Confrontations.** The human response to a polar bear attack may depend on the gender of the bear. A female with cubs is likely to respond more briefly to eliminate the perceived threat. Human response to this should be more submissive and nonthreatening, as in a grizzly bear attack. If the polar bear is roaming alone, it is more likely to be male and predatory in nature; human response in this situation should be more aggressive and defensive.

### Mountain Lion

Mountain lion attacks are infrequent but have been increasing over the last 30 years owing to increased exposure of humans to their range of movement and increasing populations.[32] Fatal and nonfatal attacks occur most often in children.[32] The mountain lion will stalk and pounce on its prey, with the goal of breaking the neck.[32] Because neck and head injuries are common, evaluation of a victim should include a trauma evaluation, especially of the neck for soft tissue and cervical spine injury. The best defense against an attack is to make oneself look large, make noise, and fight back.

### Porcupines

Porcupines do not often bite people, but rather use their quills to ward off potential offenders. A porcupine has approximately 30,000 quills, and each quill ranges in length from 1 to 4 inches.[32] The quills have a barbed feature that enables them to stay embedded in a victim. Once they penetrate the surface of the skin, they absorb fluid, expand, and work their way deeper in the tissue. This deeper penetration can cause injury to internal organs.[32]

Quills can be removed by extraction after local anesthesia. Infections are rare after a quill injury because of the antiseptic property of the quills.

### Farm Animals

#### Horses
Most horse injuries are a result of riders falling off while riding. Injuries to the head, upper extremities, and torso are common with this cause. Horses can also kick and produce significant blunt trauma to the body, causing severe internal injuries. Direct kicks to the head are frequent and tend to result in more hospitalizations and death in children than adults. Horses can also bite, but because of the flat characteristics of the teeth, they tend to result in less severe injuries. Wearing a helmet and being aware of body positioning around horses can prevent many injuries.[33]

**Management.** A victim who has fallen off from or been kicked by a horse has the potential for severe head and bodily injury and should have a thorough trauma evaluation. Bites from horses are typically polymicrobial with a mix of aerobic and anaerobic species. The *Actinobacillus* spp are gram-negative coccobacilli that are part of the normal oral flora of horses and are commonly found pathogens in infected bites. Augmentin is the first-line antibiotic treatment for horse bites.[34]

#### Cattle
Domestic cattle are large animals and can weigh up to 1300 kg. Their size and speed allow them to trample and butt victims and produce significant blunt trauma and crush injuries. Bulls can also hook victims with their horns, causing penetrating injuries to internal organs.

Attacks most commonly occur when victims are working with cattle, especially in confined spaces, such as moving cattle into pens or moving through stalls to tag or give injections. Spatial awareness and having an exit strategy is vital. Holding a long

**Table 4**
Summary of animal attacks, risk, and appropriate response

| Animal | Risk | Response to an Attack |
|---|---|---|
| Moose | Calving season<br>Provocation by dogs | Hide behind large object<br>Curl into ball & protect head if knocked to ground |
| Yak | Protecting young | Position oneself on uphill side of trail |
| Brown bear | Unexpected encounters<br>Females with cubs<br>Provoked by hunters/photographers | Make noise, avoid eye contact, remain visible, do not run/fight/climb<br>If attacked: bear spray, curl into ball & protect head |
| Black bear | Unexpected encounters<br>Females with cubs<br>Provocation<br>Unsecured food waste | Make noise, avoid eye contact, remain visible, do not run<br>If attacked: bear spray, fight back |
| Polar bear | Unexpected encounters<br>Females with cubs<br>Roaming male predator<br>Provocation | Make noise, avoid eye contact, remain visible, do not run/fight/climb<br>If attacked: bear spray, curl into ball & protect head |
| Mountain lion | Unexpected encounters<br>Activity in the proximity of the mountain lion may be seen as prey | Make noise, avoid eye contact, remain visible, do not run<br>If attacked: fight back |
| Porcupine | Unexpected encounter and direct contact with animal | Quill removal with local anesthesia and forceps |
| Horse | Ejection from horse while riding or if frightened<br>Positioning behind a horse | Wear helmet and use body awareness around horses |
| Cattle | Proximity in stalls while tagging and giving shots | Crawl to safe place |

stick can deter an approaching animal. If attacked and knocked to the ground, one should crawl to safety to try to prevent a second attack.[35]

**Management.** Traumatic wounds will need to be explored and thoroughly debrided. Trauma to the abdomen and other potential spaces can initially present as minor; however, the potential for significant internal organ damage is a possibility. Cattle can be infected with rabies, so any open wound will need to have rabies prophylaxis and tetanus vaccination updated as needed.

### Summary

Many large animal attacks in the wilderness, as well as farm animal injuries, can be prevented with knowledge of the animals and their patterns of interaction with humans. If confronted, knowing the appropriate response between a brown bear and black bear can be the difference between life and death. Patients sustaining an injury from large, wild animals must undergo a thorough trauma evaluation, with irrigation and debridement of all penetrating injuries. Rabies and tetanus prophylaxis should be considered as well (**Table 4**).

### CLINICS CARE POINTS—ANIMAL ATTACKS

- Prevention of large animal attacks starts with knowing the specific behavior patterns of the animals that may be encountered. This will help one prepare and know what to watch out for when they are in the wilderness and what to do if attacked.
- When threatened by a brown bear, one should stand their ground and not make eye contact. If attacked, one should play dead and cover their head with their hands. When threatened by a black bear or mountain lion, one should stand their ground, be loud, and fight back aggressively.
- Standard evaluation of a large animal attack in the wilderness or on the farm should include a thorough trauma evaluation for direct and indirect injuries sustained during the attack.
- Standard management of any animal injury includes copious irrigation, debridement, and postwound care, including rabies and antibiotic prophylaxis and tetanus vaccination, based on animal species and wound complexity.

### DISCLOSURE

The authors have no conflicts of interest to declare. The authors have no financial interest to report. All authors attest that this submission is original and not under review at any other publication entity.

### REFERENCES

1. U.S. pet ownership statistics. American Veterinary Medical Association. 2017-2018. Available at: https://www.avma.org/resources-tools/reports-statistics/us-pet-ownership-statistics. [Accessed 28 August 2023].
2. Walls R, Hockberger R, Gausche-Hill M, et al. Rosen's Emergency medicine - Concepts and clinical Practice E-Book: 2-volume Set. 10th edition. Elsevier; 2022. p. 659–97.
3. Phuapradit W, Saropala N. Topical application of honey in treatment of abdominal wound disruption. Aust N Z J Obstet Gynaecol 1992;32(4):381–4.

4. Tashkandi H. Honey in wound healing: An updated review. Open Life Sci 2021; 16(1):1091–100.
5. Aigner N, König S, Fritz A. Bissverletzungen und ihre besondere Stellung in der unfallchirurgischen Versorgung [Bite wounds and their characteristic position in trauma surgery management]. Unfallchirurg 1996;99(5):346–50.
6. Maimaris C, Quinton DN. Dog-bite lacerations: a controlled trial of primary wound closure. Arch Emerg Med 1988;5(3):156–61.
7. Auerbach PS, Cushing TA, Harris NS. Auerbach's wilderness medicine, 2-volume Set. 7th edition. Philadelphia, PA: Elsevier: Health Sciences Division; 2021. p. 618–44.
8. Griego RD, Rosen T, Orengo IF, et al. Dog, cat, and human bites: a review. J Am Acad Dermatol 1995;33(6):1019–29.
9. Capnocytophaga. In: Centers for Disease Control and Prevention. 2018. Available at: https://www.cdc.gov/capnocytophaga/index.html. [Accessed 28 August 2023].
10. Ordog GJ, Balasubramanium S, Wasserberger J. Rat bites: fifty cases. Ann Emerg Med 1985;14(2):126–30.
11. About Herpes B Virus. In: Centers for Disease Control and Prevention.2021. Available at: https://www.cdc.gov/herpesbvirus/about.html. [Accessed 28 August 2023].
12. Liu C, Cahill JD. Epidemiology of Rabies and Current US Vaccine Guidelines. R I Med J 2020;103(6):51–3.
13. Ma X, Monroe BP, Wallace RM, et al. Rabies surveillance in the United States during 2019. J Am Vet Med Assoc 2021;258(11):1205–20.
14. Mahadevan A, Suja MS, Mani RS, et al. Perspectives in Diagnosis and Treatment of Rabies Viral Encephalitis: Insights from Pathogenesis. Neurotherapeutics 2016;13(3):477–92.
15. Howard DR. Transplacental transmission of rabies virus from a naturally infected skunk. Am J Vet Res 1981 Apr;42(4):691–2.
16. Afshar A. A Review of Non-Bite Transmission of Rabies Virus Infection. Br Vet J 1979;135(2):142–8.
17. Qu ZY, Li GW, Chen QG, et al. Survival of a newborn from a pregnant woman with rabies infection. J Venom Anim Toxins Incl Trop Dis 2016;22:14.
18. Aguèmon CT, Tarantola A, Zoumènou E, et al. Rabies transmission risks during peripartum–Two cases and a review of the literature. Vaccine 2016 Apr 4; 34(15):1752–7.
19. Mani RS, Madhusudana SN, Mahadevan A, et al. Utility of real-time Taqman PCR for antemortem and postmortem diagnosis of human rabies. J Med Virol 2014; 86(10):1804–12.
20. Tongavelona JR, Rakotoarivelo RA, Andriamandimby FS. Hydrophobia of human rabies. Clin Case Rep 2018;6(12):2519–20.
21. Rabies. In: Centers for Disease Control and Prevention, National Center for Emerging and Zoonotic Infectious Diseases (NCEZID), Division of High-Consequence Pathogens and Pathology (DHCPP). 2022. Available at: https://www.cdc.gov/rabies/specific_groups/hcp/index.html Accessed August 10,2023. Accessed August 29, 2023.
22. Wang SY, Sun JF, Liu P, et al. Immunogenicity and safety of human diploid cell vaccine (HDCV) vs. purified Vero cell vaccine (PVRV) vs. purified chick embryo cell vaccine (PCECV) used in post-exposure prophylaxis: a systematic review and meta-analysis. Hum Vaccin Immunother 2022;18(1):2027714.

23. Ledesma LA, Lemos ERS, Horta MA. Comparing clinical protocols for the treatment of human rabies: the Milwaukee protocol and the Brazilian protocol (Recife). Rev Soc Bras Med Trop 2020;53:e20200352.
24. Moen R. Grizzly bear–human conflicts increase in Wyoming in 2014. Associated Press; 2015.
25. French S., French M., Predatory behavior of grizzly bears feeding on elk calves in Yellowstone National Park, 1986-1988. In: Proceedings of International Conference on Bear Research and Management. Victoria, British Columbia, Canada, 1989. Vol. 8, 1990. 335.
26. Gunther K, Hoekstra H. Bear-inflicted human injuries in Yellowstone, 1980-1994. Yellowstone Sci 1996;4:2.
27. Staying safe around bears, 2022. National Park Service. Available at: https://www.nps.gov/subjects/bears/safety.htm. [Accessed 29 November 2023].
28. Smith TS, Herrero S, Debruyn TD, et al. Efficacy of Bear Deterrent Spray in Alaska. J Wildl Manag 2008;2(3):640–5.
29. Freer L. Bear Behavior and Attacks. Auerbach's Wilderness Medicine 2017;682–3.
30. Herrero S. Bear attacks: their causes and avoidance. revised edition. Conn: The Lyons Press; 2002.
31. Herrero S, Fleck S. Injury to people inflicted by black, grizzly, and polar bears: Recent trends and new insights. In: Proceedings of International Conference on Bear Research and Management. Victoria, British Columbia, Canada, February 1989. Vol. 8, 1990; p. 25.
32. Phillips LL, Semple J. Bites and Injuries Inflicted by Wild and Domestic Animals. Auerbach's Wilderness Medicine 2017;637.
33. Jagodzinski T, DeMuri GP. Horse-related injuries in children: A review. Wis Med J 2005;104:50–4.
34. Elghoul N, Jalal Y, Bouya A, et al. Domestic Horse Bite: An Unusual Etiology of Crush Injury of the Fourth Finger-How to Manage? Case Rep Infect Dis 2019; 2019:2156269.
35. Centers for Disease Control and Prevention. Fatalities caused by cattle—four states, 2003-2008. MMWR (Morb Mortal Wkly Rep) 2009;58:800.

# Clinical Management of North American Snake and Marine Envenomations

Elaine Yu, DO, MS[a], Lauren Altschuh, MD[b],*

## KEYWORDS

- Snake bite • Marine envenomation • Rattlesnake • Jellyfish • Stingray

## KEY POINTS

- Establish scene safety after any envenomation to prevent additional injury.
- For crotalid snake envenomations, worsening tissue damage, hematologic abnormalities, and/or systemic symptoms are indications for antivenom administration.
- For elapid snake envenomations, prolonged observation is indicated due to possible delayed onset of neurotoxic symptoms, even with an initial asymptomatic presentation.
- For stinging marine envenomations, the treatment steps are deactivate, decontaminate, and denature.
- For puncturing marine envenomations, the treatment steps are wound care and denature.

## INTRODUCTION

North America is home to several venomous species of land and water-based creatures that deliver their venom load via biting, stinging, or puncturing the skin. The toxins produced by these creatures allow for natural predation as well as defense against predators. When humans encounter such creatures and receive a venom load, this is considered an envenomation. This article reviews common envenomations from endemic species found in the North American subcontinent. The text will be split into sections on snake envenomations and marine envenomations, with each section discussing their respective epidemiology, field management, presentation, diagnostics, and management.

---

[a] Department of Emergency Medicine, University of California San Diego, 200 W. Arbor Drive #8676, San Diego, CA 92103, USA; [b] Department of Emergency Medicine, University of California San Diego, 1501 India Street, Suite 103-147, San Diego, CA 92101, USA
* Corresponding author.
*E-mail address:* laltschuh@gmail.com

Emerg Med Clin N Am 42 (2024) 653–666
https://doi.org/10.1016/j.emc.2024.02.020
0733-8627/24/© 2024 Elsevier Inc. All rights reserved.

emed.theclinics.com

## NORTH AMERICAN SNAKE ENVENOMATIONS
### Introduction

Two subfamilies of snakes are found in North America: the crotalinae and elapidae. Crotalids include copperheads, which are responsible for the majority of bites, and rattlesnakes, which result in more morbidity and mortality.[1,2] These snakes are collectively referred to as pit vipers due to the heat-sensing pit behind their nostrils, but they also have characteristic keeled dorsal scales and undivided subcaudal scales.[3] In contrast, elapids are identified by their order of black, red, yellow, and white body rings, remembered by the mnemonic "red on yellow, kills a fellow; red on black, venom lack."[3] However, it is worth noting that this mnemonic does not apply to snakes that originate from outside of North America. The only endemic elapid species in North America is the coral snake. Coral snakes have short fangs that make it difficult to break human skin; therefore, they must latch on and "chew" rather than "bite." Due to this, there are no visible skin findings in up to 50% of elapid bites.[2]

Annually, there are an estimated 80,000 to 130,000 snake-related deaths worldwide.[4] However, North America makes up a tiny fraction of these fatalities, with only 5 to 7 annual deaths.[5] Nonetheless, snake bites are a relatively common emergency department complaint in the United States, with approximately 10,000 annual visits.[2] Of those medically evaluated bites, only one-third are from venomous species, and the reported dry bite rate (a bite without clinical evidence of envenomation) ranges from 2% to 50% depending on the study.[4,5] Crotalid bites comprise 98% of North American snake bites, and epidemiologic risk factors for exposure include males, ages 18 to 49 years, and summer months. These bites are divided into provoked or unprovoked based on whether the victim consciously aggravated the snake; provoked bites usually occur to males on their upper extremities, while unprovoked bites occur to females on their lower extremities.[4] Fortunately, only 1% of bites are to the head or neck.

### Field Management

The first step in the management of a snake bite is scene safety, and rescuers should evacuate victims away from the proximity of the offending snake, taking note of other snakes or hazards that may be locally present. If possible, identify the snake by taking photos from a distance, but never attempt to capture or kill the snake. Dead snakes or detached heads may still have an intact bite mechanism and inflict further harm if handled.[5] Larger snakes are presumed to deliver more venom; however, juveniles are still capable of inflicting injury.[5]

In the absence of proper species identification, all suspected snake bites should be treated as potential envenomations. To prevent the rapid distribution of venom from local tissues, keep the patient as calm and still as possible. Basic wound care and hemorrhage control principles apply, including the application of direct pressure for any open wounds, with tourniquets reserved only for cases of uncontrollable arterial hemorrhage. If possible, measure the circumference of the bitten extremity and mark the leading edge of erythema with a pen or marker for monitoring over time.[5] Anticipate local or regional swelling, and remove constricting clothing and/or jewelry. Splint the affected limb in a functional position, but avoid any tight constriction such as tourniquets or lymphatic wraps, as these may increase local tissue injury especially in crotalid envenomations.[6] When communicating with emergency medical services personnel, request transport to the nearest facility with access to antivenom—poison control may be a resource for identifying these facilities. Though allergic reaction is rare in first time envenomations, continue to monitor the patient for worsening local reaction or signs of systemic allergic reaction.

### Presentation

Snake bite patients may present with either immediate-onset or delayed-onset symptoms, with elapid bites potentially asymptomatic for up to 12 hours prior to the onset of neurologic deterioration (described in the following paragraphs).[2]

The most common symptoms of crotalid envenomations are local tissue injury and inflammation (90% of envenomations), hematologic abnormalities, or systemic end-organ damage.[2] A grading system has been proposed based on the severity of symptoms in crotalid envenomations:[5]

- *Minor*: local pain, mild edema, no systemic symptoms, and normal laboratory values;
- *Moderate*: severe local pain, worsening edema, non–life-threatening systemic symptoms, and abnormal laboratory values without bleeding;
- *Severe*: life-threatening systemic symptoms and abnormal laboratory values with bleeding.

Local tissue injury and inflammation can present as ecchymosis, edema, pain, hemorrhage, blistering, and/or necrosis. While this may appear to mimic compartment syndrome, there is typically only subcutaneous hypertension with normal compartment pressures, so fasciotomy should be avoided.[2,4]

Systemic symptoms are categorized by the venom's effect on the vascular, neurologic, muscular, renal, and immunologic systems. Hematologic abnormalities include consumption coagulopathy, thrombotic microangiopathy leading to myocardial infarction or cerebral ischemic infarcts, or thrombocytopenia manifesting as bleeding gums, epistaxis, or, in severe cases, intracerebral hemorrhage.

In the central nervous system, delayed-onset neurotoxicity from binding of muscarinic acetylcholine receptors leads to descending flaccid paralysis, paresthesias, altered mental status, seizures, diplopia, dysphagia, and/or respiratory failure. Muscular toxicity presents as rhabdomyolysis, although myokymia (rippling muscle movements) may be observed.[6] Renal toxicity presents as acute kidney injury and potentially progression to renal failure. Anaphylaxis or anaphylactoid reactions can occur with wheezing, dyspnea, nausea and vomiting, hypotension, and/or angioedema.

### Diagnostics

Laboratory evaluation is generally unrevealing in patients with elapid bites.[2] For crotalid bites or bites from an unknown source, broad evaluation for hematologic abnormalities and end-organ damage is warranted. Common laboratory tests include platelet count, prothrombin time (PT), international normalized ratio, and activated partial thromboplastin clotting time. Fibrinogen, D-dimer, and a 20-minute whole blood clotting test can also be used to evaluate for coagulopathies. For targeted end-organ damage, the following tests may be useful if a patient is displaying systemic symptoms:

- Renal injury: creatinine and urinalysis
- Hepatic injury: liver function panel
- Muscular injury: creatinine kinase and urine myoglobin
- Cardiac injury: electrocardiogram, chest radiography, and serial troponin
- Abdominal pain: ultrasound focused assessment with sonography for trauma examination or computed tomography (CT) to assess for occult intra-abdominal bleeding
- Neurologic injury (ie, altered mental status): CT of brain without contrast

Additionally, for any patients with suspected elapid bites who may later develop respiratory compromise as a result of diaphragmatic paralysis, a baseline negative inspiratory force (NIF) is important for ongoing monitoring.

## Management

### Monitoring and supportive care

The approach to the management of snake bite patients should follow standard trauma and emergency medicine assessment guidelines. A primary and secondary survey should be conducted, evaluating for and managing massive hemorrhage, airway compromise, breathing difficulties, circulatory dysfunction, neurologic disabilities, and exposure for additional injuries. Continuous monitoring of cardiac rhythm, blood pressure, pulse oximetry, end-tidal capnography, and limb circumference should be initiated. The leading edge of erythema should be marked every 15 to 30 minutes. Patients who are asymptomatic at the time of presentation should be observed in a monitored setting for 8 to 12 hours to ensure no development of symptoms before concluding that a dry bite has occurred.

### Antivenom

Antivenom is the mainstay of treatment for progressive local symptoms, hematologic abnormalities (PT > 15, fibrinogen<150, or platelets<150), or any systemic symptoms due to snake envenomation. There are 2 antivenoms available for crotalid bites: an equine-based F(ab')2 (Anavip) and ovine-based FabAV (CroFab).

Anavip is the current gold standard antivenom for rattlesnakes, but it is not useful for copperhead or cottonmouth bites.[4] The initial dose of Anavip is 10 vials over 60 minutes, with a repeat dose of another 10 vials if symptoms persist. If symptoms improve and then recur later, a second dose of 4 vials is indicated. Patients with pepsin, cresol, or horse allergies should be pretreated with steroids and monitored closely for anaphylaxis.

The initial dose of CroFab is 4 to 6 vials diluted in 250 mL of normal saline, or an increased dose of 8 to 12 vials for life-threatening systemic symptoms.[5,7] CroFab can be diluted in 1 L of normal saline if there is no contraindication to volume replenishment, and given as 25 mL over 10 minutes followed by 150 mL over 1 hour if there is no allergic reaction to the first 25 mL. After the first hour, an additional 4 to 6 vials can be given for persistent symptoms or hematologic abnormalities. Maintenance dosing is with 2 vials every 6 hours, for up to 3 additional rounds. An alternative regimen to the set maintenance dosing is the as-needed dosing of 2 to 4 vials for recurrent symptoms or hematologic abnormalities. Patients with papain/papaya, latex, pineapple, bromelain, and sheep allergies should be pretreated with steroids and monitored closely for anaphylaxis.

Documented side effects of crotalid antivenoms include acute hypersensitivity reactions (8%) and serum sickness (13%).[8] Laboratory tests should be repeated 18 to 24 hours after control of symptoms, prior to discharge, and at 2 to 3 days and 5 to 7 days after discharge to evaluate for delayed hematologic recurrence. There may also be recurrence of local tissue symptoms 6 to 36 hours after antivenom administration, so serial examinations are warranted.[7] For all antivenoms, children should receive the same or higher doses than adults.[4,5,7] Pregnant women with life-threatening symptoms should also receive antivenom, despite antivenom being classified as pregnancy category C (risk cannot be ruled out).[2]

The only Food and Drug Administration (FDA)–approved antivenom for elapid snakes is no longer in production in the United States. Remaining supplies of equine-based North American coral snake antivenin (NACSA) are approved for use through June

30, 2024.[9] The initial dose is 3 to 5 vials, with a repeat dose of another 3 to 5 vials if symptoms do not improve. Coralmyn, a non–FDA-approved F(ab')2 antivenom produced in Mexico, has been shown to neutralize venom from all coral snakes found in North America.[10] The initial dose is 10 vials, with a repeat dosing of 5 vials as needed.[11]

## Supplemental therapies

Though antivenom is the main treatment for snake bites, supplemental treatments may also contribute to improved patient outcomes. Of note, antivenom does not reverse hypersensitivity reactions or respiratory failure, and those must be managed separately.[2] Anaphylaxis should be managed with epinephrine and antihistamines for hypersensitivity, along with vasopressors if prolonged hypotension is present.[2] For local tissue injury, acetaminophen or opioid medications can be used for analgesia. Nonsteroidal anti-inflammatory drugs (NSAIDs) should be avoided in these patients to prevent worsening coagulopathies. Ice and/or cold therapy should be avoided, as this may increase local compartment pressures.[2] Tetanus status should be updated, as these are potentially tetanus-prone wounds. Prophylactic antibiotics are not indicated immediately after a bite, as only 3% of crotalid bites ultimately become infected.[12,13] However, if necrosis or purulence become apparent in a delayed presentation, antibiotics may be used to treat secondary cellulitis or abscess formation. Any surgical debridement of necrotic tissue or hemorrhagic blisters should be delayed 3 to 5 days from injury onset, as the wounds may evolve.[5] A summary of the treatment steps in the management of a North American snakebite can be found in **Fig. 1.**

## Controversies

There are several out-of-date and potentially harmful snake bite management strategies in popular belief that should be avoided. In the prehospital setting, suction of a snake bite to extract venom is not advised. Oral suction extracts less than 2% of venom from the wound while introducing bacteria present in normal mouth flora into the wound, increasing the risk of subsequent infection.[14] Mechanical suction products, either commercial or improvised, do not increase infection risk but do cause worsening local tissue damage with minimal benefit of venom removal.[15] Electricity, whether delivered via stun guns or car batteries, does not inactivate the venom.[16] Tourniquets to prevent systemic venom spread do not work, and have been found to increase local tissue damage; they should only be used for primary hemorrhage control in case of uncontrollable arterial hemorrhage.[5] Pressure immobilization with a lymphatic wrap is only recommended for elapids found on the Australian subcontinent (not those in North America), and studies show that most physicians and laypeople cannot do it effectively to prevent neurotoxic antivenom from reaching the systemic circulation.[17]

In the hospital setting, the treatment of coagulation abnormalities with anticoagulants should be avoided. Blood products should only be given for clinically significant bleeding as a resuscitation stopgap until antivenom can be administered.[7] Fasciotomy should be a last-resort procedure performed only if there are persistently elevated compartment pressures despite antivenom.[18] Treatment with antivenom will generally correct these abnormalities.

## NORTH AMERICAN MARINE ENVENOMATIONS
## Introduction

Annually, there are over 1200 aquatic exposures reported to US poison control centers.[1] Most life-threatening marine envenomations occur in the Indo-Pacific region, but there are many North American marine creatures that can cause significant morbidity and mortality. However, there is limited availability of marine antivenoms

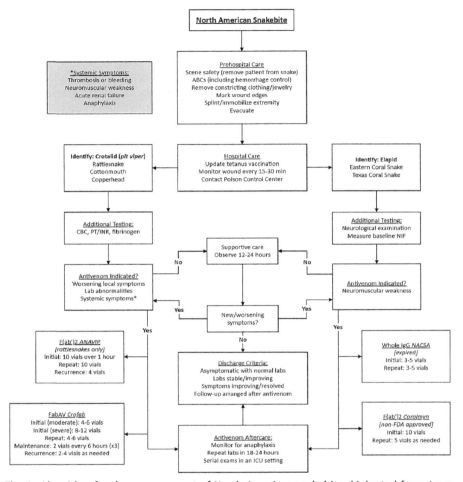

**Fig. 1.** Algorithm for the management of North American snakebite. (*Adapted from*: Lavonas EJ, et al. Unified treatment algorithm for the management of crotaline snakebite in the United States: results of an evidence-informed consensus workshop.)

in North America. Classification of marine envenomations by mechanism of envenomation guides treatment strategy, with the primary mechanisms being topical (stings) versus penetrating (bites or puncture wounds). In most cases, the management of these injuries is supportive, with different strategies for venom deactivation based on source and delivery mechanism. Of note, this review does not include toxidromes from ingested marine creatures.

### Venom delivery mechanism

Sting injuries are most commonly sustained by species in the phylum *Cnidaria*, which share pressure-activated and chemically activated nematocysts that discharge venom through a coiled barb. These nematocysts will most often cause local injury without breaking the skin. These nematocysts can be activated and provide ongoing envenomation by physical pressure or changes in temperature or acidity, which makes denaturation a critical step in the treatment of this envenomation. Commonly encountered medically relevant species within this phylum include *Carybdea alata* (Hawaiian box jellyfish), *Physalia physalis* (Portuguese man-of-war), *Chrysaora quinquecirrha* (Atlantic sea nettle), *Chiropsalmus quadrumanus* (4-handed box jellyfish), *Alata alatina* (sea wasp), *Pelagia noctiluca* (Mauve stinger), *Cyanea capillata* (lion's mane jellyfish), corals, and sea anemones.[19]

In contrast, puncture wounds seed the venom present on a spine or bristle under the skin, causing local injury. These wounds are typically sustained through accidental contact with the defensive structure of the species including miniscule chitinous bristles in Echinodermata,[20] tail barbs of stingrays, proboscis of cone snails,[21] and fin spines in Scorpaenidae.[22] These spines may be coated with venom or have venom glands which release upon mechanical pressure. Commonly encountered species displaying this envenomation mechanism include bristleworms, starfish, sea urchins, stingrays, cone snails, scorpion fish, and lion fish.[20]

The sea snake, a member of the Elapidae family typically found in Indo-Pacific waters, has also been found in Hawaii, and is worth mentioning in this North American guide. A sea snake bite is similar to that of a coral snake in that it uses its hollow fangs with attached venom glands to inject venom through a bite, although up to 80% of their bites are dry bites due to the shape and size of their fangs. These injuries are treated as any other elapid snake bite, as reviewed previously in this text.

### Field Management

### Stinging injuries

As is true in terrestrial envenomations, the first step in the management of a marine envenomation is scene safety by removing the patient from the water and distancing the patient and rescuer from the offending creature. In the event of a stinging injury, use the 3-step process of deactivate, decontaminate, and denature.

Deactivation is used to prevent any further venom discharge by nematocysts that may be present on the skin but have not yet released their venom. In Indo-Pacific waters and Australia, this is commonly accomplished by irrigation of the skin with 5% acetic acid (vinegar). In North America, deactivation is more complicated due to conflicting species-specific responses to topical solutions.[19,23,24] The American Red Cross Scientific Advisory Council recommends a location-based approach to treatment based on likely species encountered.[25] In Hawaiian waters, vinegar and copper gluconate (found in Sting No More) are most effective for the commonly encountered Hawaiian box jellyfish and Portuguese man-of-war.[26] Along the Atlantic coast and the Gulf of Mexico, topical lidocaine inhibits further nematocyst discharge in all endemic species including the Atlantic sea nettle, mauve stinger, lion's mane jellyfish, and Portuguese man-of-war while vinegar had varying results.[23]

Decontamination is the physical removal of any tentacles present on the skin, and this can be accomplished with seawater irrigation or manual removal with a blunt tool or gloved hand. Freshwater is not recommended as it may induce further nematocyst discharge. The final step is denaturation, in which any remaining heat-labile venom will be inactivated by the use of hot water immersion at temperatures up to 45°C for 30 to 90 minutes.[27] Care must be taken with prolonged immersion to avoid burns or other local injury. If hot water is not available, heat packs may also be used, although it is difficult to reach optimal temperatures with heat packs. Cold packs can be considered if heat packs are not available.[28]

### Puncture wounds

The field management of puncture wounds is similar to that of stinging wounds. Again, the first step in management of these wounds is establishing scene safety by removing the patient from the water and distancing the patient and rescuer from the offending creature. As these are wounds that break the skin, the first step is general wound care, including control of any bleeding, typically by direct pressure. In the rare case when a puncture wound is through a vascular structure, more aggressive hemorrhage control techniques such as tourniquets may be required. While pressure immobilization is not recommended for neurotoxic snake envenomations, it is recommended for neurotoxic marine envenomations such as from sea snakes and cone snails, as the venom effects are typically faster in onset.[27,29] Denaturation of the heat-labile venoms by hot water immersion is the optimal mechanism for pain control, and this may be accomplished by immersion in water at temperatures up to 45°C for 30 to 90 minutes.[30] The success of treatment may be identified by the removal of the wound from the hot water without a recurrence of pain.

### Presentation

Presenting symptoms can vary widely depending on the components of the toxin and the venom load, as well as the organ affected. Most marine venoms contain peptides and enzymes that induce pore formation and cause hemolysis, leading to the development of bullae and necrosis. Immediate skin and soft tissue injury can present as swelling, erythema, urticaria, and/or blisters. Certain species can cause pathognomonic patterns of lesions, such as the seabather's eruption from sea nettle larvae or the whiplike "frosted ladder" shape of rapid blistering with wheals and vesicles of the box jellyfish (**Fig. 2**).[31] Retained spicules from sponges develop into bullae with eventual skin necrosis, coined "sponge diver's disease."[20] Stonefish injuries classically cause significant proximal lymphedema.[22]

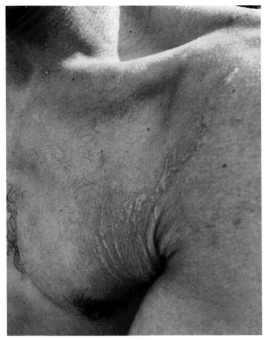

**Fig. 2.** Jellyfish envenomation. (*Courtesy of* Kirsten Hornbeak, MD and used with permission.)

Though most marine envenomations result in local skin injury, there are a few neurotoxic exposures that can cause muscle weakness, diplopia, dysarthria, and ultimately respiratory paralysis. The venom of certain species of cone snails and sea snakes is cause for concern, as it can block neuromuscular transmission.[29] Some stingrays, scorpion fish, and lionfish have venom that causes hemotoxic effects.[32,33] While Irukandji jellyfish are not found in North America, there has been an Irukandji-like syndrome described in Florida resulting in catecholamine effects such as hypertension, tachycardia, muscular cramping, anxiety, diaphoresis, lacrimation, and vomiting.[34] Severe complications can include pulmonary edema from cardiac failure and intracranial hemorrhage from hypertensive crises.

### Diagnostics

Species identification and geographic location of the envenomation are the most helpful in identifying the offending species. Physical examination of the wound may reveal a characteristic pattern or distribution of lesions that may offer clues as to the type of envenomation. Any concern for retained organic matter should prompt imaging. For example, stingray barbs are best identified with plain radiographs or MRI.[35] Residual skin findings such as the black dots indicating tattooing from a sea urchin envenomation (**Fig. 3**) may be present even without a retained foreign body, so operative exploration should be dependent on imaging confirmation and not just skin findings.

Patients with systemic symptoms should receive further workup. Neurologic deficits should be evaluated with CT of the brain as well as a measured baseline NIF if there is concern for impending respiratory compromise. Cardiopulmonary complaints should be evaluated with electrocardiography, chest radiography, and troponin testing. Any concern for impaired cardiac function should be investigated with echocardiography. Hemolytic effects of venoms may be asymptomatic and only identified with a complete blood count and coagulation studies. Rhabdomyolysis and acute kidney or liver injury can be identified with creatinine kinase and renal and liver function panel testing, respectively.

### Management

Local wound care should be performed, including updating tetanus vaccination status. Impaled foreign bodies should be stabilized, and only removed once definitive hemostasis of underlying organs and vessels can be quickly achieved, potentially in an operating room setting.[30] Analgesia can be achieved with topical medication such

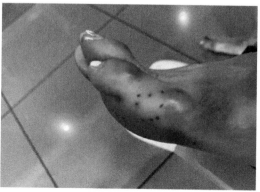

**Fig. 3.** Sea urchin tattooing. (*Courtesy of* Kirsten Hornbeak, MD and used with permission.)

lidocaine or benzocaine sprays, acetaminophen, or opioid medications. NSAIDs should be avoided if there is suspicion for hemolytic toxin effects. Local hypersensitivity reactions can be managed with topical or systemic antihistamines and steroids.

If signs of infection are present or the patient is at high risk for poor wound healing (ie, diabetes, peripheral vascular disease, or liver disease), antibiotics covering both normal skin flora (ie, *Staphylococcus* and *Streptococcus)* and marine *Vibrio* species should be initiated. Ciprofloxacin, ceftriaxone, doxycycline, or trimethoprim-sulfamethoxazole are options for coverage depending on local antibiotic resistance patterns.[30] A watchful waiting strategy may be appropriate in healthy patients, so long as the patient receives good follow-up instructions and return precautions, as local infectious symptoms may develop over 7 to 10 days.

For rare and more severe systemic reactions, specific treatments should focus on the involved organ systems. Irukandji syndrome in the Indo-Pacific is treated with magnesium, phentolamine, and clonidine, while Irukandji-like syndrome in the United States responds well to antihistamines, benzodiazepines, and opioid analgesics.[34,36] The mainstay of rhabdomyolysis treatment is intravenous hydration, with consideration of hemodialysis in cases of renal failure. Neurotoxic exposures can lead to rapid-onset respiratory failure, so close monitoring with frequent repeated neurologic examinations is paramount. Hypotension should be treated with vasopressors. Respiratory failure should prompt early intubation, and ventilatory support may be required for over 24 hours.

There are no marine antivenoms approved by the FDA. However, certain aquariums and zoos may stock antivenoms for captive species that pose a threat for handlers, such as box jellyfish and stonefish. An updated list of antivenoms available in the

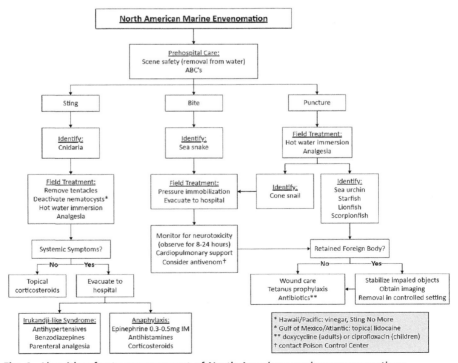

**Fig. 4.** Algorithm for te management of North American marine envenomations.

United States can be found at the Antivenom Index hosted by the University of Arizona.[37] Any antivenoms should be given in coordination with the local poison control center or your consulting toxicologist. A summary of the management of marine envenomations is found in **Fig. 4**.

## Controversies

Many popular culture treatments for jellyfish have emerged—following are some disproven techniques for the management of jellyfish envenomations. Do not use

- Urination on the area
- Ammonia
- Meat tenderizer
- Washing off tentacles with fresh water
- Scraping with a credit card or knife blade
- Shaving the area
- Rubbing with baking soda paste or sand-water slurry
- Pressure bandages to prevent venom spread
- Ice packs for pain control.

## SUMMARY

Over 35,000 envenomations are reported to US poison control centers annually. The majority of snake envenomations are from crotalids (pit vipers), that primarily cause local tissue and hemotoxic effects. Progressive symptoms, coagulopathies, and rare systemic acute kidney injury, anaphylaxis, or neuromuscular paralysis are indications for antivenom with Anavip for rattlesnakes or CroFab for any pit viper. Elapid bites are rare and may present asymptomatically for the first 12 hours before progressing to rapid respiratory failure and neuromuscular paralysis. Close observation, early intubation, and supportive treatment are mainstays of their management. Expired NACSA or foreign-produced Coralmyn may be given in consultation with poison control centers. Marine envenomations are classified as either stinging or penetrating. *Cnidaria* cause the majority of stinging injuries and display region-specific responses to first aid treatments. Hawaiian and Pacific stinging injuries respond well to vinegar and Sting No More whereas the Gulf of Mexico and Atlantic jellyfish stings show improved outcomes with topical lidocaine. Penetrating injuries require careful evaluation for retained organic matter and antibiotic prophylaxis covering marine *Vibrio* species. For all marine envenomations, hot water immersion is recommended for venom denaturation and pain control. There are no FDA-approved marine antivenoms.

## CLINICS CARE POINTS—NORTH AMERICAN SNAKE ENVENOMATIONS

- Crotalids or pit vipers—rattlesnakes, copperheads, and water moccasins/cottonmouths—produce a predominantly hemotoxic venom. Both local and systemic effects can occur.[2]

- Patients can develop coagulopathy and have occult bleeding from pit viper bites without displaying visible tissue damage.[2]

- Elapid or coral snake bites may not produce any visible signs on examination. If a coral snake is the suspected culprit, the patient should be monitored for 12 to 24 hours to ensure that delayed neurologic symptoms do not develop.[2]

- Antivenom is indicated in all bites with progressive local symptoms, hematologic abnormalities, or systemic symptoms. Antivenom does not reverse respiratory depression.

- Anavip is not useful for copperhead or cottonmouth bites; CroFab is useful for all crotalid envenomations. NACSA is no longer in production, although non-FDA-approved Coralmyn is effective for all US coral snake bites.[10]

## CLINICS CARE POINTS—NORTH AMERICAN MARINE ENVENOMATIONS

- If it stings, decontaminate (removal); deactivate (Hawaii/Pacific—vinegar and copper gluconate; Gulf of Mexico/Atlantic—topical lidocaine); and denature (heat).[25]
- If it stabs or bites, wound care and heat immersion. Apply pressure immobilization for sea snake or cone snail envenomations.[29]
- Patients presenting after possible exposure and envenomation by sea snakes, cone snails, scorpion fish, and sea urchins are at risk for the development of neurologic symptoms and respiratory failure. Close observation periods are recommended for these patients.
- For the antibiotic treatment of wounds resulting from marine envenomations, make sure to cover for marine *Vibrio* species.[30] Doxycycline is a reasonable choice in children; fluoroquinolones are often used in adults.[27]

## DISCLOSURE

The authors declare that they do not have a current financial relationship with any non-eligible entities (commercial interests) that may have a direct interest in the subject matter of the continuing medical education program.

## REFERENCES

1. Gummin DD, Mowry JB, Beuhler MC, et al. 2021 Annual Report of the National Poison Data System. Clin Toxicol 2022;60(12):1381–643.
2. Sheikh S, Leffers P. Emergency department management of North American snake envenomations. Emerg Med Pract 2018;20(9):1–26.
3. Cardwell MD. Recognizing dangerous snakes in the United States and Canada: a novel 3-step identification method. Wilderness Environ Med 2011;22(4):304–8.
4. Seifert SA, Armitage JO, Sanchez EE. Snake Envenomation. N Engl J Med 2022; 386(1):68–78.
5. Kanaan NC, Ray J, Stewart M, et al. Wilderness Medical Society Practice Guidelines for the Treatment of Pitviper Envenomations in the United States and Canada. Wilderness Environ Med 2015;26(4):472–87.
6. Greene S, Cheng D, Vilke GM, et al. How Should Native Crotalid Envenomation Be Managed in the Emergency Department? J Emerg Med 2021;61(1):41–8.
7. Lavonas EJ, Ruha AM, Banner W, et al. Unified treatment algorithm for the management of crotaline snakebite in the United States: results of an evidence-informed consensus workshop. BMC Emerg Med 2011;11:2.
8. Schaeffer TH, Khatri V, Reifler LM, et al. Incidence of immediate hypersensitivity reaction and serum sickness following administration of Crotalidae polyvalent immune Fab antivenom: a meta-analysis. Acad Emerg Med 2012;19(2): 121–31.
9. Notification of Shelf *life Extension for North American coral snake Antivenin 10 mL vial*, 2021, Pfizer Inc. Available at: https://www.pfizerhospitalus.com/sites/default/files/news_announcements/coral_snake_antivenin_extended_use_dating_4-27-21.pdf.

10. Sánchez EE, Lopez-Johnston JC, Rodríguez-Acosta A, et al. Neutralization of two North American coral snake venoms with United States and Mexican antivenoms. Toxicon 2008;51(2):297–303.
11. Anonymous A. Joint Trauma System Clinical Practice Guideline: Global Snake Envenomation Management. J Spec Oper Med 2020;20(2):43–74.
12. August JA, Boesen KJ, Hurst NB, et al. Prophylactic Antibiotics Are Not Needed Following Rattlesnake Bites. Am J Med 2018;131(11):1367–71.
13. LoVecchio F, Klemens J, Welch S, et al. Antibiotics after rattlesnake envenomation. J Emerg Med 2002;23(4):327–8.
14. Alberts MB, Shalit M, LoGalbo F. Suction for venomous snakebite: a study of "mock venom" extraction in a human model. Ann Emerg Med 2004;43(2):181–6.
15. Bush SP. Snakebite suction devices don't remove venom: they just suck. Ann Emerg Med 2004;43(2):187–8.
16. Ben Welch E, Gales BJ. Use of stun guns for venomous bites and stings: a review. Wilderness Environ Med 2001;12(2):111–7.
17. Norris RL, Ngo J, Nolan K, et al. Physicians and lay people are unable to apply pressure immobilization properly in a simulated snakebite scenario. Wilderness Environ Med 2005;16(1):16–21.
18. Darracq MA, Cantrell FL, Klauk B, et al. A chance to cut is not always a chance to cure- fasciotomy in the treatment of rattlesnake envenomation: A retrospective poison center study. Toxicon 2015;101:23–6.
19. Ward NT, Darracq MA, Tomaszewski C, et al. Evidence-based treatment of jellyfish stings in North America and Hawaii. Ann Emerg Med 2012;60(4):399–414.
20. Hornbeak KB, Auerbach PS. Marine Envenomation. Emerg Med Clin North Am 2017;35(2):321–37.
21. Halford ZA, Yu PY, Likeman RK, et al. Cone shell envenomation: epidemiology, pharmacology and medical care. Diving Hyperb Med 2015;45(3):200–7.
22. Diaz JH. Marine Scorpaenidae Envenomation in Travelers: Epidemiology, Management, and Prevention. J Travel Med 2015;22(4):251–8.
23. Birsa LM, Verity PG, Lee RF. Evaluation of the effects of various chemicals on discharge of and pain caused by jellyfish nematocysts. Comp Biochem Physiol C Toxicol Pharmacol 2010;151(4):426–30.
24. Lakkis NA, Maalouf GJ, Mahmassani DM. Jellyfish Stings: A Practical Approach. Wilderness Environ Med 2015;26(3):422–9.
25. Scientific Advisory Council Scientific Review Jellyfish Stings. 2016.
26. Yanagihara AA, Wilcox C, King R, et al. Experimental Assays to Assess the Efficacy of Vinegar and Other Topical First-Aid Approaches on Cubozoan (Alatina alata) Tentacle Firing and Venom Toxicity. Toxins 2016;8(1). https://doi.org/10.3390/toxins8010019.
27. Spyres MB, Lapoint J. Identification and management of marine envenomations in pediatric patients. Pediatr Emerg Med Pract 2020;17(4):1–24.
28. Wilcox CL, Yanagihara AA. Heated Debates: Hot-Water Immersion or Ice Packs as First Aid for Cnidarian Envenomations? Toxins 2016;8(4):97.
29. Kohn AJ. Human injuries and fatalities due to venomous marine snails of the family Conidae. Int J Clin Pharmacol Ther 2016;54(7):524–38.
30. DiTullio A, Auerbach P. Marine Envenomations. 2014. Harwood-nuss' clinical Practice of emergency medicine.
31. Balhara KS, Stolbach A. Marine envenomations. Emerg Med Clin North Am 2014;32(1):223–43.

32. Kirchhoff KN, Billion A, Voolstra CR, et al. Stingray Venom Proteins: Mechanisms of Action Revealed Using a Novel Network Pharmacology Approach. Mar Drugs 2021;20(1). https://doi.org/10.3390/md20010027.
33. Yazawa K, Wang JW, Hao LY, et al. Verrucotoxin, a stonefish venom, modulates calcium channel activity in guinea-pig ventricular myocytes. Br J Pharmacol 2007;151(8):1198–203.
34. Grady JD, Burnett JW. Irukandji-like syndrome in South Florida divers. Ann Emerg Med 2003;42(6):763–6.
35. Docter TA, Altschuh LB, Medak AJ, et al. Comparison of Radiographic, Ultrasound, and Magnetic Resonance Imaging for the Detection of Retained Stingray Barb: A Cadaveric Study. Wilderness Environ Med 2021;32(3):302–7.
36. Fernandez I, Valladolid G, Varon J, et al. Encounters with venomous sea-life. J Emerg Med 2011;40(1):103–12.
37. Johnson B. Antivenom Index. Silver Spring, MD: Association of Zoos & Aquariums; 2023.

# Lightning Strike Injuries

Eric Hawkins, MD, MPH, FAEMS, FAWM*, Gabrielle Gostigian, MD,
Sofiya Diurba, MD

## KEYWORDS

- Lightning • Lightning strike injuries • Wilderness medicine

## KEY POINTS

- Lightning is incredibly common and lightning strike injuries are best addressed with early recognition, action, and planning.
- Most lightning-related injuries are nonfatal and most sequelae are temporary, but it is important to know which chronic complications to be vigilant of when caring for these patients long term.
- Use a reverse triage process to address multiple lightning victims, as those who appear deceased may instead have temporary respiratory paralysis and respond well to resuscitative care.
- It is critical to screen all lightning strike victims for associated traumatic injuries (including penetrating trauma and blast injuries).
- Prevention is the best way to avoid lightning strike injuries.

## INTRODUCTION

Lightning strikes are an uncommon but potentially significant environmental cause of fatal and nonfatal injuries. Overall, most lightning incidents are not lethal but require prompt recognition of life-threatening emergencies to prevent death on-scene and mitigate significant long-term complications. This text serves as a review of the pathophysiology, injury patterns, evaluation, treatment, and prevention strategies of lightning strike injuries.

## EPIDEMIOLOGY

Lightning is incredibly common and is thought to occur almost 50 to 100 times per second worldwide, with 20% of those leading to a ground strike.[1,2] It is a significant cause of global mortality with an estimated 24,000 fatalities per year, though data from developing countries are often difficult to obtain.[3,4] Contrary to common perceptions, most lightning strikes are nonlethal, and approximately, 10 nonfatal victims are

Department of Emergency Medicine, Atrium Health Carolinas Medical Center Main, Wake Forest University School of Medicine, Charlotte, NC, USA
* Corresponding author. 1604 Scott Avenue, Charlotte, NC 28203.
E-mail address: eric.hawkins@atriumhealth.org

Emerg Med Clin N Am 42 (2024) 667–678
https://doi.org/10.1016/j.emc.2024.02.021
0733-8627/24/© 2024 Elsevier Inc. All rights reserved.

**emed.theclinics.com**

seen for every fatality reported.[2] In the United States specifically, there was an average of 27 deaths per year from 2009 to 2018, with an annual odds of being struck by lightning of approximately 1 in 1.22 million.[5] Most deaths occur in males, in younger populations between the ages of 20 and 45, and cluster between the warmer months of May to September.[3,4,6–8]

Geographically, lightning is most common in the mid-latitudes, in areas of the world near warm coastal waters or mountains. Worldwide, sub-Saharan Africa has the most lightning strikes per year, followed by the Himalayan region. Both of these regions have adjacent warm ocean regions that bring in moisture that rapidly rises against ascending mountain ranges.[3,9] These regions also have the highest rates of lightning mortality, mostly due to the outdoor lifestyles of inhabitants and barriers to seeking shelter when needed.[4] In contrast, lightning is rare in both the North and South poles, given their dry climate and colder air. In the United States, Florida leads the country in annual lightning strikes and deaths, with over 2000 lightning strike injuries over the last 50 years.[7] States like North Carolina, Georgia, Alabama, and Texas have analogous proximity to warm currents from both the Gulf of Mexico and the Atlantic, combined with populations that frequently participate in outdoor industries and recreational activities like boating, golf, and fishing, and thus have similarly elevated rates of lightning exposure and injuries.[6,7] Outside the southeastern United States, other high-risk states include Colorado, New Jersey, Missouri, and Pennsylvania.[6,7]

## BACKGROUND
### Physics of Lightning and Thunder

Lighting is caused by the mixing of unstable layers of moist warm and cold air. This creates an updraft of humid air, which leads to the formation of clouds of condensation and ice, as water vapor rises, cools, and freezes at higher atmospheric levels.[10] The formation of ice and condensed water particles at higher elevations creates an electrical gradient, with upper levels of the cloud containing positively charged ice particles, and lower levels of the cloud filled with more negative charge. Lightning then forms as this electrical gradient is dissipated, restoring equilibrium to the system.[2,10–12] This discharge may also occur from lower levels of the cloud to the ground, which tends to be positively charged relative to the negatively charged layers above. A single flash can generate between 100 million to 1 billion volts of electricity, and may contain as many as 30 strokes, which contributes to the flickering characteristic of lightning.[2]

Lightning discharge creates a stroke of charged particles up to 2 to 3 cm in diameter with estimated temperatures as high as 50,000 °C, which is 4 times hotter than the surface of the sun. This rapidly generated heat creates shockwaves of ionized and superheated air that quickly expand and explode to cause thunder and may be heard as far as 10 miles away from the lightning strike.[12,13] Sound travels at a speed of 5 s/mile, which is significantly less than the speed of light (and visualization of the lightning bolt); this may be used to estimate the distance from the observer to the origin of the sound and lightning, forming the basis for the rule of thumb used to determine safe lightning distance. However, it should be noted that the ability to hear thunder may be decreased by surrounding formations like mountains and vegetation, related storm wind or rain, or man-made noise like traffic or industrial activities.[14] In general, more abrupt and jarring lightning cracks signify closer proximity to the lightning strike, whereas more rumbling and deeper-toned thunder suggests that lightning is farther in the distance.

## *Types of Lighting Injury*

Contact with and subsequent injury from a lightning strike can occur by 5 main mechanisms. The most common is called a ground current, which occurs when lightning strikes a nearby object or ground and travels through the ground to the victim.[14,15] Accounting for nearly half of lightning strike injuries, this is a significant risk to both humans and livestock who are frequently exposed in open terrain. A side splash mechanism, the second most common type of lightning injury, occurs when lightning hits an object and then jumps to a nearby person without traveling through the ground.[14] Similarly, contact injuries occur when an object touching the victim is struck by lightning, and the current immediately transmits through their body before leaving to the ground or another object.[15] An upward streamer mechanism may also occur when current flows up from the ground and exits the body, meeting charged particles above with subsequent lightning discharge.[15,16] In this scenario, the current serves as a conduit for the lightning strike, sending it straight toward the individual. Finally, a direct strike occurs when a victim is hit by a continuous and uninterrupted lightning strike.[14] Based on case reports and principles of electric energy transmission, this is thought to be the most dangerous mechanism of injury, but still only accounts for 3% to 5% of all lightning fatalities due to it being a relatively rare occurrence.[3]

## CLINICAL FEATURES
### *Pathophysiology*

Lightning can harm the human body in a variety of ways. The primary injury mechanism occurs through the generation of heat as massive electrical current rapidly passes over and through body tissue, which may cause superficial burns in a flashover mechanism or more internal damage with deeper current penetration.[14] This deeper tissue injury can cause significant detriment to neurologic, cardiac, and respiratory functions. Finally, a lightning strike can also cause a concussive force that may precipitate blast injury and significant subsequent trauma.

### *Injury Patterns by Organ System*

#### *Cardiopulmonary*

The most severe complication after a lightning strike is cardiopulmonary arrest. This occurs via direct damage to the cardiac electrical activity of the heart, leading to ventricular fibrillation or asystole, or via a secondary cardiopulmonary arrest from loss of ventilatory drive and subsequent respiratory failure and hypoxia.[17–19] Most will not survive without immediate intervention; however, if they do survive, almost all have an excellent chance of recovery.[15,20] In the case of cardiac arrest caused by a lightning-induced primary dysrhythmia, cardiopulmonary resuscitation (CPR) and defibrillation will aid in restarting the heart's native conduction, pacing, and mechanical functions. If instead the cardiac arrest is secondary to respiratory stunning and hypoxia, rescue breathing may help restore normal cardiopulmonary activity. Respiratory failure from lightning strikes is often temporary and transient if the victim receives ventilatory support until normal central respiratory drive resumes. Overall, the mortality of cardiopulmonary arrest secondary to lightning strikes tends to have a better prognosis than arrests caused by more traditional etiologies such as coronary artery disease, heart failure, or other cardiac risk factors.[20]

Other cardiac complications from lightning can range from benign to severe arrythmias, hypertension, or functional problems secondary to excessive stimulatory autonomic activation or catecholamine effects. These can include sinus tachycardia, atrial fibrillation, idioventricular rhythms, temporary ST or QT segment changes, bundle branch blocks, and further conduction defects.[17,21–24] Most arrythmias tend to be transient and resolve within a week of the precipitating event, but may occasionally persist and become a chronic disorder. Cardiac ventricular function may be impaired and decompensate into cardiomyopathy, but this also tends to be transient and self-limited.[24–27] Temporary hypertension after a lightning strike is common, and is likely secondary to increased circulating catecholamines.[28] Coronary vasospasm has also been reported and can exhibit electrocardiographic (ECG) patterns suggestive of cardiac ischemia, generally with spontaneous resolution not long after the primary electrical injury.[29]

### Neurologic

In addition to damaging the brain centers responsible for central neurologic respiratory drive, lightning strikes can cause a wide range of central or peripheral neurologic issues, mostly occurring in the period immediately following the initial injury. These may include altered mental status, seizures, amnesia, temporary blindness or deafness, numbness, and headache.[12,30–32] These tend to resolve within a few hours of onset, though some may persist long term.

Lightning strikes are also uniquely associated with condition called keraunoparalysis, which is a condition that causes immediate but temporary paralysis and weakness of 1 or multiple extremities.[30,31,33] The current theory is that spinal artery vasospasm and peripheral vasoconstriction from increased catecholamine release and adrenergic surge lead to associated skin mottling, cyanosis, and decreased or absent pulse in the affected limb.[34] In general, lower extremities are affected more than upper extremities. Though these findings should not be confused with direct spinal cord injury or vascular arterial occlusion, appropriate trauma precautions should be taken if the situation is unclear. Keraunoparalysis generally resolves spontaneously soon after initial injury without any indicated treatments, although there is a slight increase in the development of chronic pain syndromes in these patients.[18,30]

Despite the relatively low overall mortality, many lightning strike victims go on to develop chronic neurologic and/or psychiatric problems. If the patient survives an initial cardiac arrest, post-ischemic encephalopathy may be seen if there was a prolonged resuscitation or period of hypoxia.[31] The primary event may also result in associated traumatic brain injury such as subarachnoid hemorrhage, epidural hematoma, or subdural hematoma, each of which may have varied short-term and long-term complications and should be treated with standard post-traumatic care. Other prolonged and often delayed neurologic issues may include dystonia, neuromuscular movement disorders, amyotrophic lateral sclerosis, and Parkinson-like syndromes.[34] Long-term neuropsychiatric issues have also been well documented and may include memory difficulties, sleep disturbances, personality changes, post-traumatic stress disorder, anxiety, or depression.[12,31,32,35,36] Neuropsychiatric syndromes are often the most significant chronic issues from lightning strike injuries, warranting consultation and treatment. Similarly, chronic headaches or chronic pain syndromes from neuropathy may develop and require referral to neurology or pain management.[37]

### Cutaneous

Lightning strikes can cause various types of cutaneous burns and skin changes. Most are superficial, with deep burns representing less than 5% to 10% of reported injuries (because of the incredibly short exposure of the lightning strike and energy transfer involved).[38,39] Many of these deeper full-thickness burns are due to contact with overlying synthetic clothing or metal (in jewelry, belts, or other accessories) that becomes superheated from the lighting strike; this can be especially damaging when the skin is wet.[14,37,40]

Superficial or partial-thickness burns present with a few characteristic patterns.[12] Linear burns occur when water vapor or sweat on the skin vaporizes from the heat of the lighting strike and burns underlying cutaneous tissues. Punctate burns are small focal circular sites of skin incineration ranging from a few millimeters to a centimeter in diameter, thought to be caused by current entering and exiting the body.[9]

Special skin findings called Lichtenberg figures represent a unique cutaneous phenomenon seen only with lightning strikes.[41–44] These are feathering patterns that occur just after injury, may be pink or brown in tone, and may or may not have a raised texture. These are not burns. Rather, it is theorized these may be caused by capillary damage and dilation in the affected dermal layer, resulting in subsequent red blood cell extravasation into the underlying tissue.[45] They are self-limited, usually resolving within a few hours to days of initial injury.

### Ocular

Eye injuries are common in lightning strikes and can be caused by a variety of mechanisms including thermal damage, electrical injury, or blunt force. Cataracts are the most common ocular complication and may form anytime from immediately post-injury to months later.[12,46–49] Other potential ocular complications include iritis, uveitis, retinal detachment, and associated traumatic injuries like hyphema, corneal abrasions or lesions, or a ruptured globe.[50] Photophobia, nonreactive or dilated pupils, or even transient blindness may also occur, either as a result of the intense light exposure of the lightning strike or from subsequent autonomic dysfunction of the eye. Because of this potential finding, it is not recommended that pupillary reactivity be used to gauge brainstem function or used in the acute evaluation of brain death.[51]

### Trauma

Traumatic injuries from lightning typically occur from blunt force mechanisms. Akin to a primary blast injury, a concussive wave from the explosive force of the lighting strike may cause barotrauma and damage to air-filled cavities such as the inner ears, lungs, or gastrointestinal tract. Examples here can include ruptured tympanic membranes, pneumothorax, pneumomediastinum, and pneumoperitoneum.[52–54] Other blunt and penetrating injuries may occur as the victim is thrown from the blast, including traumatic brain injuries, fractures (including of the skull, spine, and extremities), dislocations, or injuries to muscles or tendons from subsequent impact.[28] Muscle myonecrosis and compartment syndrome may also result from the initial traumatic injury. However, these are seen with significantly less frequency in lightning injuries compared to high-voltage injuries sustained in industrial or residential settings.[12,31]

## PREHOSPITAL EVALUATION
### Scene Safety

Scene safety is always important in the wilderness/environmental setting, especially when evaluating and treating lightning strike victims. Hazardous surrounding weather may require a rapid evacuation to a more sheltered area if possible, or even a delay in rescue efforts until the dangerous conditions pass.[13,14] Initial respondents should also activate the emergency response system, who may have more information about surrounding conditions. Once the ongoing safety of the patient and rescuers is ensured, focus moves to initial evaluation, identification of life-threatening injuries, emergent stabilization, and eventual movement to a more definitive care site.

### Reverse Triage

In a potential mass casualty incident (MCI) from a lightning strike, the process of triage and reverse triage are important concepts for consideration. In standard MCIs, rescuers seek to help those who have survived, and may forgo treatment of those who are already deceased or have non-viable injuries in order to maximize resources for the survivors.[55] In contrast, the concept of reverse triage just after a lightning strike prioritizes the initial treatment and resuscitation of individuals without palpable pulse or spontaneous respirations.[20] As described previously, these patients may have a transient arrhythmia or temporary interruption of their normal respiratory drive (in the medulla); providing rescue breathing, CPR, and defibrillation to lightning strike victims can lead to return of normal respirations and spontaneous circulation at higher rates compared to cardiopulmonary arrest in the general population.[3,14] Those who are already breathing or who are conscious are highly likely to survive the event, allowing more effort to be focused on those who are found in cardiopulmonary arrest. During assessment, pulses for these patients should be palpated centrally due to peripheral vasospasm and autonomic dysfunction associated with lightning injuries.[15] Contrary to some public misperceptions, these victims do not pose a threat of carrying residual electrical charge, and resuscitation should not be delayed unless other environmental factors impact scene safety.[3]

### Primary and Secondary Surveys

Further efforts should focus on a complete primary survey, with emphasis on hemorrhage control and then full assessment of circulation, airway, breathing, and disability.[12] If no immediate life threats are identified, a secondary survey is then performed, concentrating on a full history and physical examination as well as identification of any burns, traumatic injuries, or further issues. A thorough evaluation for evidence of lightning strikes (such as a subtle burn mark, burned clothing, or unexplained alterations in mental status) should occur because the mechanism of injury is not always obvious.[13] Lightning strike patients should all be assessed and stabilized as if they have blunt traumatic injury, with transport as soon as possible to more definitive care.

### Prehospital Resuscitation

If the patient is found to have a pulse and spontaneous respirations, they should be placed in a rescue position with protection of their cervical spine, and kept warm to prevent complications of hypothermia.[13] Any obvious sites of bleeding should receive application of direct pressure or a tourniquet (if available). If the patient has a pulse but inadequate respirations, rescue breaths should be given every 5 to 6 seconds. If CPR is needed, all available resuscitative efforts should be employed with standard compressions and rescue breathing. An automated electronic defibrillator should be used if available to analyze any possible arrythmia and deliver a shock if needed, which is especially important given the high rate of ventricular tachycardia or ventricular fibrillation in this population. In the event of return of spontaneous circulation, special care must be given to continue rescue breathing so that any residual brain stem malfunction does not cause subsequent respiratory depression and secondary hypoxic cardiac arrest.[13]

### Termination of Resuscitation

There is a paucity of evidence-based guidelines to direct the termination of CPR and the resuscitative efforts of lightning strike victims who require prolonged resuscitation in the field. Most prehospital experts advocate for 20 to 30 minutes of full resuscitative measures before CPR termination and declaration of death under general circumstances.[12,14] However, these recommendations may not apply to more remote or wilderness settings, where there may be even less resources available and greater transport distances to definitive care. As noted earlier, traditional methods of viability in the field (such as pupillary response or distal pulses) may be unreliable given the frequently encountered autonomic instability after lightning strike, and should not be used to guide decisions regarding the termination of resuscitative efforts.[12] As noted earlier, cardiac arrest from lightning strikes has higher potential survival than standard causes of cardiac arrest in the general population, but there is no evidence that these victims benefit from prolonged CPR or resuscitative measures.[56]

## HOSPITAL EVALUATION
### History and Examination

Once a lightning strike victim has arrived to definitive care, prehospital resuscitative efforts can be helpful in guiding further evaluation and treatment. Any information from on-scene witnesses or emergency medical services is important, as the patient may exhibit altered mental status or confusion regarding the events leading up to and including the injury. A full examination is necessary, especially focusing on the neurologic, cardiovascular, and respiratory systems, as well as a full head-to-toe examination of the skin to look for burns or further evidence of injury.

### Diagnostics

Laboratory and radiographic testing depends on the severity of the injuries involved and the overall stability of the patient. All patients should undergo ECG testing to evaluate for signs of arrythmia, changes in QT intervals, or signs of cardiac ischemia.[3,12,24] Depending on patient presentation, laboratory tests such as a complete blood count, comprehensive metabolic panel, cardiac enzymes, and creatinine kinase (CK) may be indicated.[13] Rhabdomyolysis, which causes elevated CK levels and can lead to renal impairment, is uncommonly seen in lightning strike injuries when compared with high-voltage industrial injuries. While the utility of total CK levels and cardiac enzymes is somewhat limited in the assessment for skeletal and myocardial damage according to recent guidelines, these tests may still be warranted given specific clinical scenarios and patient presentations.[3] Radiographic studies also depend on patient examination findings, but should at minimum include a chest X ray to evaluate for lung injury or signs of pneumothorax. Other X rays of the extremities or pelvis should be considered if there is clinical concern for fractures or dislocations. Computed tomography scanning may be indicated if there are signs of altered mental status or head injury, or if there are concerns for more significant spinal, intrathoracic, or intraabdominal injuries.

### Treatment

Given the wide range of presentations from lightning strikes, the treatment of individual patients depends on their specific identified injuries. In general, standard trauma and burn protocols should be followed.[12,13] If the patient is significantly altered, special attention should be paid to their airway and breathing status, as they may require aggressive interventions if their mentation deteriorates further. Persistent disorientation requires good intravenous (IV) access and likely IV fluid therapy with crystalloid fluids, especially if hypotension is present.[14] If significant burns or lacerations are noted, tetanus prophylaxis is also warranted; however, antibiotics are generally not indicated without significant wound contamination or open fractures. Other more advanced therapies such as blood products for associated hemorrhage, antiepileptics for seizures, or antiarrhythmics for persistent cardiac dysrhythmias should follow standard protocols for the individual issue at hand. One exception is that the pulseless and paralyzed extremity should not be assumed to have compartment syndrome and receive fasciotomy, as it is more likely to represent keraunoparalysis (described previously). Keraunoparalysis should be managed expectantly given the transient and self-resolving nature of this unique lightning strike pattern of injury.[12]

### Disposition

Patients who have been evaluated and been deemed high risk should be admitted and observed in a hospital setting.[3,13] This includes a minimum of 24 hours of observed cardiac telemetry monitoring for patients who have survived a direct strike, have chest pain or persistent dyspnea, or who have abnormal ECGs or heart function on echocardiogram.[3,23–25,57,58] Other high-risk patients who should be observed include those who have had a loss of consciousness, any focal neurologic complaints, and any significant burns to the head or extremities. Pregnant women at greater than 20 weeks gestation are another high-risk group and should also undergo fetal monitoring for greater than 24 hours, with an obstetric consultation to help guide further disposition decisions. Although reports of maternal fatality from lightning strikes are low in the literature, fetal mortality risk is higher due to the fetus being surrounded by highly conductive amniotic fluid.[59] Fetal and maternal complications related to lighting strikes include induction of labor, primary electrical injury including fetal demise, and placental abruption (which can occur as far out as 24 hours after a lightning injury).[3,60] It has also been recommended that a fetal Doppler be performed 1 to 2 weeks after lightning injury to assess for fetal demise.[60]

## PREVENTION

Safe practices, such as developing a safety plan and understanding preventive measures, are paramount for reducing the likelihood of injuries from lightning strikes. A pre-established safety plan while outdoors can help prepare for rapidly changing environmental conditions and reduce chaos during evacuation of individuals or large groups. These plans should consist of current weather forecasts, predetermined shelter locations, evacuation routes, and an understanding of local weather pattern and terrains.[3]

Individuals should enact their safety plan as soon as they hear thunder. There are many methods of estimating a storm's distance by timing lightning flashes with thunder; however, these techniques are prone to inter-operator variability and can create a false sense of security. After the storm has seemingly passed, people should wait a minimum of 30 minutes after the last thunderclap before returning to their outdoor activities.[3]

When an individual identifies the risk of imminent lightning, they should seek shelter immediately. The safest protections are solid fully enclosed buildings followed by hardtop vehicles.[3,61] Open shelters such as dugouts, bus stops, or picnic shelters should be avoided due to the risk of side splash and ground current.[3,62] If an individual is in a remote location, they should seek safety in a cave, dense forest, or deep ravine, which tend to be safer than open or exposed areas.[3,14] If an individual does not have access to such areas, they should immediately leave elevated areas (such as ridgelines or summits) and avoid tall isolated objects or trees.[63] If an individual suspects an imminent strike, they should sit or crouch with their knees and feet close together, or lift their feet off the ground if seated, in order to create only 1 point of contact with the ground.[64]

If there is a group of individuals, they should separate by approximately 20 feet or more to reduce the likelihood of multiple injuries from a single lightning strike.[14]

Special consideration should be given to individuals participating in water sports during a storm. If swimming or kayaking near the shore, they should immediately exit the water and seek shelter.[3] When boating, individuals should seek shelter in the cabin of the boat (if able), or stay as low as possible within the vessel.

## SUMMARY

Lightning is a significant environmental cause of death, both in the United States and worldwide. There are unique aspects of lightning strike injuries that necessitate deviations from standard care, which can improve their survival and overall outcomes. Reverse triage is an especially important concept, as it runs counter to traditional MCI response methods, and must be undertaken immediately to ensure maximal resuscitative success. Common injury patterns are also important to review, as some injuries are pathognomonic for lightning strikes while others are subtle and require heightened awareness for proper detection. While most lightning-related injuries resolve spontaneously, it is important to remember that some may have significant long-term symptoms; patients should be provided with anticipatory guidance and appropriately referred for specialist follow-up, evaluation, and treatment.

## CLINICS CARE POINTS

- Lightning is incredibly common and lightning strike injuries are best addressed with early recognition, action, and planning.
- Most lightning-related injuries are nonfatal and most sequelae are temporary, but it is important to know which chronic complications to be vigilant of when caring for these patients long term.
- Reverse triage is important to apply to lightning strike victims because those who appear deceased may instead have only temporary respiratory paralysis.
- It is important to screen all lightning strike victims for associated traumatic injuries.
- Prevention is the best way to avoid lightning strike injuries.

## DISCLOSURE

The authors have no financial disclosures.

## REFERENCES

1. Geographic N. Lightning. 2023. Available at: https://www.nationalgeographic.com/environment/article/lightning#:~:text=Cloud%2Dto%2Dground%20lightning%20boltsyet%20their%20power%20is%20extraordinary. [Accessed 12 September 2023].
2. NOAA. Frequently Asked Questions About Lightning. 2023. Available at: https://www.nssl.noaa.gov/education/svrwx101/lightning/faq/. [Accessed 12 September 2023].
3. Davis C, Engeln A, Johnson EL, et al. Wilderness Medical Society practice guidelines for the prevention and treatment of lightning injuries: 2014 update. Wilderness Environ Med 2014;25(4 Suppl):S86–95.

4. Holle R. Annual rates of lightning fatalities by country.. 20th Annual International Lightning Detection Conference. 2008. Available at: http://www.vaisala.com/Vaisala%20Documents/Scientific%20papers/Annual_rates_of_lightning_fatalities_by_country.pdf. [Accessed 9 September 2023].

5. NWS. How Dangerous is Ligtning. Available at: https://www.weather.gov/safety/lightning-odds. [Accessed 10 September 2023].

6. Adekoya N, Nolte KB. Struck-by-lightning deaths in the United States. J Environ Health 2005;67(9):45–50, 58.

7. Control CfD. Data. 2022. Available at: Lightning Strike Victim 2022; https://www.cdc.gov/disasters/lightning/victimdata.html. [Accessed 20 September 2023].

8. Gasser B. Cases of Lightning Strikes during Mountain-Sports Activities: An Analysis of Emergencies from the Swiss Alps. Int J Environ Res Public Health 2022;19(7).

9. Ritenour AE, Morton MJ, McManus JG, et al. Lightning injury: a review. Burns 2008;34(5):585–94.

10. Uman M. Lightning. New York, NY: Dover Publications; 2017.

11. NOAA. Severe Weather 101: Lightning Basics. 2023. Available at: https://www.nssl.noaa.gov/education/svrwx101/lightning/. [Accessed 12 September 2023].

12. O'Keefe Gatewood M, Zane RD. Lightning injuries. Emerg Med Clin North Am 2004;22(2):369–403.

13. Nelson RD. M.H., Management of Lightning Injuries and Severe Storms. In: S H, editor. Wilderness EMS. Lippncott, Williams and Williams; 2017.

14. Mary Ann Cooper. C.J.A., Ronald L. Holle, Ryan Blumenthal, Norberto Navarrete Aldana, Lightning-related injuries and safety. In: Auerbach P, editor. Auerbach's wilderness Medicine. Elsevier; 2017.

15. van Ruler R, Eikendal T, Kooij FO, et al. A shocking injury: A clinical review of lightning injuries highlighting pitfalls and a treatment protocol. Injury 2022; 53(10):3070–7.

16. Cooper MA. A fifth mechanism of lightning injury. Acad Emerg Med 2002;9(2): 172–4.

17. Christophides T, Khan S, Ahmad M, et al. Cardiac Effects of Lightning Strikes. Arrhythm Electrophysiol Rev 2017;6(3):114–7.

18. Jost WH, Schönrock LM, Cherington M. Autonomic nervous system dysfunction in lightning and electrical injuries. NeuroRehabilitation 2005;20(1):19–23.

19. Kim YM, Jeong JH, Kyong YY, et al. Use of cold intravenous fluid to induce hypothermia in a comatose child after cardiac arrest due to a lightning strike. Resuscitation 2008;79(2):336–8.

20. Vanden Hoek TL, Morrison LJ, Shuster M, et al. Part 12: cardiac arrest in special situations: 2010 American Heart Association Guidelines for Cardiopulmonary Resuscitation and Emergency Cardiovascular Care. Circulation 2010;122(18 Suppl 3):S829–61.

21. Dronacahrya L, Poudel R. Lightning induced atrial fibrillation. Kathmandu Univ Med J 2008;6(24):514–5.

22. Leiria TL, Pires LM, Kruse ML, et al. Struck by lightning: a case of nature-induced pre-excited atrial fibrillation. Circ Arrhythm Electrophysiol 2013;6(2). e20-1.

23. Palmer AB. Lightning injury causing prolongation of the Q-T interval. Postgrad Med J 1987;63(744):891–4.

24. Lichtenberg R, Dries D, Ward K, et al. Cardiovascular effects of lightning strikes. J Am Coll Cardiol 1993;21(2):531–6.

25. Rivera J, Romero KA, González-Chon O, et al. Severe stunned myocardium after lightning strike. Crit Care Med 2007;35(1):280–5.

26. Dundon BK, Puri R, Leong DP, et al. Takotsubo cardiomyopathy following lightning strike. BMJ Case Rep 2009;2009.
27. Ritchie D, Trott T, Bryant J, et al. Takutsubo cardiomyopathy and flash pulmonary edema in a trauma patient. J Emerg Med 2013;45(4):530–2.
28. Epperly TD, Stewart JR. The physical effects of lightning injury. J Fam Pract 1989; 29(3):267–72.
29. McIntyre WF, Simpson CS, Redfearn DP, et al. The lightning heart: a case report and brief review of the cardiovascular complications of lightning injury. Indian Pacing Electrophysiol J 2010;10(9):429–34.
30. Cherington M. Spectrum of neurologic complications of lightning injuries. Neuro-Rehabilitation 2005;20(1):3–8.
31. Cherington M. Neurologic manifestations of lightning strikes. Neurology 2003; 60(2):182–5.
32. Primeau M, Engelstatter GH, Bares KK. Behavioral consequences of lightning and electrical injury. Semin Neurol 1995;15(3):279–85.
33. Naik SB, Murali Krishna RV. M.K.R., A Case of Keraunoparalysis: A Bolt from the Blue. Indian J Crit Care Med 2018;22(11):804–5.
34. Kumar A, Srinivas V, Sahu BP. Keraunoparalysis: What a neurosurgeon should know about it? J Craniovertebral Junction Spine 2012;3(1):3–6.
35. Duff K, McCaffrey RJ. Electrical injury and lightning injury: a review of their mechanisms and neuropsychological, psychiatric, and neurological sequelae. Neuropsychol Rev 2001;11(2):101–16.
36. Primeau M. Neurorehabilitation of behavioral disorders following lightning and electrical trauma. NeuroRehabilitation 2005;20(1):25–33.
37. Cooper MA. Emergent care of lightning and electrical injuries. Semin Neurol 1995;15(3):268–78.
38. Selvaggi G, Monstrey S, Van Landuyt K, et al. Rehabilitation of burn injured patients following lightning and electrical trauma. NeuroRehabilitation 2005;20(1): 35–42.
39. Maghsoudi H, Adyani Y, Ahmadian N. Electrical and lightning injuries. J Burn Care Res 2007;28(2):255–61.
40. Herrero F, García-Morato V, Salinas V, et al. An unusual case of lightning injury: a melted silver necklace causing a full thickness linear burn. Burns 1995;21(4): 308–9.
41. Cherington M, McDonough G, Olson S, et al. Lichtenberg figures and lightning: case reports and review of the literature. Cutis 2007;80(2):141–3.
42. Cherington M, Olson S, Yarnell PR. Lightning and Lichtenberg figures. Injury 2003;34(5):367–71.
43. Domart Y, Garet E. Images in clinical medicine. Lichtenberg figures due to a lightning strike N Engl J Med 2000;343(21):1536.
44. Raniero D, Uberti A, Del Balzo G, et al. Unusual Lichtenberg figures in a lightning strike's victim: Case report and literature review. Leg Med (Tokyo) 2022;56: 102028.
45. Byard RW. Lichtenberg figures-morphological findings. Forensic Sci Med Pathol 2023;19(2):269–72.
46. Espaillat A, Janigian R , To K. Cataracts, bilateral macular holes, and rhegmatogenous retinal detachment induced by lightning. Am J Ophthalmol 1999;127(2): 216–7.
47. Cazabon S, Dabbs TR. Lightning-induced cataract. Eye (Lond) 2000;14(Pt 6): 903–4.

48. Alexík M, Stubna M, Kácerik M. [Cataract after lightning injury–case report]. Cesk Slov Oftalmol 2011;67(1):27–9.
49. Dinakaran S, Desai SP, Elsom DM. Telephone-mediated lightning injury causing cataract. Injury 1998;29(8):645–6.
50. Norman ME, Albertson D, Younge BR. Ophthalmic manifestations of lightning strike. Surv Ophthalmol 2001;46(1):19–24.
51. Hanson GC, McIlwraith GR. Lightning injury: two case histories and a review of management. Br Med J 1973;4(5887):271–4.
52. Habarth-Morales TE, Rios-Diaz AJ, Isch E, et al. Incidence and Epidemiology of Traumatic Tympanic Membrane Rupture: A National Trauma Data Bank Analysis. J Craniofac Surg 2023;34(1):168–72.
53. Halldorsson A, Couch MH. Pneumomediastinum caused by a lightning strike. J Trauma 2004;57(1):196–7.
54. Moulson AM. Blast injury of the lungs due to lightning. Br Med J 1984;289(6454):1270–1.
55. Lerner EB, McGovern JE SR. Prehospital triage for mass Casualties. In: e Cone DC, editor. Emergency medical services clinical practice and systems oversignt. United Kingdom: John Wiley & Sons; 2015.
56. Campbell-Hewson G, Egleston CV, Robinson SM. Diagnosing death. Death after electric shock and lightning strike is more clear cut than suggested. Bmj 1997;314(7078):442–3.
57. Saglam H, Yavuz Y, Yurumez Y, et al. A case of acute myocardial infarction due to indirect lightning strike. J Electrocardiol 2007;40(6):527–30.
58. Dundon BK, Puri R, Leong DP, et al. Takotsubo cardiomyopathy following lightning strike. Emerg Med J 2008;25(7):460–1.
59. García Gutiérrez JJ, Meléndez J, Torrero JV, et al. Lightning injuries in a pregnant woman: a case report and review of the literature. Burns 2005;31(8):1045–9.
60. Fish RM. Electric injury, part III: cardiac monitoring indications, the pregnant patient, and lightning. J Emerg Med 2000;18(2):181–7.
61. Blumenthal R. Injuries and deaths from lightning. J Clin Pathol 2021;74(5):279–84.
62. Walsh KM, Cooper MA, Holle R, et al. National Athletic Trainers' Association position statement: lightning safety for athletics and recreation. J Athl Train 2013;48(2):258–70.
63. Zafren K, Durrer B, Herry JP, et al. Lightning injuries: prevention and on-site treatment in mountains and remote areas. Official guidelines of the International Commission for Mountain Emergency Medicine and the Medical Commission of the International Mountaineering and Climbing Federation (ICAR and UIAA MEDCOM). Resuscitation 2005;65(3):369–72.
64. WP R. Backcountry Lightning Risk Reduction—Lightning Crouch Versus Standing with Feet Together. Tuscon, AZ: 23rd International Lighting Detection Conference; 2014.

# Climate Change

Christopher Lemon, MD[a],*, Nicholas Rizer, MD[b],
Jace Bradshaw, MD[b,c]

## KEYWORDS

- Emergency medicine • Climate change • Health impacts • Vulnerable populations

## KEY POINTS

- Although climate change is already unfolding, there is still time for prompt and decisive action to limit the extent of negative health consequences.
- To facilitate meaningful discussions with colleagues and patients about the health impacts of climate change, emergency providers must possess a basic understanding of climate science.
- While no one is entirely immune to the health impacts of climate change, certain populations tend to be more vulnerable than others—and tend to have less responsibility in creating the problem.
- Climate change can be considered a "threat multiplier" in the contexts of physical and mental heath, as well as social unrest.
- Emergency medicine stands uniquely qualified to lead the health sector's response to climate change through its expertise in disaster preparedness and response, collaborative research, innovative medical education, and familiar interdepartmental working relationships upon which to build comprehensive hospital mitigation efforts.

## INTRODUCTION

In a letter intended for his great-granddaughter in the year 2100, United Nations Secretary-General António Guterres wrote:

*"Today, our world stands at a crossroads, with two paths before us that will have a direct impact on your future.*

The first leads to a future of relentless temperature increase, deadly droughts and famines, melting glaciers, and rising seas. Communities ravaged and erased by floods and wildfires. Extinction and biodiversity loss on an epic scale.

[a] Department of Emergency Medicine, Johns Hopkins School of Medicine, The Johns Hopkins University School of Medicine, Davis Building, Suite 3220, Smith Avenue, Baltimore, MD 21209, USA; [b] Department of Emergency Medicine, Johns Hopkins Medicine, The Johns Hopkins University School of Medicine, Davis Building, Suite 3220, Smith Avenue, Baltimore, MD 21209, USA; [c] Department of Anesthesiology and Critical Care Medicine, Johns Hopkins Medicine
* Corresponding author. Johns Hopkins Department of Emergency Medicine, 5801 Smith Avenue, Davis Building, Suite 3220, Baltimore, MD 21209.
*E-mail address:* clemon1@jh.edu

Emerg Med Clin N Am 42 (2024) 679–693
https://doi.org/10.1016/j.emc.2024.02.022
0733-8627/24/© 2024 Elsevier Inc. All rights reserved.

emed.theclinics.com

In short, a trail of destruction.

The second path leads to the legacy you deserve… [inclusive of] better health…"[1]

Emergency medicine (EM) stands with humanity at this crossroads. The effects of climate change are far-reaching and are already affecting human health and health care delivery systems.[2] Manifestations of climate change such as unprecedented heatwaves, devastating wildfires, and extreme flooding events have direct clinical implications for public health. The health care sector, whose vulnerabilities were exposed by the COVID-19 pandemic, will be burdened with responding to these effects. Furthermore, current social, economic, political, and energy insecurity threatens to increase the proportion of vulnerable populations. As a leader in disaster medicine and acting as a health care safety net for a potentially growing portion of society, EM will be forced to adapt to care for the adverse clinical impacts of climate change on human health.[3] At this climate crossroads, EM must choose to use its distinctive potential to forge a path toward adaptation and climate change mitigation for the health care sector.

This article will begin by providing a concise overview of climate science to set the stage for the pressing climate health challenges we face today. Second, it will describe how salient features of climate change can have an impact on human health, exploring various climate susceptible diseases and exposures likely to become increasingly frequent in the practice of EM. Third, it will consider the indirect impacts of climate change on health, discussing the vulnerability of specific populations and specific aspects of our health care system that are prone to climate-induced disruption. Finally, it will highlight how the field of EM, given its scope of practice, patient demographics, and its integral role within local communities, is uniquely positioned to lead the health care sector in responding to the challenges posed by climate change.

## BACKGROUND: CLIMATE SCIENCE
### Basic Concepts

In EM, we routinely react to the health impacts of isolated extreme events (floods, heat waves, and so forth); however, it is important to recognize that climate change refers to a longer-term average of weather patterns. Looking retrospectively, we can appreciate the gradual climate changes that have occurred across many millennia, as well as observe examples of natural climate variability—and yet, now we are witnessing these changes within a single lifetime as a result of human activity.[4(p26)]

### Greenhouse Effect and Global Warming Potential

The energy balance of solar energy entering Earth's systems and energy being radiated back out to space is what provides homeostasis for habitable planetary temperatures—like a greenhouse.[4] This greenhouse effect (GHE) intensifies as human activity emits more greenhouse gasses (GHG) into the atmosphere, which absorb and reradiate heat back to Earth's surface, leading to increased global warming.[5]

Not all GHGs are created equally (or naturally). Their chemical composition and respective "half-life" in the atmosphere determine their global warming potential (GWP).[6] Carbon dioxide, a natural byproduct of combustion, is the reference metric and one ton of carbon dioxide has a GWP = 1.[6] By comparison, other gases trap more heat: methane's GWP = 27 to 30, nitrous oxide = 273, and engineered fluorinated gases (some used in anesthesia) can have a GWP = 1,00s-10,000s.[6]

Despite its comparatively low GWP, carbon dioxide is the primary contributor to climate change due to the incomprehensively gigantic volumes released into the atmosphere from the burning of fossil fuels and land use practices, rising from 280 parts per million (ppm) prior to the industrial revolution to 420 ppm as of August 2023.[4(p27),7]

The health care sector is responsible for 4.4% of net global emissions, and if it were a country, it would be the world's fifth-largest emitter of GHGs—United States health care is responsible for just over a quarter of those emissions.[8]

### Climate Modeling and Projections

A climate tipping point signifies an abrupt shift from a period of climate stability, and such a transition could have catastrophic implications for our health, as further explored later in discussion.[5] Climatologists research a myriad of interconnected feedback systems accelerating the threat of this phenomenon. For example, glaciers and snow reflect solar energy but on a warming planet, sea ice melts to reveal a darker ocean below, leading to more planetary heat absorption, more warming, and thus, more ice melt, with consequential sea level increase.[5]

When the Paris Agreement on climate change was internationally adopted in 2015, expert consensus aimed to limit warming to a $< 2°C$ increase above preindustrial levels to avoid unleashing the worst climate impacts on the world.[9] With more data, that critical threshold has now dropped to a $< 1.5°C$ increase.[10] The ocean has effectively masked more rapid changes in climate by absorbing 91% of the excess heat trapped by GHGs and 31% of our carbon dioxide emissions to date; however, effective "momentum" of climate change implies that even when we eliminate emissions, the planet will continue to warm for an unspecified period.[11]

According to the United Nations Intergovernmental Panel on Climate Change (UN IPCC), the planet is more likely than not to cross that 1.5°C threshold of warming in the near term—likely by the early 2030s, and possibly even sooner.[12(p12)] Our relative position on either side of this number should not equate to a binary outcome of "win" or "loss" for humanity. Rather, each incremental increase in warming introduces the potential for more severe and extreme climate conditions, resulting in increasingly dire consequences. Human activity created the current climate crisis, and it also remains the most unpredictable variable in projecting how bad it will become.[4(p34)]

## CONNECTING CLIMATE CHANGE TO HUMAN HEALTH AND VULNERABILITY

A projected 3.3 to 3.6 billion people are already highly vulnerable to the impacts of climate change.[12(p5)] Environmental degradation from human activities including habitat loss, overexploitation of bioresources, and climate change, is leading to mass extinction and compromising ecosystems upon which human welfare depends.[13] Climate-related changes in heat stress, diarrhea, malnutrition, and infections such as malaria, are expected to cause a quarter of a million additional deaths annually from 2030 to 2050.[14] Climate change will amplify vulnerability, as its impacts will not be equitably experienced across gender, income, class, ethnicity, age, or physical abilities.[12]

Entire regions of low and middle-income countries (LMICs) are susceptible to climate-induced surges in health care demand.[15] Minority, low-income, and indigenous populations face heightened climate-induced health risks due to poverty, geography, and limited access to care—they simultaneously live in regions highly likely to be affected by extreme weather events while lacking the resources to respond and adapt to new climate challenges.[16–20]

The emergency department (ED), "the de facto safety net for the health care system," is a critical access point to care for all segments of society, especially the most vulnerable.[3] During the COVID-19 pandemic in 2020, the Centers for Disease Control and Prevention (CDC) reported 131 million ED visits in the U.S., with the highest rates among infants, adults over 75 years of age, non-Hispanic Black individuals, and those with Medicaid or state-based programs.[21] These statistics reinforce the need to explore the reliance of vulnerable populations on EM during times of crises, especially when considering the health impacts of climate change.

## SALIENT FEATURES OF CLIMATE CHANGE AND HEALTH IMPACTS
### A Warming Planet

The United Nations World Meteorologic Organization confirmed that 2023 was the warmest year on human record, with temperatures tracking 1.4°C ± 0.12°C more than preindustrial levels.[22] In terms of health consequences, climate change contributed to 37% of heat-related deaths across 43 countries in 2021.[23] Since the 1960s, major U.S. cities are experiencing longer, more intense, and three-times more frequent heat waves.[24] One study explored the relationships between the historical discriminatory practice of redlining, intraurban heat conditions, and heat-related ED visits, finding such neighborhoods had elevated heat-related outpatient visits and inpatient admission rates.[25]

Even places not accustomed to heat are experiencing their share of health impacts. Anchorage, Alaska reached 32°C (90°F) in 2019; in 2023, the first study to assess the health impacts of extreme temperature in Alaska suggested that even at a heat index ("how hot it feels," taking into account air temperature and humidity) as low as 21.1°C (70°F), Alaskans may be at increased risk of heat illness and cardiopulmonary effects.[26]

Populations at the extremes of age are also particularly vulnerable. Between 2000 and 2004 and 2017 to 2021, heat-related mortality increased by 68% for individuals more than 65 year old, with higher-than-average rates in non-Hispanic Black individuals.[27,28] Children are susceptible to heat-related illness for several reasons, including their inability to understand the risk of heat, their inability to adequately thermoregulate, their higher metabolisms, and their increased likelihood to participate in physical activities outdoors.[29] One study of more than 3.8 million ED visits by children and adolescents found a link between higher maximum daily temperatures during the warm season and an increased relative risk of ED visits.[30]

The continuum of heat-related illness, as well as prehospital and ED treatment, has been described in the literature.[31,32] While the EM curriculum addresses the management of heat-related illness, it is essential to recognize the *indirect* burden in emergency health care. Higher temperatures exacerbate common emergency ED presentations, particularly cardiovascular disease, stroke, and renal disease due to factors such as dehydration, hypercoagulability, electrolyte disturbances, and systemic inflammatory response.[33,34] Climate change can be viewed as a "threat multiplier," exacerbating disease presentations already familiar to the practice of emergency medicine—this concept will reemerge as a theme in psychiatric and societal contexts later in discussion.[14]

### Degrading Air Quality

Air pollution and climate change are interconnected. Fossil fuel combustion releases ozone precursors, and increasing temperatures catalyze *ground-level* ozone formation (different than the "ozone layer" in the stratosphere).[3] By 2030, the climate-associated formation of ground-level ozone is anticipated to cause tens of thousands more deaths annually in the United States.[35]

The Air Quality Index (AQI) combines ozone measurements with other pollutants including fine particulate matter, carbon monoxide, sulfur, and nitrogen dioxide to assess the potential health risks. A higher AQI signifies an increased risk to health, particularly for vulnerable groups such as the elderly, children, and individuals with pre-existing pulmonary conditions.[36] These pollutants inflame the airways, enter the blood stream, and exacerbate underlying cardiopulmonary disease.[3]

Hazardous air quality was the hallmark of summer 2023 in the Northern Hemisphere – approximately 45 million acres (18 million hectares) of Canadian forests burned, with smoke pollution tracking to Northwest Europe.[37] One study chronicled the association between Canadian wildfire smoke and asthma-related problems in New York City EDs, hundreds of miles away.[38]

Global trends reveal an increase in very-high or extremely high fire danger days in 61% of countries since the beginning of this century.[27] Poor wildfire management practices and climate change-induced factors, such as drought and heat, contribute to more severe fires with significant impacts on environmental and human health.[39,40] There has been a call for research on the long-term health effects of repeated smoke exposures, particularly for children and firefighters, and there is also emerging research into the potential link between wildfire exposure and preterm birth.[41,42]

Emergency providers may also encounter novel respiratory impacts from climate change. For example, although pollen is a recognized aeroallergen causing rhinitis and asthma exacerbations, research is now investigating the connection between climate change, extended pollen seasons, and allergic sensitization.[43,44] Children's health problems associated with pollen exposure are projected to increase by 17% at 2°C due to global warming.[41]

### Shifting Hydrologic Cycles

Please provide author name and publisher location for Ref. 56.Climate change profoundly impacts the hydrologic cycle, influencing both marine and freshwater ecosystems, and the people who depend upon them. Water scarcity already impacts 1 to 2 billion people annually, and associated health implications are compounded by the fact that 70% of these "drylands" are in developing regions prone to poverty, food insecurity, inadequate infrastructure, and poor access to health care.[45]

As previously discussed, human-induced warming is also a key driver of glacier retreat, sea ice reduction, and the accelerated increase in annual sea levels. A warmer atmosphere has greater capacity to hold moisture, and thus, greater potential for extreme precipitation events; between 1970 and 2019, 44% of disasters were related to flooding.[10]

These regions will be prone to waterborne hazards. This could take the form of viral, bacterial, and protozoan infections, as well as toxin exposure from cyanobacteria and specific algae types, manifesting in a wide array of symptoms such as fever, flu-like symptoms, diarrhea, neurologic issues, and liver injury.[35,46]

Despite a traditionally low incidence rate, *Vibrio vulnificus* carries a significantly high wound infection fatality rate of approximately 18%.[47] Cases surged eightfold between 1988 and 2018, coinciding with a notable geographic expansion in brackish and saltwater environments.[47]

Waterborne illnesses can also result from exposure to byproducts of human land use which encompasses residential and agricultural runoff, industrial practices, and other forms of contamination.[35] These challenges strain the infrastructure for drinking water, wastewater, and stormwater management, particularly when compounded by the more frequent and intense precipitation, hurricanes, and storm surges associated with climate change.[3,35]

### Changing Ecosystems

The concept of "One Health" has been adopted by groups such as the World Health Organization (WHO): the health of people, domestic and wild animals, plants, and ecosystems are interdependent as are health challenges.[48] In 2016, the United Nations Conference on Biodiversity recognized a link between ecosystem degradation and the emergence of pandemics. Several years later, the outbreak of COVID-19 drew greater attention to the concept that the same human activities propelling climate change are also hastening biodiversity loss and driving zoonotic disease.[49]

The emergence of the Zika virus in the Americas in 2016 was linked to thousands of birth defects, prompting physicians to publish an editorial entitled, "Zika Virus: A Call to Action for Physicians in the Era of Climate Change."[50] Climate change not only has the potential to expand the geographic reach of vector-borne diseases, but also serves as a catalyst for their resurgence.[51] Regions with shifting land-use patterns or insufficient vector control and public health initiatives may face elevated susceptibility to these diseases.[25,34] With a high level of confidence, the UN IPCC reported that the incidence of vector-borne diseases has risen in recent decades.[10] Without adaptive measures and reinforced control strategies, diseases such as malaria, Lyme disease, West Nile virus (WNV), and dengue are projected to continue to increase.[10]

Emergency departments play a crucial role in the local detection of vector-borne disease. Emergency physicians should remain vigilant for an anticipated increase in cases and transmission seasons, stay informed about local disease emergence, and focus on travel histories and potential exposures when addressing seemingly nonspecific clinical complaints.[52]

### Intensifying Weather Patterns

From 2010 to 2020, communities classified as highly vulnerable to climate change by the UN IPCC experienced an alarming 15-fold increase in mortality rates during floods, droughts, and storms, in stark contrast to those in regions deemed to have very low vulnerability.[12] Moreover, many of these highly vulnerable communities are also the least responsible for causing these climate disasters.[12]

The risk posed by extreme weather hinges upon several factors including the nature of the hazard, level of exposure, community vulnerability, and the capacity to prepare for, manage, and recover from such events.[53] *Compound* weather events can further amplify risk as 2 or more events intersect in terms of timing or location—like sequential heatwaves or the combination of drought and sudden severe precipitation, respectively.[53,54]

EDs must adapt to handle increased volume surges postnatural disasters.[53] While many health systems already have plans in place to address climate risks, these plans may prove insufficient to cope with the increased frequency and magnitude of climate-related impacts.[27,53] Furthermore, such plans may fail to anticipate other sources of displaced patient volume after a disaster, such as from the lack of access to primary care, other hospital systems, or pharmacies.[55]

Coastal communities are particularly at risk for sea level rise, extreme weather events, and resource disruption.[56] In more vulnerable regions such as South Pacific Island communities, it was found that 62% of all health care facilities were within 500m of the coast and particularly susceptible to sea level increase.[57] In 2017, an estimated 5740 excess deaths were attributed to Hurricane Maria; of these deaths, approximately one-third stemmed from the inability to access medical care.[58]

There is a pressing need to enhance the resilience of health care systems to meet the growing demands arising from climate change.[59,60] Increasing physical damage to hospitals is anticipated to jeopardize transportation, water supplies, and operations.[53,61] Loss of power can result in wide-ranging disruptions to critical machinery and infrastructure such as intravenous pumps, ventilators, refrigeration (laboratory specimens and temperature-sensitive medications), and communications.[62]

*Mental Health Impacts*

The IPCC, with a high level of confidence, highlights the multifaceted mental health impacts stemming from various complex climate-related challenges, encompassing extreme weather events, famine, health care system breakdowns, displacement, migration, and heightened anxiety/distress.[10] Elevated temperatures, heatwaves, and humidity are linked to worsened mental health outcomes and even increased suicidality.[27] A meta-analysis found that with every 1°C increase in ambient temperature, there is a 2.2% increase in mental health-related mortality and a 0.9% increase in mental health related morbidity.[39] Even certain medications commonly used to treat mental illness can pose a hazard during heat stress as they can impede the body's central thermoregulation.[35]

The direct and indirect stressors of climate change are anticipated to create and exacerbate vulnerabilities for those with mental health probems.[27] Globally, 50% of individuals with mental health disorders receive no treatment, climbing to nearly 90% in resource-limited settings.[63] A comprehensive literature review of climate change impacts on mental health referred to the problem as a "risk [threat] multiplier," noting that many of the disadvantages that create poor mental health are the same issues driving problems amplified by climate change—poor governance, social inequalities, poverty, and pollution.[64]

*Driving Displacement*

In the era of climate change, displaced individuals will represent a massive and growing vulnerable population with the potential to rely heavily upon acute care resources.[65,66] As of 2021, 149.6 million people resided less than a meter above sea level, threatened not just by eventual inundation, but also by interim instability related to severe storms and flooding, erosion, infectious diseases, and salinization of water and soil.[27] In 2022, 98% of the recorded 32.6 million internal displacement events were caused by weather-related hazards including floods, storms, wildfires, and droughts—60% of these displaced individuals and refugees now live in countries that are among the most vulnerable to climate change.[67]

The 1951 Refugee Convention provides protections only for those seeking safety from war, violence, conflict, or prosecution when crossing an international border—"climate refugees" are not formally recognized and do not qualify for protection under international law.[68] However, once again, climate change is frequently referred to as a "threat multiplier"—in this case exacerbating resource limitations, poverty, and social unrest that drive migration.[69] The United Nations Higher Commission for Refugees (UNHCR) is analyzing gaps in applying refugee protections specifically to those people fleeing from conflict and/or violence that is *linked to* disaster events and/or the adverse effects of climate change.[70] Nevertheless, there is a need for additional research to understand the impact that the increasing number of internally and internationally displaced and migrating people will have on acute care health systems.

## OPPORTUNITIES FOR EMERGENCY MEDICINE ACTION

It is easy to feel overwhelmed and powerless when contemplating the wide-ranging impacts that climate change will have on humanity and our health. However, the recent COVID-19 pandemic proved that EM can and must function in seemingly unimaginable circumstances. A common approach to undertaking action on climate change is often framed as *adaptation—managing the unavoidable* through preparation, as well as *mitigation—avoiding the unmanageable* by preventing the situation from degrading further.[71(p86)] The sentiments should resonate with EM pedagogy. Many efforts to act on climate change dovetail with routine EM activities including patient care, research, collaboration, and education.

### Climate Adaptation

The United Nations introduced the Sendai Framework for Disaster Risk Reduction in 2015, the same year as the Paris Agreement for global climate action. This framework serves as a comprehensive guide for managing disaster risk across various hazards, recognizing the pivotal role of climate change as a key driver of these risks.[72] Emergency physicians, often at the forefront of disaster medicine, lead disaster fellowships and training programs, fostering international collaboration.[73] EM is often also responsible for coordinating hospital preparedness drills and overseeing interagency cooperation involving emergency medical services and fire response, law enforcement, public health systems, and government infrastructure.

Local EDs, attuned to local politics, socioeconomics, and social determinants of health, play a crucial role in framing climate-related health care in their communities—and this includes their health care systems. To comprehensively address the intricate risks posed by climate change on health care systems, it is essential to conduct thorough vulnerability assessments and explore respective adaptation strategies. The literature offers guidance and methodologies for conducting climate and health stress tests, aiming to bolster health systems' capabilities in managing both acute and chronic impacts tied to climate events.[74]

### Climate Mitigation

The U.S. health care sector alone contributes to 10% of the country's total greenhouse gas (GHG) emissions.[75] Ironically, according to the WHO, the direct damage costs from climate change to health are estimated to be between \$2 to 4 billion annually by 2030; yet, enhancing operational and equipment efficiency in energy use has the potential to save US hospitals \$1 billion over a span of 5 years.[14,75]

The concept of "Climate-Smart Healthcare," coined in a collaborative report by the World Bank Group and associates, emphasizes low-carbon and resilience strategies for the health sector.[76] This includes investing in renewable and efficient energy sources, minimizing waste, implementing sustainable health care waste management, and building resilience strategies to withstand extreme weather events.[76] A thorough review of these approaches titled "The Climate-Smart Emergency Department," focused on these and other considerations such as water management and sustainable transportation, is available in the literature.[75] Given its broad reach in facilitating interdepartmental patient care and outpatient follow up, EM is uniquely positioned to identify, advocate for, and champion climate mitigation strategies throughout the health care sector.

### Patient Care

Every encounter in the ED represents an opportunity to consider whether climate change is impacting a patient's health. Consolidated clinical practice improvements and interventions to address climate-related health threats in EM were outlined by Sorensen and colleagues[3] Free programs, such as Climate for Health Ambassador Training, are available to compliment the training of emergency health care workers.[77] The innovative Climate Rx program fosters connections among patients and colleagues, guiding them on how to address the health risks associated with climate change by simply scanning a QR code on a badge worn during shifts.[78]

## Research and Collaboration

In 2018, the American College of Emergency Physicians (ACEP) formulated a policy promoting *interdisciplinary* collaboration with public health agencies and various stakeholders in addressing health implications resulting from climate change, including emphasis on the ED's importance in participating in epidemiologic research, expanding disease surveillance systems, and considering early warning systems.[79]

Furthermore, EDs bring a distinctive understanding of local health determinants and the impacts of climate events on their communities. The integration of these diverse perspectives into national and international EM frameworks creates substantial opportunities to foster a comprehensive outlook. This can be achieved through the establishment of collaborative working groups, research platforms, and publications.

## Education

EM, as a specialty, holds the responsibility for both formal and informal education across various domains, reaching medical students, residents, faculty, and the entire ED team, including nurses, techs, and administrative staff. Importantly, education extends to patients, who play a crucial role in informing our understanding of climate impacts on health.

Often student initiated, medical school curricula are adapting to include climate considerations, incorporating relevant elective courses aligned with the goals and objectives set by the American Association of Medical Colleges (AAMC).[3,80–83]

The Journal of Graduate Medical Education quoted the WHO regarding climate change as "the single biggest threat facing humanity."[14] Citing a lack of climate change-related educational tools for preparing future physicians and health professionals, it issued a "Call for Articles on Climate and Graduate Medical Education."[84]

Innovative approaches are emerging to address the climate and health education gap on multiple levels. This includes the establishment of formalized fellowships in health and climate at institutions such as the University of Colorado and Harvard, as well as broadly accessible continuing medical education (CME) content and open-access online curricula.[3,85–88]

## SUMMARY

Author, geophysicist, and climatologist Michael E. Mann recently wrote:

> *"It is also important to recognize that climate change isn't a cliff that we go off at certain thresholds of planetary warming such as the oft-discussed 1.5°C (2.7°F) warming level, though it is often framed that way. Climate action isn't a binary case of "success" or "failure."*

> *A better analogy is that it's a dangerous highway we're going down. We need to take the earliest exit ramp possible."*[89]

U.N. Secretary-General Guterres rightly describes humanity as standing at a "climate crossroad."[1] However, Mann's analogy is more accurate in the sense that climate change is already in motion, and perhaps, relatable to the emergency medicine mindset. The EM approach to climate change should mirror EM training – quickly recognize the dangerous nature of the situation, respond swiftly and judiciously to the currently available information, and remain prepared to consider new data and adapt to evolving circumstances. The unstable vital signs of a critical patient would compel the EM physician to work hard at stabilization—*should the unstable vitals of our planet be treated any differently?*

## CLINICS CARE POINTS

---

- Optimize Protocols: Continuously refine and practice emergency protocols to mitigate and adapt to climate-related health challenges. For example, consider enhancing heat stroke treatment through triage protocols that prioritize it as vigorously as stroke and STEMI. Strengthen emergency preparedness and surge capacity response to match frequency and intensity of extreme weather events.
- Monitor Infectious Disease Trends: Stay alert to trends in infectious disease patterns, emphasizing the importance of travel and exposure histories in clinical evaluations.
- Ensure Medication Safety: Collaborate with pharmacy teams to address and mitigate medication-related risks. This includes ensuring patients have access to essential medications like insulin during disasters, and educating them about the potential impact of certain medications (e.g., antipsychotics, beta-blockers, diuretics, anticholinergics) on the body's ability to thermoregular during heatwaves. Aim to integrate such precautions into electronic medical records, prompting advisories for best practices, similar to those for Qt prolongation.
- Strengthen Support Networks: Collaborate closely with case management, social work, and psychiatry colleagues to bolster support frameworks for those patients who are most vulnerable, acknowledging the heightened risks of social stressors, domestic violence, neglect, non-accidental trauma, and mental health emergencies driven by climate change.

---

## DISCLOSURE

None of the authors have any relevant financial disclosures.

## REFERENCES

1. Guterres, António. The Head of the United Nations Makes a Climate-Change Apology to His Future Great-Great-Granddaughter. Time. Published online April 20, 2023. Available at: https://time.com/collection/earth-awards-2023/6272884/antonio-guterres-climate-change-apology-great-great-granddaughter/. [Accessed 11 September 2023].
2. Haines A, Ebi K. The Imperative for Climate Action to Protect Health. N Engl J Med 2019;380(3):263–73. https://doi.org/10.1056/NEJMra1807873.
3. Sorensen CJ, Salas RN, Rublee C, et al. Clinical Implications of Climate Change on US Emergency Medicine: Challenges and Opportunities. Ann Emerg Med 2020;76(2):168–78.
4. Lemery J, Knowlton K, Sorensen C, editors. Global climate change and human health: from science to practice. 2nd edition. San Fransisco: Jossey-Bass; 2020.
5. The Study of Earth as an Integrated System. NASA Global Climate Change: Vital Signs of the Planet. Available at: https://climate.nasa.gov/nasa_science/science/. [Accessed 14 September 2023].
6. Greenhouse Gas Emisions: Understanding Global Warming Potentials. United States Environmental Protection Agency. Available at: https://www.epa.gov/ghgemissions/understanding-global-warming-potentials#:~:text=Chlorofluorocarbons%20(CFCs)%2C%20hydrofluorocarbons%20(,more%20heat%20than%20CO2. [Accessed 15 September 2023].
7. Trends in Atmospheric Carbon Dioxide. NOAA: Global Monitoring Laboratory: Earth System Research Laboratories. Published September 5, 2023. Available at: https://gml.noaa.gov/ccgg/trends/. [Accessed 14 September 2023].

8.  How the Health Sector Contributes to the Global Climate Crisis and Opportunities for Action. 2019. Available at: https://noharm-global.org/sites/default/files/documents-files/5961/HealthCaresClimateFootprint_090619.pdf. [Accessed 29 September 2023].

9.  The Paris Agreement. Available at: https://unfccc.int/process-and-meetings/the-paris-agreement. [Accessed 15 September 2023].

10. IPCC. Climate Change 2022: Impacts, Adaptation and Vulnerability. Contribution of Working Group II to the Sixth Assessment Report of the Intergovernmental Panel on Climate Change. Cambridge, UK and New York, NY, USA: Cambridge University Press. Cambridge University Press; 2022. p. 3056. https://doi.org/10.1017/9781009325844.

11. Li Z, England MH, Groeskamp S. Recent acceleration in global ocean heat accumulation by mode and intermediate waters. Nat Commun 2023;14(1):6888.

12. Calvin K, Dasgupta D, Krinner G, et al. IPCC, 2023: Climate Change 2023: Synthesis Report. Contribution of Working Groups I, II and III to the Sixth Assessment Report of the Intergovernmental Panel on Climate Change [Core Writing Team. In: Lee H, Romero J, editors. IPCC. Geneva, Switzerland: First. Intergovernmental Panel on Climate Change (IPCC); 2023. https://doi.org/10.59327/IPCC/AR6-9789291691647.

13. Shivanna KR. The Sixth Mass Extinction Crisis and its Impact on Biodiversity and Human Welfare. Resonance 2020;25(1):93–109.

14. Climate change and health. World Health Organization. 2023. Available at: https://www.who.int/news-room/fact-sheets/detail/climate-change-and-health.

15. Theron E, Bills CB, Calvello Hynes EJ, et al. Climate change and emergency care in Africa: A scoping review. Afr J Emerg Med 2022;12(2):121–8.

16. Ford JD, Berrang-Ford L, King M, et al. Vulnerability of Aboriginal health systems in Canada to climate change. Glob Environ Change 2010;20(4):668–80.

17. Schramm PJ, Al Janabi AL, Campbell LW, et al. How Indigenous Communities Are Adapting To Climate Change: Insights From The Climate-Ready Tribes Initiative: Analysis examines how indigenous communities are adapting to climate change. Health Aff 2020;39(12):2153–9.

18. Lansbury Hall N, Crosby L. Climate Change Impacts on Health in Remote Indigenous Communities in Australia. Int J Environ Health Res 2022;32(3):487–502.

19. Jones M, Mills D, Gray R. Expecting the unexpected? Improving rural health in the era of bushfires, novel coronavirus and climate change. Aust J Rural Health 2020;28(2):107–9.

20. Levy BS, Patz JA. Climate Change, Human Rights, and Social Justice. Ann Glob Health 2015;81(3):310.

21. Cairns C, Ashman J, King JM. Emergency department visit rates by Selected Characteristics: United States, 2020. National Center for Health Statistics (U.S.); 2022. https://doi.org/10.15620/cdc:121837.

22. WMO Confirms That 2023 Smashes Global Temperature Record. 2024. Available at: https://wmo.int/news/media-centre/wmo-confirms-2023-smashes-global-temperature-record. [Accessed 26 January 2024].

23. Vicedo-Cabrera AM, Scovronick N, Sera F, et al. The burden of heat-related mortality attributable to recent human-induced climate change. Nat Clim Change 2021;11(6):492–500.

24. Climate change Indicators: heat waves. United States Environmental Protection Agency. Available at: https://www.epa.gov/climate-indicators/climate-change-indicators-heat-waves. [Accessed 11 September 2023].

25. Li D, Newman GD, Wilson B, et al. Modeling the Relationships Between Historical Redlining, Urban Heat, and Heat-Related Emergency Department Visits: An Examination of 11 Texas Cities. Environ Plan B Urban Anal City Sci 2022;49(3):933–52.

26. Hahn MB, Kuiper G, Magzamen S. Association of Temperature Thresholds with Heat Illness– and Cardiorespiratory-Related Emergency Visits during Summer Months in Alaska. Environ Health Perspect 2023;131(5):057009.

27. Romanello M, Di Napoli C, Drummond P, et al. The 2022 report of the Lancet Countdown on health and climate change: health at the mercy of fossil fuels. Lancet 2022;400(10363):1619–54.

28. Climate Change Indicators: Heat-Related Deaths. United States Environmental Protection Agency. Available at: https://www.epa.gov/climate-indicators/climate-change-indicators-heat-related-deaths. [Accessed 25 September 2023].

29. Xu Z, Sheffield PE, Su H, et al. The impact of heat waves on children's health: a systematic review. Int J Biometeorol 2014;58(2):239–47.

30. Bernstein AS, Sun S, Weinberger KR, et al. Warm Season and Emergency Department Visits to U.S. Children's Hospitals. Environ Health Perspect 2022;130(1):017001.

31. Lipman GS, Gaudio FG, Eifling KP, et al. Wilderness Medical Society Clinical Practice Guidelines for the Prevention and Treatment of Heat Illness: 2019 Update. Wilderness Environ Med 2019;30(4):S33–46.

32. Rublee C, Dresser C, Giudice C, et al. Evidence-Based Heatstroke Management in the Emergency Department. West J Emerg Med 2021;22(2):186–95.

33. Basu R, Pearson D, Malig B, et al. The effect of high ambient temperature on emergency room visits. Epidemiol Camb Mass 2012;23(6):813–20.

34. Desai Y, Khraishah H, Alahmad B. Heat and the Heart. Yale J Biol Med 2023;96(2):197–203.

35. USGCRP, et al. The Impacts of Climate Change on Human Health in the United States: A Scientific Assessment. Washington, DC: U.S. Global Change Research Program; 2016. p. 312. http://dx.doi.org/10.7930/J0R49NQX.

36. Air Quality Index (AQI) Basics. AirNow. Available at: https://www.airnow.gov/aqi/aqi-basics/. Accessed September 10, 2023.

37. Northern Hemisphere Wildfires: A Summer of Extremes. 2023. Available at: https://atmosphere.copernicus.eu/northern-hemisphere-wildfires-summer-extremes. [Accessed 2 January 2024].

38. Chen K, Ma Y, Bell ML, et al. Canadian Wildfire Smoke and Asthma Syndrome Emergency Department Visits in New York City. JAMA 2023;330(14):1385.

39. D'Evelyn SM, Jung J, Alvarado E, et al. Wildfire, Smoke Exposure, Human Health, and Environmental Justice Need to be Integrated into Forest Restoration and Management. Curr Environ Health Rep 2022;9(3):366–85.

40. Abatzoglou JT, Williams AP. Impact of anthropogenic climate change on wildfire across western US forests. Proc Natl Acad Sci U S A 2016;113(42):11770–5.

41. Climate change and Children's health and well-being in the United States. Environmental Protection Agency; 2023. Available at: https://www.epa.gov/system/files/documents/2023-04/CLiME_Final%20Report.pdf. [Accessed 11 September 2023].

42. Rice MB, Henderson SB, Lambert AA, et al. Respiratory Impacts of Wildland Fire Smoke: Future Challenges and Policy Opportunities. An Official American Thoracic Society Workshop Report. Ann Am Thorac Soc 2021;18(6):921–30.

43. Singh AB, Kumar P. Climate change and allergic diseases: An overview. Front Allergy 2022;3:964987.

44. Climate Change Indicators: Ragweed Pollen Season. United States Environmental Protection Agency. Available at: https://www.epa.gov/climate-indicators/climate-change-indicators-ragweed-pollen-season. [Accessed 19 September 2023].

45. Stringer LC, Mirzabaev A, Benjaminsen TA, et al. Climate change impacts on water security in global drylands. One Earth 2021;4(6):851–64.

46. Levy K, Smith SM, Carlton EJ. Climate Change Impacts on Waterborne Diseases: Moving Toward Designing Interventions. Curr Environ Health Rep 2018;5(2): 272–82.

47. Archer EJ, Baker-Austin C, Osborn TJ, et al. Climate warming and increasing Vibrio vulnificus infections in North America. Sci Rep 2023;13(1):3893.

48. Mackenzie JS, Jeggo M. The One Health Approach-Why Is It So Important? Trop Med Infect Dis 2019;4(2):88.

49. Wyns A. Global biodiversity deal is not pandemic proof. Lancet Planet Health 2023;7(3):e185–6.

50. Yang YT, Sarfaty M. Zika virus: A call to action for physicians in the era of climate change. Prev Med Rep 2016;4:444–6.

51. Rocklöv J, Dubrow R. Climate change: an enduring challenge for vector-borne disease prevention and control. Nat Immunol 2020;21(5):479–83.

52. Thomson MC, Stanberry LR. Climate Change and Vectorborne Diseases. N Engl J Med 2022;387(21):1969–78.

53. Ebi KL, Vanos J, Baldwin JW, et al. Extreme Weather and Climate Change: Population Health and Health System Implications. Annu Rev Public Health 2021;42: 293–315.

54. Zscheischler J, Martius O, Westra S, et al. A typology of compound weather and climate events. Nat Rev Earth Environ 2020;1(7):333–47.

55. Radcliff TA, Chu K, Der-Martirosian C, et al. A Model for Measuring Ambulatory Access to Care Recovery after Disasters. J Am Board Fam Med 2018;31(2):252–9.

56. Hess JJ, Malilay JN, Parkinson AJ. Climate Change. Am J Prev Med 2008;35(5): 468–78.

57. Taylor S. The Vulnerability of Health Infrastructure to the Impacts of Climate Change and Sea Level Rise in Small Island Countries in the South Pacific. Health Serv Insights 2021;14. 117863292110208.

58. Kishore N, Marqués D, Mahmud A, et al. Mortality in Puerto Rico after Hurricane Maria. N Engl J Med 2018;379(2):162–70.

59. Paterson J, Berry P, Ebi K, et al. Health Care Facilities Resilient to Climate Change Impacts. Int J Environ Res Public Health 2014;11(12):13097–116.

60. Biddle L, Wahedi K, Bozorgmehr K. Health system resilience: a literature review of empirical research. Health Policy Plan 2020;35(8):1084–109.

61. Paterson DL, Wright H, Harris PNA. Health Risks of Flood Disasters. Clin Infect Dis 2018;67(9):1450–4.

62. Klinger C, Landeg O, Murray V. Power Outages, Extreme Events and Health: a Systematic Review of the Literature from 2011-2012. PLoS Curr 2014. https://doi.org/10.1371/currents.dis.04eb1dc5e73dd1377e05a10e9edde673.

63. Roland J, Lawrance E, Insel T, Christensen H. The digital mental health revolution: Transforming care through innovation and scale-up. Doha, Qatar: World Innovation Summit for Health; 2020.

64. Lawrance EL, Thompson R, Newberry Le Vay J, et al. The Impact of Climate Change on Mental Health and Emotional Wellbeing: A Narrative Review of Current Evidence, and its Implications. Int Rev Psychiatry 2022;34(5):443–98.

65. Keizer E, Senn O, Christensen MB, et al. Use of acute care services by adults with a migrant background: a secondary analysis of a EurOOHnet survey. BMC Fam Pract 2021;22(1):119.
66. Markkula N, Cabieses B, Lehti V, et al. Use of health services among international migrant children – a systematic review. Glob Health 2018;14(1):52.
67. Seigfried K. Climate Change and Displacement: The Myths and The Facts. The UN Refugee Agency. 2023. Available at: https://www.unhcr.org/us/news/stories/climate-change-and-displacement-myths-and-facts.
68. Apap J, Harju SJ. The Concept of "Climate Refugee": Towards A Possible Definition. 2023. Available at: https://www.europarl.europa.eu/RegData/etudes/BRIE/2021/698753/EPRS_BRI(2021)698753_EN.pdf. [Accessed 2 January 2024].
69. Huber J, Madurga-Lopez I, Murray U, et al. Climate-related migration and the climate-security-migration nexus in the Central American Dry Corridor. Clim Change 2023;176(6):79.
70. Weerasinghe S. Overview of UNHCR Study, 'In Harm's Way: International Protection in the Context of Nexus Dynamics between Conflict or Violence and Disaster or Climate Change.'. Int J Refug Law 2019;31(1):149–60.
71. Myers S, Frumkin H. Planetary health. Washington, DC: Island Press; 2020. https://doi.org/10.5822/978-1-61091-966-1.
72. What is the Sendai Framework for Disaster Risk Reduction? United Nations Office for Disaster Risk Reduction. Available at: https://www.undrr.org/implementing-sendai-framework/what-sendai-framework. [Accessed 29 September 2023].
73. Disaster Medicine Fellowships and Other Training Programs. ACEP Disaster Medicine Section. 2021. Available at: https://www.acep.org/disastermedicine/resources/disaster-medicine-fellowships-and-other-training-programs. [Accessed 27 September 2023].
74. Ebi K, Berry P, Hayes K, et al. Stress Testing the Capacity of Health Systems to Manage Climate Change-Related Shocks and Stresses. Int J Environ Res Public Health 2018;15(11):2370.
75. Linstadt H, Collins A, Slutzman JE, et al. The Climate-Smart Emergency Department: A Primer. Ann Emerg Med 2020;76(2):155–67.
76. Climate-Smart Healthcare. Low-Carbon and Resilience Strategies for the Health Sector. 2017. Available at: https://documents1.worldbank.org/curated/en/322251495434571418/pdf/113572-WP-PUBLIC-FINAL-WBG-Climate-smart-Healthcare-002.pdf. [Accessed 22 September 2023].
77. Climate for Health Ambassador Training. Climate for Health. Available at: https://climateforhealth.org/ambassadors-training/. [Accessed 2 January 2024].
78. Climate Rx: Care for your health, care for our climate. Climate Rx: Care for your health, care for our climate. Available at: https://www.climaterx.org. [Accessed 2 January 2024].
79. Impact of Climate Change on Public Health and Implications for Emergency Medicine. American College of Emergency Physicians. 2018. Available at: https://www.acep.org/patient-care/policy-statements/impact-of-climate-change-on-public-health-and-implications-for-emergency-medicine. [Accessed 25 September 2023].
80. Liu I, Rabin B, Manivannan M, et al. Evaluating strengths and opportunities for a co-created climate change curriculum: Medical student perspectives. Front Public Health 2022;10:1021125.
81. Navarrete-Welton A, Chen JJ, Byg B, et al. A grassroots approach for greener education: An example of a medical student-driven planetary health curriculum. Front Public Health 2022;10:1013880.

82. Pillai P, Patz JA, Seibert CS. Climate Change and Environmental Health Must Be Integrated Into Medical Education. Acad Med 2021;96(11):1501–2.

83. Gomez J, Goshua A, Pokrajac N, et al. Teaching medical students about the impacts of climate change on human health. J Clim Change Health 2021;3:100020.

84. Sullivan GM, Simpson D, Yarris LM, et al. A Call for Articles on Climate and Graduate Medical Education-JGME Supplement Issue. J Grad Med Educ 2023;15(2): 143–5.

85. Lemery J, Sorensen C, Balbus J, et al. Science Policy Training for a New Physician Leader: Description and Framework of a Novel Climate and Health Science Policy Fellowship. AEM Educ Train 2019;3(3):233–42.

86. Medicine for A Changing Planet. Medicine for A Changing Planet. Available at: https://www.medicineforachangingplanet.org. [Accessed 11 September 2023].

87. Climate & Health Program. University of Colorado Anschutz Medical Campus. Available at: https://medschool.cuanschutz.edu/climateandhealth/diploma-in-climate-medicine. [Accessed 29 September 2023].

88. Lemery J, Balbus J, Sorensen C, et al. Training Clinical And Public Health Leaders In Climate And Health: Commentary explores training clinical and public health leaders in climate and health. Health Aff (Millwood) 2020;39(12):2189–96.

89. Mann ME. Opinion: Climate Doomism Disregards the Science. APS News 2023; 32(10). Available at: https://www.aps.org/publications/apsnews/202310/back page.cfm. [Accessed 1 October 2023].

# Spaceflight Environment

Samantha A. King, MD*, Craig J. Kutz, MD, MPH, PhD,
Natacha G. Chough, MD, MPH

## KEYWORDS

- Aerospace medicine • Spaceflight • Microgravity • Extreme environments

## KEY POINTS

- Microgravity has multiple system implications, with many related to the cephalad fluid shift.
- Available medical care and resources in the spaceflight environment are currently limited by mass and volume constraints, thereby focusing on stabilization and evacuation.
- With the boom in commercial spaceflight and opportunities for orbital and suborbital flight, emergency medicine physicians may start to see spaceflight participants in their terrestrial patient population.

## INTRODUCTION

Spaceflight encompasses multiple different environments and is defined as travel beyond the von Karman Line, located 100 km above sea level. This travel can include:

1. Suborbital flight, which is generally short in duration (minutes) and does not result in an orbit of the Earth;
2. Low-earth orbit (LEO), which currently ranges in duration from several hours to a year, and includes operational activities of the International Space Station (ISS);
3. Exploration missions, which include travel to the moon and Mars.[1]

Risk is inherent in human spaceflight exploration and involves physiologic and performance hazards. Thus, risk mitigation is a key focus of the National Aeronautics and Space Administration's (NASA) Human Research Program and related risk management boards. In general, these risks consist of reduced gravity, radiation, isolation, remote location, behavioral and human factors, and unique environmental stressors. Spaceflight research has been ongoing since Yuri Gagarin launched into space in 1961.[2] Yet, the relative overall paucity of humans traveling into space limits the breadth of knowledge on the risks and outcomes of spaceflight. Terrestrial analogs

University of Texas Medical Branch (UTMB), Division of Aerospace Medicine, Department of Global and Emerging Diseases, School of Public and Population Health, 301 University Boulevard, Health Clinics, 4.208, Galveston, TX 77555-1150, USA
* Corresponding author.
*E-mail address:* samanthaking.1531@gmail.com

Emerg Med Clin N Am 42 (2024) 695–709
https://doi.org/10.1016/j.emc.2024.02.023
0733-8627/24/© 2024 Elsevier Inc. All rights reserved.

emed.theclinics.com

are used as alternatives, including extreme isolation (eg, Human Research Exploration Analog, or HERA), alternobaric environments (eg, NASA Extreme Environment Mission Operations, or NEEMO), head-down tilt bed rest, limited microgravity exposure (ie, parabolic flights), and austere environments (eg, polar operations). The field continues to evolve as more knowledge gaps are investigated.

This article is meant to provide a high-level overview of the spaceflight environment for the general awareness of emergency medicine physicians. It does not serve as a comprehensive guide, nor is it a substitute for ACGME-accredited Aerospace Medicine training programs or other physician specializations, qualifications, or credentialing in Aerospace Medicine.

## SCREENING AND PREVENTION

Prevention of illness and injury continues to be essential to crew health and safety due to the multitude of challenges in the spaceflight environment. As the expansion and frequency of space travel have increased in the past two decades, so has the spectrum of medical conditions that have flown in space, highlighting the importance of *prevention* as part of the Aerospace Medicine risk mitigation model. Prevention of injury and illness not only benefits individuals, but also the entire crew and mission. Disability, incapacitation, or loss of life by a crew member can lead to substantial consequences for mission success and safety. As a result, medical screening and guidelines have been created for both professional astronauts and spaceflight participants, in conjunction with protocols for acute medical conditions and emergency scenarios that cannot be prevented.[3–5] While there are restrictions for astronaut selection (generally any medical condition that could interfere with the performance of duties or cause sudden incapacitation), an increasing number of medical conditions have been evaluated and risks mitigated through screening and guidelines with successful spaceflight participation.

## ENVIRONMENTAL FACTORS AND THEIR HEALTH IMPLICATIONS
### Microgravity

Microgravity is colloquially referred to as weightlessness, or "0 G," although the latter is not technically accurate. Due to the constant free fall of objects orbiting the Earth, a gravitational force of $1 \times 10^{-6}$ times normal Earth gravity is exerted upon all objects in this state, thus conferring a "micro" degree of gravitational pull toward the Earth. Microgravity has impacts on every human physiologic system, ranging from minor nuisances to significant health impacts if not counteracted with appropriate mitigations, known as *countermeasures*. Physiologic changes to microgravity do not occur at the same rate between organ systems, nor equally between individuals.[6]

### Cardiovascular

With the transition from normal gravity (1-G on Earth) to microgravity, physiologic fluid distribution from the lower extremities shifts to accumulate in the torso and head, with an approximate cephalad fluid shift of 1 to 2 L (**Fig. 1**).[6,7] As a result, cardiac output increases, attributed to increased preload and stroke volume, with a maintenance of heart rate and an increase in cardiac chamber size.[6,8] Plasma volume loss occurs, in part, due to decreased water intake, related to mission timeline constraints and possible decreased thirst sensation, and upper body fluid redistribution.[9] The volume loss was initially thought to be due to a fluid shift-related diuresis, though that has not been supported in later studies.[6] Fluid shifts result in increased jugular venous diameter and can result in decreased or retrograde blood flow.[6,10] It is proposed that this

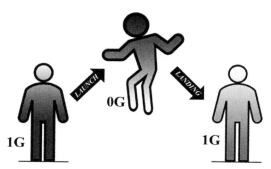

**Fig. 1.** Representation of fluid shift from 1-G to 0-G environment.

decreased flow, in addition to changes in coagulopathy, contributed to the development of an internal jugular thrombus in an astronaut while onboard the ISS.[10] Orthostatic intolerance upon return to the 1-G environment is attributed, in part, to fluid shifts returning to their preflight baseline.[6] Decreased body mass, venous valvular changes, and alterations in baroreceptor sensitivity have also been reported as contributing factors.[6,8]

Astronauts have also been noted to have cardiac atrophy during the course of spaceflight, as well as a more spherically shaped heart noted on in-flight ultrasounds.[8] In addition to structural changes, cardiac dysrhythmias, though brief, have also been noted during spaceflight.[6] The exact cause of dysrhythmias is unknown, though potential structural changes, electrolyte disturbances, and alterations in the autonomic nervous system have been postulated as factors.[6–8]

In order to maintain cardiovascular and musculoskeletal health, astronauts aboard the ISS follow a rigorous exercise protocol. This countermeasure has significantly decreased the muscle atrophy and bone demineralization effects of microgravity.[11]

### Neurologic and ophthalmic
Exposure to microgravity induces alterations to the neurovestibular system. Astronauts often experience space motion sickness (SMS), characterized by symptoms such as nausea, vomiting, dizziness, malaise, and disorientation due to conflicting sensory inputs in the absence of gravity.[6] These symptoms are typically transient, resolving within the first few days of exposure to microgravity. Upon return to 1-G, astronauts, and spaceflight participants may temporarily experience disorientation and postural instability related to the neurovestibular readaptation.[12,13]

In addition, neuro-ophthalmic symptoms may emerge, involving a spectrum of findings collectively known as spaceflight-associated neuro-ocular syndrome (SANS).[14] While no astronaut has been found to have permanent visual or cognitive deficits as a result of SANS, permanent structural changes have been noted.[14] Changes include hyperopic shifts, optic disc edema, chorioretinal folds, and globe flattening.[15] The etiology of SANS is not fully understood and continues to be a primary focus of spaceflight research. Current understanding indicates fluid shifts may be contributory, yet pathophysiology is still presumed to be multifactorial.[14] Unfortunately, no current countermeasure is available to reverse the structural changes noted, though in-flight corrective lenses can be used for a hyperopic shift.

Separately, given the lack of gravitational force, there is an increased risk for floating debris, thus increasing the risk of ocular foreign bodies, corneal abrasions, and eye irritation.[16]

### Musculoskeletal

In the microgravity environment, individuals invariably adopt an overall neutral body posture with a semicrouched torso, flexed limbs, and forward leaning of the neck.[6,17] Low back pain is a common complaint among astronauts during the early in-flight phase, and is part of the spectrum of space adaptation syndrome (SAS).[18] Individuals experience spinal elongation, atrophy of the paraspinal musculature, and decreased lumbar lordosis.[18] In addition, there is decreased bone and muscular loading, which, without countermeasures, can lead to demineralization and atrophy, respectively.[19] Bone loss is not homogenous, often varying both anatomically and between individuals. To help counter these changes and maintain cardiovascular health, astronauts are required to perform daily resistive and aerobic exercises along with nutritional countermeasures.[20]

### Pulmonary

Physiologic pulmonary changes in microgravity can be observed, though they are rarely of operational or clinical significance. As previously discussed, microgravity leads to a cephalad fluid shift, which causes fluid to accumulate in the apices, leading to changes in lung mechanics.[21] There is an increase in the recruitment of abdominal musculature in the breathing cycle and changes in the relative ratios of ventilation/perfusion.[21] The redistribution of fluids does not appear to impact pulmonary gas exchange efficiency, and these changes return to baseline, even after 6 months of microgravity exposure.[21] Vital capacity transiently reduces during spaceflight, but also returns to baseline after several days.[22]

Due to increased foreign object debris, individuals are at increased risk of accidental foreign body inhalation.[6] Air composition changes are also a consideration and will be discussed later in this article.

### Gastrointestinal

Overall, the process of eating is unaffected by microgravity.[23] Yet, studies indicate that microgravity can lead to changes in gastric motility, resulting in slower transit times, reduced nutrient absorption, and changes to the gut microbiome.[24] Astronauts often experience a blunted sense of taste and smell due to headward fluid shifts and consequent congestion. In combination with a decreased variety of food options, this can often decrease appetites.[25] Thus, it is challenging to maintain balanced diets with sufficient macro- and micronutrients. Nutritional deficiencies can potentially contribute to alterations in bone metabolism and muscle mass.[26] Current understanding indicates that no clinically significant increase in symptoms of gastrointestinal reflux, distention, or other gastrointestinal-related complaints occurs in astronauts, aside from occasional constipation.[6]

### Genitourinary

Cephalad fluid shifts result in the increased activation of the renin-angiotensin-aldosterone system, leading to sodium retention, edema, decreased plasma volume, and increased sympathetic tone.[27] However, as previously noted, there is no resultant diuresis-related volume loss related to microgravity. During preparation and launch, prolonged near-supine positioning and decreased oral intake may contribute to these findings.[6] In addition, the increased excretion of calcium and other substrates has been theorized to lead to an increased risk of nephrolithiasis.[28]

Astronauts have reported urinary symptoms during space missions, including decreased urine output, increased residual urine volume, and a sensation of incomplete bladder emptying. The physiologic mechanisms behind urinary retention in microgravity are complex and not yet fully understood. However, it is believed that factors such as changes in fluid dynamics, altered bladder mechanics, and disrupted sensory input from gravity contribute to this issue, as well as anticholinergic side effects from any medications taken for SMS.[27]

### Hematologic and immunologic

Astronauts have been noted to have decreased red blood cell mass when exposed to microgravity, resulting in a relative anemia upon landing.[29] While not fully understood, the current proposed mechanism is due to a microgravity-related hemolysis.[30] In addition, changes to T-cell function, NK-cell function, and alterations in plasma cytokine concentrations have been identified, with relatively few changes to B-cell function.[31] These changes are suspected to lead to the reactivation of latent viruses such as herpes virus, and allergic responses such as dermatitis.[32] Upon return, individuals are considered temporarily immunosuppressed for approximately 7 to 10 days.[6]

### Radiation

Individuals are exposed to increasing amounts of radiation as they leave the protective atmosphere and magnetic fields of Earth. In the spaceflight environment, individuals may be exposed to high energy particles trapped in Earth's electromagnetic field, solar particle events (SPE, also known as "solar flares"), and galactic cosmic radiation (GCR).[33] The amount of radiation exposure will increase with SPEs, and while vehicle and operational protective measures attempt to attenuate radiation exposure, these do not fully eliminate the risk.[33] Mission events, such as extravehicular activities, may increase the risk of exposure from an SPE.[33] Exposure to radiation has potential impacts on all human physiologic systems. Acute high radiation exposure can have particularly detrimental neurologic, hematologic, and mucosal impacts.[34] Individuals with chronic radiation exposure are at risk of the development of cancer, detrimental neurologic effects, and tissue damage, including cardiovascular damage.[33] NASA has radiation exposure limits for astronauts, who are considered radiation workers per occupational guidelines.

### Extravehicular Activity

Extravehicular activity (EVA), commonly known as a "spacewalk," is one of the highest risk activities performed in spaceflight. EVA involves an individual leaving the safety of their vehicle, or spacecraft, to perform activities in the vacuum of space in a multi-layer pressurized suit. As missions transition to involving more exploration, EVAs will increase in frequency for lunar and Martian habitats.

Prior to the execution of an EVA, US astronauts undergo suited training in the Neutral Buoyancy Lab (NBL), a large pool whereby procedures are rehearsed for the EVA planned in-flight.[6] During this training, they are exposed to diving operations and are at risk of decompression sickness (DCS), arterial gas embolism, barotrauma, and musculoskeletal injuries.[6,35]

EVAs in space are performed at lower suit pressure than in the spacecraft cabin.[6] Leaving the vehicle puts individuals at greater risk of radiation exposure, and, as with NBL operations, DCS and barotrauma.[6] Various prebreathe protocols have been used to reduce DCS risk, whereby astronauts breathe 100% O2 prior to EVA or ambient pressure changes in an attempt to eliminate saturated blood nitrogen.[36]

Though decompression sickness and treatment are not covered in detail in this review, DCS can be challenging to treat in spaceflight, with no access to a hyperbaric chamber. Instead, overpressurization of an EVA suit can be used, yet is limited by its inability to reach therapeutic hyperbaric oxygen levels.[6] These limitations underscore the importance of preventive safety and medical measures such as robust prebreathe protocols.

In addition to the risk of DCS, musculoskeletal injuries and other injuries, such as fingernail delamination, have been reported from EVA.[35] During EVAs, an individual's life support system is provided by the spacesuit. Similar to environmental controls within the ISS, considerations for temperature, moisture, waste, and other environmental variables such as $CO_2$ need to be controlled.[6]

### Isolation and Behavioral Health

Individuals in spaceflight are exposed to increased psychosocial stressors including small enclosed spaces, delayed communications, and a limited number of individuals for social interaction. The environment of spaceflight has been shown to lead to increased fatigue, difficulty with concentration, and sleep disturbance.[6] Environmental stressors are also likely to have an impact on mental health, given that individuals experience changes to circadian patterns, increased noise, and decreased personal space.[37] Particularly as missions lengthen in distance, communications will continue to have increasing time delays, which may exacerbate stressors.[38] An increase in adaptive countermeasures will be essential.[38] Interpersonal issues may also develop between crew or with mission control, even without underlying psychological illnesses.[39]

Despite these increased stressors and environmental changes, astronauts have reported fewer behavioral health issues than comparative analog studies, and report overall positive experiences.[6] A range of countermeasures have been implemented for professional astronauts to combat the potential behavioral health impacts of spaceflight. The primary mitigation strategy focuses on early screening and prevention through training and team dynamic exercises.[6] During missions, routine private psychological conferences and cognitive screening occur with psychiatrists and psychologists for behavioral health monitoring and support.[6] Family support and communication are also a crucial component of behavioral health.

## LAUNCH AND LANDING CONSIDERATIONS

In order to leave and return to Earth, significant force and acceleration are required. Individuals traveling to and from space experience significant gravitational forces (G-forces) depending on the flight profile and vehicle (**Table 1**).[6] Current capsule-based systems, whereby crew are recumbent for launch and landing, experience G-forces predominantly in the $+G_x$ direction. However, these forces are different in a fixed-wing vehicle, particularly upon landing.[40]

Significant $+G_x$ exposure can result in decreased pulmonary function and reserve.[40] Cardiac effects have also been noted, including electrocardiographic changes and dysrhythmias.[40] Additionally, due to increased gravitational force, limitations in the ability to lift one's arm or leg would be noticeable, as extremities would be perceived as significantly heavier by the individual.

**Table 1**
**Direction and perception of gravitational forces**

| Force Vector | Body Perceives | Direction of Force | Example |
| --- | --- | --- | --- |
| $+ G_x$ | Pushed into seat back | Back to Front | Step on gas |
| $- G_x$ | Pushed into seat belt | Front to Back | Step on brake |
| $+ G_y$ | Pressure on left | Left to Right | Bank/turn right |
| $- G_y$ | Pressure on right | Right to left | Bank/turn left |
| $+ G_z$ | Pushed into ground | Bottom to top | Going up in elevator |
| $- G_z$ | Pushed to ceiling | Top to Bottom | Going down in elevator |

$+G_z$ forces may be experienced in fixed-wing vehicles upon landing, which can lead to decreased brain perfusion.[40] This decreased blood flow can have substantial operational effects, including gray-outs, almost loss of consciousness (A-LOC), and G-force induced loss of consciousness (G-LOC).[40] Countermeasures include antigravity straining maneuvers (AGSMs) and repeated exposures to increase tolerance.[41]

High $\pm$ $G_y$ exposures can have substantial shearing forces and may need to be taken into consideration during trauma assessments in an off-nominal launch or landing situation.[40]

Similar to any other transportation industry, spaceflight is subject to accidents and close calls. Not every launch or landing will go according to plan, and there is a risk of both nonfatal and fatal injuries. As with other high-velocity, combustion-propelled vehicles, individuals may suffer traumatic injuries, toxic inhalations, and burns in the setting of a launch or landing.

## RETURN AND REHABILITATION

The spaceflight environment continues to have physiologic impacts even after return to a terrestrial environment. The duration and extent of these effects are dependent upon the length of time spent in space, as well as the individual.[6] As previously noted, individuals experience a fluid shift and perturbations of the nervous and cardiovascular systems that lead to neurovestibular symptoms and orthostatic intolerance upon return to 1-G. Astronauts generally salt load prior to return to Earth and may be given IV fluids to help re-establish terrestrial fluid balance norms.[6]

Some musculoskeletal deconditioning is notable upon return, despite exercise countermeasures to minimize this impact during spaceflight.[6] Upon return, astronauts undergo a rehabilitation program to recondition and minimize potential long term health impacts, such as bone demineralization and muscle atrophy.[6] In addition, significant neurovestibular effects such as vertigo and disequilibrium are noted upon return, persisting for as long as 11-days postlanding.[6,42]

Ultimately, short-duration orbital or suborbital flights may require little to no observation periods upon landing. However, for longer duration missions and travel, individuals likely require a period of extensive monitoring and rehabilitation, as well as temporary limitations on driving and flying as pilot-in-command.[6]

## MEDICAL EMERGENCIES IN SPACEFLIGHT
### Current Medical Operational Model

Due to volume and mass constraints resulting in relatively limited resources in spaceflight, emergency medical treatment focuses on stabilization and evacuation for complex interventional needs. Crew have access to multiple medical kits, which include medications such as analgesics and antibiotics, injectable and topical medications, intravenous (IV) therapies, supraglottic and definitive airways, medical diagnostic hardware, and medical supplies such as various wound closure modalities, syringes, needles, and bandage supplies.[6] However, resupply capabilities are limited. Therefore, after the initial treatment of a condition that requires a higher level of care, current operations dictate evacuation back to Earth as opposed to definitive intervention in orbit. As missions increase in duration and distance, this operational model will continue to evolve and adapt.

### Cardiopulmonary Resuscitation

While no astronaut or spaceflight participant has experienced cardiac arrest in space, there is research on how to resuscitate an incapacitated individual given the remote environment of spaceflight.[7] Defibrillation has been successfully tested on parabolic flights, and an automated external defibrillator is available aboard the ISS.[43] Care must be taken to ensure that the electrical charge delivered by such devices remains isolated from other hardware. There have also been studies on how to best perform chest compressions in space, with several proposed methods (**Fig. 2**). The current recommended technique is the handstand technique (see **Fig.** 2D), which involves strapping the patient to a hard surface with the responder floating above them. The responder keeps their hands in the American Heart Association (AHA)-recommended position, with the chest compression force being generated by the responder pushing their legs against an opposing surface.[43] This requires the responder to have a surface on which to place their feet at a reasonable distance. The use of automated compression devices has been proposed, but use may be limited by the ability to transport

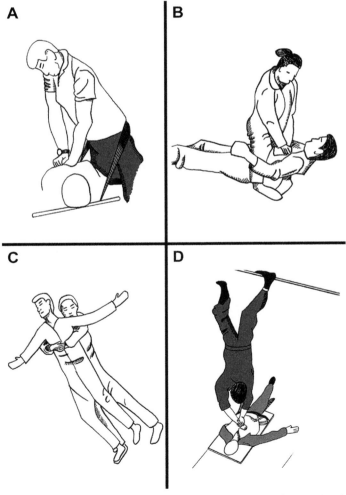

**Fig. 2.** Cardiopulmonary resuscitation methods in microgravity. (*A*) Restrained, (*B*) Evetts-Russomano, (*C*) Reverse Bear Hug (RHB), (*D*) Handstand. (Image credit: Thomas del Ninno, MD.)

such a device due to mass-volume constraints, and the impacts of the unisolated force causing vibration to the vehicle.[44]

### Airway Management

Though an unlikely scenario, intubation in microgravity has been researched in analog environments, with increased success using video laryngoscopy compared with direct laryngoscopy.[45] However, upon intubation, challenges remain with maintaining ventilation and intravenous medications administration (including sedation) due to restricted resource volume. In addition to intubation, automated ventilation and oxygen delivery via nasal cannula, nonrebreather face mask, or bag-valve mask are available and may be considered, though research is minimal. Astronauts and spaceflight participants are at an increased risk of respiratory issues due to the inhalation of foreign objects in the setting of reduced gravity, and potential increased environmental exposures on planetary surfaces.[21,46] Individuals may have difficulty with the clearance of inhaled particles.[21]

### Traumatic Injury and Imaging

While musculoskeletal complaints are common in spaceflight, severe traumatic injury has so far been avoided due to appropriate safety measures. There may be a higher risk potential for major trauma in future missions, particularly as planetary surface exploration frequency and gravitational forces increase relative to microgravity.[47] In case of such injuries, the current medical model supports stabilization and evacuation. For traumatic resuscitation, IV fluids, but not blood products, are available. From an imaging standpoint, ultrasound is currently the only capability.[48] While ultrasound is diagnostic for a large range of conditions, examinations performed in spaceflight have considerations related to microgravity. For instance, a remote-guided FAST examination can be performed, but fluid and air will collect differently than on Earth, and potential differences should be taken into account during interpretation.[49]

### Infections, Medications, and Surgery

Spaceflight confers a slight increased risk of infections due to relative, reversible immunosuppression. Since the 1960s, NASA has implemented a preflight quarantine program to mitigate the risk of pathogen introduction and subsequent risk to crew health and mission objectives.[6]

In-flight infections have occurred in astronauts, including pyelonephritis. Symptomatology does not differ appreciably from terrestrial cases.[50] Such infections can be attributed to inciting factors such as the design of a urine collection device or changes in hygiene, and are not considered occult or opportunistic in origin, as is often the case with terrestrial immunocompromised patients. In addition, changes to bacterial virulence have been noted in microgravity, although the direct risk of these changes is not fully understood nor known to be clinically significant.[51] Antibiotics are available, although limited data suggests that changes occur in pharmacokinetics and pharmacodynamics of these medications, as well as many others, when used in the spaceflight environment.[52]

As mission profiles continue to lengthen in duration and distance, making evacuation difficult or impossible, the potential for surgical intervention in microgravity has been considered.[53] No documented human surgical intervention has been performed in space, although multiple studies continue to investigate the potential volume and logistical considerations required.[53] Concerns including the ability to maintain a clear and sterile field need to be considered. Body fluids, including blood, can stay in place due to surface tension and would not spontaneously clear from a surgical field of view.[6] Large volumes of free-floating bodily fluids present a biohazard risk in excess of terrestrial norms.

### Toxicologic Exposures

Astronauts are at risk of toxic exposure during all phases of spaceflight. Multiple potential toxic sources include, but are not limited to, payload chemicals, propellants, fire, and system contaminants.[54] Multiple crew exposures to various compounds have been previously reported, spurring the development of guidelines and procedures to reduce exposure risk and to handle actual exposures.[54] Air quality is constantly monitored, and allowable limits of various compounds have been studied and reported, known as Spacecraft Maximum Allowable Concentrations (SMACs).[54]

One particular air quality concern is $CO_2$. While there are $CO_2$ scrubbers aboard the ISS, vehicle design constraints limit their ability to replicate terrestrial $CO_2$ levels. Consequently, astronauts are exposed to a concentration of $CO_2$ approximately ten times that of Earth. NASA currently sets a limit on the ISS of a 1-hr average atmospheric $CO_2$ exposure level of 3.0 mm Hg, as measured by the life support system.[55] The development of $CO_2$ "pockets" due to the lack of gravitational air flow can also occur, resulting in a more localized area of concentrated exposure (eg, if a crewmember is working in one area for a prolonged period of time).[56] Persistently elevated $CO_2$ has been associated with headaches and cognition changes.[57]

Another toxic concern is potential ammonia exposure. At present, ammonia is used as part of the cooling system aboard the ISS. Inhalation of ammonia at lower concentrations can be an irritant, but at higher concentrations puts crew at risk for significant respiratory distress and possible laryngospasm.[54] Current treatment of an exposure includes supportive measures including decontamination, bronchodilation, and airway management.[58] Given the significant risk to crew health and cabin exposure, emergency response protocols have been developed should a leak occur.[59] If adequate ventilation is not achieved, these protocols dictate undocking and return.

At launch and landing, astronauts and ground personnel are at risk of exposure to hypergolic propellant fuels, such as nitrogen tetroxide and monomethylhydrazine. Accidental exposure has occurred in the history of spaceflight.[60] Exposure to these fuels can be lethal, and lower concentration exposures put individuals at risk for mucosal/skin irritation and hematologic, gastrointestinal, and respiratory symptoms. Prolonged exposure can lead to pulmonary edema.[61,62] Combustion of these propellants puts individuals at risk for burns and blast injuries. These chemicals can impregnate suit material and later be released into the surrounding environment, putting rescue crews at risk.[63] Despite the risks, these propellants have predominantly been safely used, but do require safety education.[60]

## IMPLICATIONS FOR EMERGENCY MEDICINE

While the average emergency medicine physician may not care for a patient who has been exposed to the spaceflight environment, recent exponential growth in the commercial spaceflight industry has resulted in an increase in launches from US soil, and an increasing number of spaceflight participants. It may not be long before one could encounter a spaceflight participant, ground support personnel, or launch spectator in the Emergency Department in the wake of a spaceflight mass casualty incident, particularly in areas whereby there are frequent launches and landings. Knowing about the spaceflight environment will allow a physician to more readily care for these patients.

Further, the impacts of the spaceflight environment overlap with other Emergency Medicine health care arenas, such as hyperbaric medicine, toxicology, and point-of-care ultrasound.

Of note, prior to pursuing civilian Aerospace Medicine residency, Emergency Medicine is one of the many primary medical specialties undertaken by prospective applicants to Aerospace Medicine training programs. Training for civilian Aerospace Medicine physicians requires the completion of an Accreditation Council of Graduate Medical Education (ACGME)-accredited residency or fellowship.[64] At the time of this article, there are currently 2 civilian and 3 military ACGME-accredited Aerospace Medicine residency training programs within the United States. Having an introductory understanding of the field will allow Emergency Medicine physicians to better advise interested applicants and promote competent background training in one's chosen primary specialty, including those coming from an Emergency Medicine residency.

## UPCOMING CHALLENGES

Aerospace medicine and the spaceflight environment are not without their continued challenges. Despite more than 60 years of successful human spaceflight and research, there are many questions still unanswered. For instance, conditions such as SANS do not currently have a countermeasure or mitigation strategy in exploration missions.[14] As the distance between Earth and astronauts increases through lunar and Martian exploration, communication delays will increase, with one-way lags of up to 20 minutes. This will impact the ability of ground-based intervention and medical guidance.[65] Additionally, current treatment models involve the condition stabilization and evacuation of critical patients, which will not be feasible in transit to Mars. Continued research into spaceflight human physiology, as well as preventive care to mitigate risk, will likely have great impacts on safe and successful missions.

In addition to exploration missions, there is an anticipated increase in commercial spaceflight and spaceflight participants who will not have undergone the rigorous screening and preventive strategies of NASA's current astronaut corps. As such, there will need to be continued understanding of the impacts of abnormal environments on baseline pathophysiology. Different risk mitigation strategies, and the longitudinal care of these individuals, will be paramount.

## CLINICS CARE POINTS

- Preventive medicine is the foundation of care for astronauts and spaceflight participants. Planning for and minimizing health complications has allowed for 60+ years of successful spaceflight.

- Spaceflight has impacts on every physiologic system due to changes brought on by microgravity, radiation, and other environmental factors.

- Definitive emergency treatment in spaceflight focuses on stabilization and evacuation.

- Upon return, spaceflight participants will have notable effects on their cardiovascular, neurovestibular, and musculoskeletal systems that could impact acute care.

- Treatment of spaceflight participants in the terrestrial Emergency Department setting involves understanding the physiologic changes and environmental exposures caused by the spaceflight environment.

## DISCLOSURE

The authors declare that they do not have any relevant financial and/or nonfinancial relationships to disclose.

## REFERENCES

1. Hodkinson PD, Anderton RA, Posselt BN, et al. An overview of space medicine. Br J Anaesth 2017;119:i143–53.
2. Williams DR. A Historical Overview of Space Medicine. McGill J Med 2020;6(1).
3. Baisden DL, Beven GE, Campbell MR, et al. Human health and performance for long-duration spaceflight. Aviat Space Environ Med 2008;79(6):629–35.
4. Law J, Mathers CH, Fondy SRE, et al. NASA's human system risk management approach and its applicability to commercial spaceflight. Aviat Space Environ Med 2013;84(1):68–73.
5. Aerospace Medical Association Task Force on Space Travel. Medical guidelines for space passengers. Aerospace Medical Association Task Force on Space Travel. Aviat Space Environ Med 2001;72(10):948–50.
6. Barratt MR, Baker E, Pool SL. *Principles of Clinical Medicine for Space Flight.* Second edition. New York, NY: Springer; 2019.
7. Vernice NA, Meydan C, Afshinnekoo E, et al. Long-term spaceflight and the cardiovascular system. Precis Clin Med 2020;3(4):284–91.
8. Baran R, Marchal S, Garcia Campos S, et al. The Cardiovascular System in Space: Focus on In Vivo and In Vitro Studies. Biomedicines 2021;10(1):59.
9. Olde Engberink RHG, van Oosten PJ, Weber T, et al. The kidney, volume homeostasis and osmoregulation in space: current perspective and knowledge gaps. npj Microgravity 2023;9:29.
10. Kim DS, Vaquer S, Mazzolai L, et al. The effect of microgravity on the human venous system and blood coagulation: a systematic review. Exp Physiol 2021; 106(5):1149–58.
11. English KL, Downs M, Goetchius E, et al. High intensity training during spaceflight: results from the NASA Sprint Study. Npj Microgravity 2020;6(1):21.
12. Shishkin N, Kitov V, Sayenko D, et al. Sensory organization of postural control after long term space flight. Front Neural Circuits 2023;17:1135434.
13. Macaulay TR, Peters BT, Wood SJ, et al. Developing Proprioceptive Countermeasures to Mitigate Postural and Locomotor Control Deficits After Long-Duration Spaceflight. Front Syst Neurosci 2021;15:658985.
14. Lee AG, Mader TH, Gibson CR, et al. Spaceflight associated neuro-ocular syndrome (SANS) and the neuro-ophthalmologic effects of microgravity: a review and an update. Npj Microgravity 2020;6(1):7.
15. Mader TH, Gibson CR, Pass AF, et al. Optic Disc Edema, Globe Flattening, Choroidal Folds, and Hyperopic Shifts Observed in Astronauts after Long-duration Space Flight. Ophthalmology 2011;118(10):2058–69.
16. Meer E, Grob S, Antonsen EL, et al. Ocular conditions and injuries, detection and management in spaceflight. Npj Microgravity 2023;9(1):37.
17. Han Kim K, Young KS, Rajulu SL. Neutral Body Posture in Spaceflight. Proc Hum Factors Ergon Soc Annu Meet 2019;63(1):992–6.
18. Penchev R, Scheuring RA, Soto AT, et al. Back Pain in Outer Space. Anesthesiology 2021;135(3):384–95.
19. Stavnichuk M, Mikolajewicz N, Corlett T, et al. A systematic review and meta-analysis of bone loss in space travelers. Npj Microgravity 2020;6(1):13.

20. Genah S, Monici M, Morbidelli L. The Effect of Space Travel on Bone Metabolism: Considerations on Today's Major Challenges and Advances in Pharmacology. Int J Mol Sci 2021;22(9):4585.
21. Prisk GK. Pulmonary challenges of prolonged journeys to space: taking your lungs to the moon. Med J Aust 2019;211(6):271–6.
22. Prisk GK. Microgravity and the respiratory system. Eur Respir J 2014;43(5): 1459–71.
23. Yang JQ, Jiang N, Li ZP, et al. The effects of microgravity on the digestive system and the new insights it brings to the life sciences. Life Sci Space Res 2020;27: 74–82.
24. Siddiqui R, Qaisar R, Goswami N, et al. Effect of Microgravity Environment on Gut Microbiome and Angiogenesis. Life Basel Switz 2021;11(10):1008.
25. Olabi AA, Lawless HT, Hunter JB, et al. The effect of microgravity and space flight on the chemical senses. J Food Sci 2002;67(2):468–78.
26. Baba S, Smith T, Hellmann J, et al. Space Flight Diet-Induced Deficiency and Response to Gravity-Free Resistive Exercise. Nutrients 2020;12(8):2400.
27. Baran C, Erkoç M, Ötünçtemur A. The Place of Urology in Aerospace Medicine; A New Horizon. Eur Arch Med Res 2022;38(1):1–4.
28. Patel SR, Witthaus MW, Erturk ES, et al. A history of urolithiasis risk in space. Can J Urol 2020;27(3):10233–7.
29. Trudel G, Shafer J, Laneuville O, et al. Characterizing the effect of exposure to microgravity on anemia: more space is worse. Am J Hematol 2020;95(3):267–73.
30. Trudel G, Shahin N, Ramsay T, et al. Hemolysis contributes to anemia during long-duration space flight. Nat Med 2022;28(1):59–62.
31. Crucian BE, Choukèr A, Simpson RJ, et al. Immune System Dysregulation During Spaceflight: Potential Countermeasures for Deep Space Exploration Missions. Front Immunol 2018;9:1437.
32. Rooney BV, Crucian BE, Pierson DL, et al. Herpes Virus Reactivation in Astronauts During Spaceflight and Its Application on Earth. Front Microbiol 2019; 10:16.
33. Chancellor JC, Scott GBI, Sutton JP. Space Radiation: The Number One Risk to Astronaut Health beyond Low Earth Orbit. Life Basel Switz 2014;4(3):491–510.
34. Clements BW, Casani JAP. Nuclear and Radiological Disasters. In: *Disasters and Public Health*. Oxford, UK: Butterworth-Heinemann; 2016. p. 357–83.
35. Dunn J, Benson E, Norcross J, et al. Risk of injury and Compromised performance due to EVA operations. Houston, TX: National Aeronautics and Space Administration; 2021.
36. Conkin J. Report NASA/TP-2011-216147: Preventing decompression sickness over three decades of extravehicular activity. Houston, TX: National Aeronautics and Space Administration; 2011.
37. Arone A, Ivaldi T, Loganovsky K, et al. The Burden of Space Exploration on the Mental Health of Astronauts: A Narrative Review. Clin Neuropsychiatry 2021; 18(5):237–46.
38. Patel ZS, Brunstetter TJ, Tarver WJ, et al. Red risks for a journey to the red planet: The highest priority human health risks for a mission to Mars. Npj Microgravity 2020;6(1):33.
39. Kanas NA, Salnitskiy VP, Boyd JE, et al. Crewmember and mission control personnel interactions during International Space Station missions. Aviat Space Environ Med 2007;78(6):601–7.
40. Pollock RD, Hodkinson PD, Smith TG, et al. The x, y and z of human physiological responses to acceleration. Exp Physiol 2021;106(12):2367–84.

41. Whitley PE. Pilot performance of the anti-G straining maneuver: respiratory demands and breathing system effects. Aviat Space Environ Med 1997;68(4):312–6.
42. Homick JL, Reschke MF. Postural equilibrium following exposure to weightless space flight. Acta Otolaryngol 1977;83(5–6):45 5–64.
43. Hinkelbein J, Kerkhoff S, Adler C, et al. Cardiopulmonary resuscitation (CPR) during spaceflight - a guideline for CPR in microgravity from the German Society of Aerospace Medicine (DGLRM) and the European Society of Aerospace Medicine Space Medicine Group (ESAM-SMG). Scand J Trauma Resusc Emerg Med 2020; 28(1):108.
44. Forti A, Van Veelen MJ, Scquizzato T, et al. Mechanical cardiopulmonary resuscitation in microgravity and hypergravity conditions: A manikin study during parabolic flight. Am J Emerg Med 2022;53:54–8.
45. Hinkelbein J. Spaceflight: the final frontier for airway management? Br J Anaesth 2020;125(1):e5–6.
46. Pohlen M, Carroll D, Prisk GK, et al. Overview of lunar dust toxicity risk. Npj Microgravity 2022;8(1):55.
47. Kirkpatrick AW, Ball CG, Campbell M, et al. Severe traumatic injury during long duration spaceflight: Light years beyond ATLS. J Trauma Manag Outcomes 2009;3(1):4.
48. Law J, Macbeth PB. Ultrasound: from Earth to space. McGill J Med MJM Int Forum Adv Med Sci Stud 2011;13(2):59.
49. Hamilton DR, Sargsyan AE, Kirkpatrick AW, et al. Sonographic detection of pneumothorax and hemothorax in microgravity. Aviat Space Env Med 2004;75(3): 272–7.
50. Johnston RS, Dietlein LF, Berry CA. Biomedical results of Apollo. Washington, DC: National Aeronautics and Space Administration, Scientific and Technical Report Office; 1975.
51. Taylor PW. Impact of space flight on bacterial virulence and antibiotic susceptibility. Infect Drug Resist 2015;8:249–62.
52. Blue RS, Bayuse TM, Daniels VR, et al. Supplying a pharmacy for NASA exploration spaceflight: challenges and current understanding. Npj Microgravity 2019; 5(1):14.
53. Rajput S. A review of space surgery - What have we achieved, current challenges, and future prospects. Acta Astronaut 2021;188:18–24.
54. NASA Office fo the Chief Health & Medical Officer. NASA-STD-3001 Technical Brief: Spaceflight toxicology, Revision B. Washington, DC: National Aeronautics and Space Administration; 2023.
55. NASA Office of the Chief and Health Medical Officer.*NASA Spaceflight Human-System Standard Volume 2: Human Factors, Habitability, and Environmental Health Revision D*, National Aeronautics and Space Administration; Washington, DC, 2023.
56. Georgescu MR, Meslem A, Nastase I. Accumulation and spatial distribution of $CO_2$ in the astronaut's crew quarters on the International Space Station. Build Environ 2020;185:107278.
57. NASA Office of the Chief Health & Medical Officer. NASA-STD-3001 technical brief: Carbon Dioxide ($CO_2$) Revision C. Washington, DC: National Aeronautics and Space Administration; 2023.
58. Padappayil R, Borger J. Ammonia Toxicity. In: StatPearls Publishing. 2023. Available at: https://www.ncbi.nlm.nih.gov/books/NBK546677/. [Accessed 22 July 2023].

59. Duchesne S, Sweterlitsch PhD J, Son PhD C, et al. In: Impacts of an Ammonia Leak on the Cabin Atmosphere of the International Space Station. San Diego: California:American Institute of Aeronautics and Astronautics; 2012.

60. Nufer B. In: A Summary of NASA and USAF Hypergolic Propellant Related Spills and Fires, In: *SpaceOps 2010 conference*. Huntsvill, AL: American Institute of Aeronautics and Astronautics; 2010.

61. National Research Council (US) Subcommittee on Acute Exposure Guideline Levels. Acute Exposure Guideline Levels for Selected Airborne Chemicals: Volume 1. National Academies Press (US); Washington (DC), 2000. 3, Monomethylhydrazine.

62. National Center for Biotechnology Information. PubChem Compound Summary for CID 25352, Dinitrogen tetroxide. 2003. Available at: https://pubchem.ncbi.nlm.nih.gov/compound/Dinitrogen-tetroxide. [Accessed 22 July 2023].

63. Schwertz H, Roth LA, Woodard D. Propellant Off-Gassing and Implications for Triage and Rescue. Aerosp Med Hum Perform 2020;91(12):956–61.

64. Thamer SB, Bello J, Stevanovic M, et al. Nationwide survey of medical student interest in and exposure to aerospace medicine. Npj Microgravity 2023;9(1):44.

65. Drake BG., Exploration of Mars Design Reference Architecture 5.0 Addendum, *National Aeronautics and Space Administration*, 2009.

# Moving?

## Make sure your subscription moves with you!

To notify us of your new address, find your **Clinics Account Number** (located on your mailing label above your name), and contact customer service at:

Email: **journalscustomerservice-usa@elsevier.com**

**800-654-2452** (subscribers in the U.S. & Canada)
**314-447-8871** (subscribers outside of the U.S. & Canada)

Fax number: **314-447-8029**

**Elsevier Health Sciences Division**
**Subscription Customer Service**
**3251 Riverport Lane**
**Maryland Heights, MO 63043**

*To ensure uninterrupted delivery of your subscription, please notify us at least 4 weeks in advance of move.